A MASSAGE THERAPIST'S GUIDE TO

Pain management

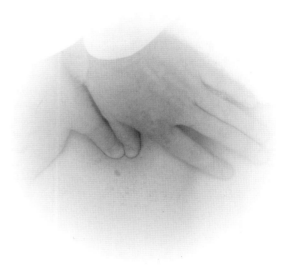

Commissioning Editor: Alison Taylor
Development Editor: Carole McMurray
Project Manager: Nancy Arnott
Designer: Stewart Larking
Illustration Manager: Merlyn Harvey
Illustrators: Graeme Chambers

A MASSAGE THERAPIST'S GUIDE TO

Pain management

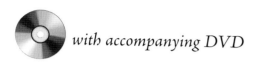

with accompanying DVD

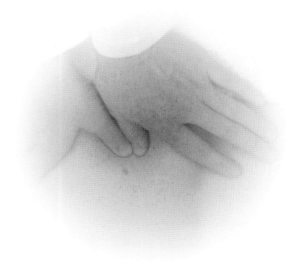

Sandy Fritz BS MS

*Director, Health Enrichment Center,
School of Therapeutic Massage, Lapeer, MI, USA*

Leon Chaitow ND DO

*Osteopathic Practitioner and Honorary Fellow,
University of Westminster, London, UK*

Foreword by

Diana Thompson

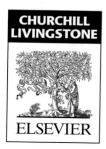

CHURCHILL
LIVINGSTONE

ELSEVIER

EDINBURGH LONDON NEW YORK OXFORD PHILADELPHIA ST LOUIS SYDNEY TORONTO 2011

CHURCHILL
LIVINGSTONE
ELSEVIER

ISBN 978-0-443-06947-5

British Library Cataloguing in Publication Data
A catalogue record for this book is available from the British Library

Library of Congress Cataloging in Publication Data
A catalog record for this book is available from the Library of Congress

Notices

Knowledge and best practice in this field are constantly changing. As
new research and experience broaden our understanding, changes in
research methods, professional practices, or medical treatment may
become necessary.

Practitioners and researchers must always rely on their own experience
and knowledge in evaluating and using any information, methods,
compounds, or experiments described herein. In using such information
or methods they should be mindful of their own safety and the
safety of others, including parties for whom they have a professional
responsibility.

With respect to any drug or pharmaceutical products identified,
readers are advised to check the most current information provided
(i) on procedures featured or (ii) by the manufacturer of each product
to be administered, to verify the recommended dose or formula, the
method and duration of administration, and contraindications. It is
the responsibility of practitioners, relying on their own experience and
knowledge of their patients, to make diagnoses, to determine dosages
and the best treatment for each individual patient, and to take all
appropriate safety precautions.

To the fullest extent of the law, neither the Publisher nor the authors,
contributors, or editors, assume any liability for any injury and/
or damage to persons or property as a matter of products liability,
negligence or otherwise, or from any use or operation of any methods,
products, instructions, or ideas contained in the material herein.

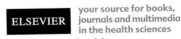
Printed in China

Contents

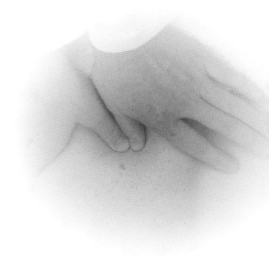

The DVD accompanying this text includes video sequences of all the techniques indicated in the text by the icon. To look at the video for a given technique, click on the relevant icon in the contents list on the DVD. The DVD is designed to be used in conjunction with the text and not as a stand-alone product.

Foreword

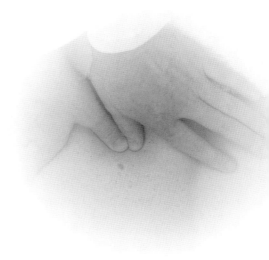

After 30 years in this profession, one might think they have seen it all. But as the health and wellness field becomes increasingly enlightened and science better informs our practices, familiar conditions become newly defined and differentiated. As a result, we become better equipped to assess and treat conditions, and more importantly, better able to offer compassion, hope and relief to those afflicted.

Chronic pain is one of those newly defined and differentiated conditions. Acute pain remains a fair bit easier to comprehend: a symptom, a therapeutic response to injury and illness that has a purpose and is typically responsive to treatment. Chronic pain, as so deftly described in this book, is now considered a disease in and of itself, a complex pathology, and a contributor to multiple pathologies. It is most likely a dysfunction of the nervous system, impacting many other systems of the body, and is no longer productive, lingering long after the original infliction is resolved. As such, treatment cannot mirror traditional approaches to acute pain conditions. To complicate matters, chronic pain presents itself in ways unique to each individual, and may require a multiple-disciplinary team to achieved desired results. To effectively manage chronic pain conditions, massage therapists must master critical thinking skills, implement clinical decision-making strategies, and work as a part of integrative medical teams.

I treat a patient with chronic pain associated with Lyme disease. Having treated complicated types of chronic pain, I was disconcerted when this patient's presentation was different and baffling. First, I was unaware that neurological complications of untreated Lyme disease existed, were so severe and so prevalent. Second, I was perplexed by my patient's pain: his pain sensitivity is heightened not only to one type of pain but to multiple types of pain, encompassing different systems in the body. After reading this book, I have a much deeper and broader understanding of the complexities of chronic pain and its many faces. I am better equipped to recognize, assess and treat the vast array of complications, and complement the approaches of other members of his health care team. I also understand that his diagnosis is the current diagnosis and that new information may present itself and send us in another direction. And if it does, I have strategies to help me adapt due to Sandy Fritz and Leon Chaitow's outcomes-based approach to treatment planning.

The book's content is exquisite. At a time when many texts and courses lack adequate scientific citations, this book dedicated an entire chapter to the research, going beyond the citations by providing pages of research summaries (abstracts). It is imperative that massage therapists become research literate in order to be more fully integrated into healthcare and be a part of health care reform, and Fritz and Chaitow provide the teaching moments. The information is balanced, combining the science and the art with a healthy dose of personality, assisting all levels and styles of learners in comprehending complicated details and concepts. In addition to understanding the complex origins of pain, the authors teach us to listen and respond to our patients, assess their unique expression of pain, and design a treatment approach that addresses the vast array of pathologies and symptoms associated with this baffling and confounding condition.

The timing of this book is impeccable. Current research on chronic pain is sufficient enough to give us insights into the mechanisms of chronic pain and the clinical effectiveness of a variety of manual therapy treatments. The National Center for Complementary and Alternative Medicine (NCCAM) has expressed their commitment to investigating massage as a treatment for managing pain. President Obama has called for a committee to investigate and design a prevention and wellness approach to healthcare to move us away from a system driven solely by illness and disease, an approach massage therapists apply every day. Massage has a foothold in the integrative health care movement due to the efficacy, safety and cost-effectiveness demonstrated by early research results. Pain is our raison d'être. It is important that we do all we can to master our craft and manage this pervasive condition.

I invite you in with my favorite quote from this book, "It hurts to be in pain whether that pain is acute or chronic, physical, emotional or spiritual, helpful or harmful. Massage therapists must appreciate the mechanisms causing, enhancing and creating the pain experience to competently use massage to help those experiencing pain."

Diana Thompson

Acknowledgements

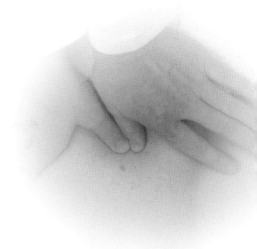

I would like to acknowledge my assistant, Amy Husted, for all her dedicated work on this text. Additionally, the editorial and production staff at Elsevier have been helpful, supportive and patient as this text was developed. Even though Dr. Chaitow is a co-author for this texts, I personally acknowledge his guidance, mentoring, and friendship, as well as his contributions.

CHAPTER ONE
Understanding pain

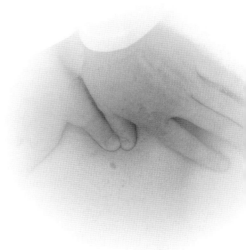

CHAPTER CONTENTS

INTRODUCTION

This first chapter provides an overview of various types of pain. The content establishes a language for discussing pain and creates the structure for the following chapters. Massage therapy applied to address the symptoms and causes of pain can be very beneficial as long as the treatment is based on accurate information and safe and best practices. Bond (1984) describes pain as being a personal and unique experience which arises in the brain due to injury to the body tissue, disease, or due to biochemical changes in the body. Productive pain is an important protective mechanism when the pain response mechanism is working appropriately. The pain response can become maladaptive and therefore nonproductive.

PAIN OVERVIEW

Pain can be caused or exacerbated by stress, muscle tension, nerve damage, chemical imbalance, disordered breathing syndromes, nutritional disruption, side effects from medication, vascular dysfunction, sinus disorders, tumors, and many more internal and external influences. Pain management methods are targeted to alter these influences or shift the pain sensations. Research indicates potential for therapeutic massage to decrease stress and muscle tone, support more normal circulation of body fluids, and support effective breathing function. Massage may be able to reduce some side effects from pain medication. Massage therapy can also be used in a palliative manner substituting pleasurable sensations for the pain response. In Chapter 2 the research will be explored to support the benefits of massage.

The degree to which a person reacts to pain comes from biological, psychological and cultural makeup. Past encounters with painful illness and injury can influence pain sensitivity. People who are prone to recurring illness and injury in the same area can experience increasing pain sensation for the same or even less degree of pathology.

Pain is caused by the stimulation of nociceptors. These receptors are usually stimulated by chemicals such as substance P, bradykinin, and histamine, which excite the nerve endings. Pain is elicited by three different classes of stimuli: mechanical, chemical, and thermal. Soft tissue pain is caused by the chemicals released from illness, injury, or from mechanical irritation caused by cumulative stress, microinflammation, or extreme hot or cold. Emotional or psychological stress, called autonomic disturbances, can cause pain by causing hypertonic muscles and shifts in fluid flow affecting oxygen and nutrient delivery and waste removal.

People associate pain to actual or potential tissue damage. Pain is unpleasant and therefore an emotional experience. This situation becomes problematic when individuals are unable to separate hurt from actual biological tissue harm. Chronic pain is not typically related to tissue damage yet those experiencing it need to learn the difference.

Pain of somatic origin and from the viscera sends impulses to the limbic and hypothalamus areas of the brain and may be responsible for emotional reactions of anxiety, fear, anger, and depression. Also, the brain inhibits or enhances a reaction to pain. This can explain how people can sometimes ignore pain and why fear and anxiety can exaggerate pain. How a person responds to pain is called pain tolerance. How a person interprets the pain sensation increases or decreases tolerance. Interventions that change perception and meaning of pain can increase tolerance allowing an individual to have better coping strategies in response to pain stimuli.

Many people report pain in the absence of tissue damage or any likely pathophysiological cause. This situation mystifies the health care community and is difficult to treat. There is usually no way to distinguish this type of pain experience from that caused by tissue damage based on subjective reporting. Regardless of the known or unknown cause of pain, if an individual claims to be in pain it should be accepted as pain. We also need to remember that successful management of pain requires multiple support professionals that attend to the physical, psychological and spiritual components of the pain experience. The massage therapist must understand pain and use massage methods effectively to manage pain to be part of a multidisciplinary team.

TAXONOMY (THE SCIENCE OF CLASSIFICATION) FOR PAIN

Pain, according to the International Association for the Study of Pain, is an unpleasant sensory and emotional experience associated with actual or potential tissue damage, or described in terms of such damage.

To understand treatment processes that target pain, it is necessary to delve deeper into pain mechanisms and pain management. As in many areas, the terminology that describes pain processes is confusing. The International Association for the Study of Pain supports a taskforce that is working on a more concise taxonomy (the science of classification) for pain (http://www.iasppain.org//AM/Template.cfm? Section=Home). See Box 1.1. The taxonomy for massage therapy is also confusing. Box 1.2 provides guidelines for massage therapy methods classifications.

CAUSAL FACTORS OF PAIN

Pain receptors are found in almost every tissue of the body and may respond to any type of stimulus. Because of their sensitivity to all stimuli, pain receptors perform a protective function by identifying changes that may endanger the body.

> When stimuli for other sensations, such as touch, pressure, heat, and cold, reach a certain intensity, they stimulate the sensation of pain as well. Excessive stimulation of a sensory organ causes pain. Additional stimuli for pain receptors include excessive distension or dilation of a structure, prolonged muscular contractions, muscle spasms, inadequate blood flow to tissues, or the presence of certain chemical substances. (Meldrum 2003)

Pain receptors can become sensitized which results in fewer stimuli necessary to cause pain sensation.

Sensitized receptors = fewer stimuli create more pain

Injured tissue may release prostaglandins, making peripheral nociceptors more sensitive to the normal pain response (hyperalgesia). Aspirin and other nonsteroidal anti-inflammatory drugs (often referred to as NSAIDs) inhibit the action of prostaglandins and reduce pain.

PAIN SENSATION

The point at which a stimulus is perceived as painful is called the pain threshold. This varies somewhat from individual to individual. One factor affecting the pain threshold is perceptual dominance, in which the pain felt in one area of the body diminishes or

Box 1.1 IASP pain terminology

These definitions have been reproduced with permission of the International Association for the Study of Pain® (IASP®). The definition may not be reproduced for any other purpose without permission.

Allodynia

Pain due to a stimulus which does not normally provoke pain. It is important to recognize that allodynia involves a change in the quality of a sensation, whether tactile, thermal, or of any other sort. The original modality is normally non-painful, but the response is painful.

Analgesia

Absence of pain in response to stimulation which would normally be painful.

Anesthesia dolorosa

Pain and numbing in an area or region after it has been anesthetized.

Causalgia

A syndrome of sustained burning pain, allodynia, and hyperpathia after a traumatic nerve lesion, often combined with vasomotor and sudomotor dysfunction and later trophic changes.

Central pain

Pain initiated or caused by a primary lesion or dysfunction in the central nervous system.

Dysesthesia

An unpleasant abnormal sensation, whether spontaneous or evoked.

Hyperalgesia

An increased response to a stimulus which is normally painful. Current evidence suggests that hyperalgesia is a consequence of perturbation of the nociceptive system with peripheral or central sensitization, or both.

Hyperesthesia

Increased sensitivity to stimulation, excluding the special senses.

Hyperpathia

A painful syndrome characterized by an abnormally painful reaction to a stimulus, especially a repetitive stimulus, as well as an increased threshold.

Hypoalgesia

Diminished pain in response to a normally painful stimulus.

Hypoesthesia

Decreased sensitivity to stimulation, excluding the special senses.

Neuralgia

Pain in the distribution of a nerve or nerves.

Neuritis

Inflammation of a nerve or nerves.

Neurogenic pain

Pain initiated or caused by a primary lesion, dysfunction, or transitory perturbation in the peripheral or central nervous system.

Neuropathic pain

Pain initiated or caused by a primary lesion or dysfunction in the nervous system.

Neuropathy

A disturbance of function or pathological change in a nerve: in one nerve, mononeuropathy; in several nerves, mononeuropathy multiplex; if diffuse and bilateral, polyneuropathy.

Nociceptor

A receptor preferentially sensitive to a noxious stimulus or to a stimulus which would become noxious if prolonged.

Noxious stimulus

A noxious stimulus is one which is damaging to normal tissues.

Pain

An unpleasant sensory and emotional experience associated with actual or potential tissue damage, or described in terms of such damage.

(Continued)

Box 1.1 (Continued)

Pain threshold
   The least experience of pain which a subject can recognize.

Pain tolerance level
   The greatest level of pain which a subject is prepared to tolerate.

Paresthesia
   An abnormal sensation, whether spontaneous or evoked.

Peripheral neurogenic pain
   Pain initiated or caused by a primary lesion or dysfunction or transitory perturbation in the peripheral nervous system.

Peripheral neuropathic pain
   Pain initiated or caused by a primary lesion or dysfunction in the peripheral nervous system.

NOTE: The pain terminology was modified and approved for publication by the IASP Council in Kyoto, November 29–30, 2007. The above pain terminology is reproduced with permission from Merskey H, Bogduk N (eds) 1994 Part III: Pain terms, a current list with definitions and notes on usage (pp 209–214). Classification of chronic pain, 2nd edn. IASP Task Force on Taxonomy, IASP Press, Seattle ®1994.

Box 1.2 Proposed taxonomy of massage practice

Principal goals of treatment	Relaxation massage	Clinical massage	Movement re-education	Energy work
Intention	Relax muscles, move body fluids, promote wellness	Accomplish specific goals such as releasing muscle spasms	Induce sense of freedom, ease, and lightness in body	Hypothesized to free energy blockages
Commonly used styles (examples*)	Swedish/Classic massage, spa massage Sports massage	Myofascial trigger point therapy Myofascial release Strain–counterstrain	Proprioceptive Neuromuscular Facilitation Strain–counterstrain Trager	Acupressure Reiki Polarity Therapeutic Touch Tuina
Commonly used techniques (examples**)	Gliding Kneading Friction Holding Percussion Vibration	Direct pressure Skin rolling Resistive stretching Stretching – manual Cross-fiber friction	Contract–relax Passive stretching Resistive stretching Rocking	Direction of energy Smoothing Direct pressure Holding Rocking Traction

*While some styles of massage are commonly used in addressing one of the four principal treatment goals, some may be used to address several distinct treatment goals.
**By varying the intent (or purpose) for a technique, many of them can be used in massages with different principal treatment goals.
Sherman et al 2006 BMC Complementary and Alternative Medicine 6:24 doi:10.1186/1472-6882-6-24.

obliterates the pain felt in another area. Not until the most severe pain is diminished does the person perceive or acknowledge the other pain. This mechanism is often activated with massage application that produces a 'good hurt.'

Pain tolerance refers to the length of time or intensity of pain that the person endures before acknowledging it and seeking relief. Unlike the pain threshold, pain tolerance is more likely to vary from one individual to another. A person's tolerance to pain is influenced by a variety of factors, including personality type, psychological state at the onset of pain, previous experiences, socio-cultural background, and the meaning of the pain to that person (e.g. the ways in which it affects the person's lifestyle). Factors that decrease pain tolerance include repeated exposure to pain, fatigue, sleep deprivation, and stress. Warmth, cold, distraction, alcohol consumption, hypnosis, and strong spiritual beliefs or faith, all act to increase pain tolerance.

PAIN TYPES

There are different types of pain and multiple ways to describe pain.

The three basic categories of pain are somatic, visceral, and neuropathic which can be experienced at the same time.

Somatic and visceral

Somatic pain is caused by the activation of pain receptors in either the cutaneous (body surface) or deep tissues (musculoskeletal and fascial tissues).

- Surface somatic pain is perceived as sharp and may have a burning or pricking quality.
- When pain occurs in the musculoskeletal and fascial tissues, it is called deep somatic pain. Deep somatic pain is usually described as dull or aching but localized.
- Visceral pain is pain that originates in the organs of the body. It is often felt on the body surface in the classical referred pain patterns. It tends to be episodic and poorly localized (see Fig 1.1).

Nociceptive, neuropathic pain and mixed category pain

Pain can also be classified as nociceptive, neuropathic pain and mixed category pain.

Nociceptive pain occurs with damage to tissues that contain nociceptors, which are the nerves that sense and respond to parts of the body which suffer from damage. Nociceptors transmit pain signals to the brain. Pain due to tissue injury is usually experienced as local, constant, and throbbing.

Examples include sprains, bone fractures, burns, bruises, inflammation from an infection or arthritic disorder, obstructions, and myofascial pain. Visceral pain is a type of nociceptive pain that involves the internal organs.

Nociceptive pain is usually time limited, meaning that when the tissue damage heals, the pain typically goes away. Arthritis is an exception since it can last indefinitely. Nociceptive pain tends to respond well to treatment with opioid medication. Because nociceptive pain is opiate-responsive it is logical to expect that massage methods that encourage endogenous

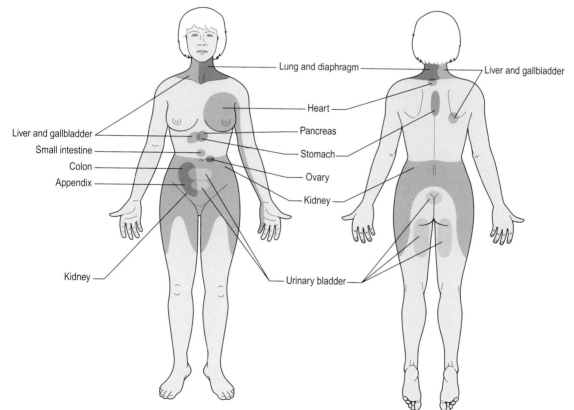

Figure 1.1 Referred pain. The diagram indicates cutaneous areas to which visceral pain may be referred. If pain is encountered in these areas during a massage, the massage practitioner needs to refer the client to a physician for diagnosis to rule out visceral dysfunction.

opiates such as endorphins would be effective in the management of this type of pain.

Neuropathic pain occurs in response to injury or malfunction in the peripheral or central nervous system. The pain is experienced as burning, cutting, piercing, or stabbing. Usually the pain is triggered by an injury: nerves can be infiltrated or compressed by tumors, strangulated by scar tissue, or inflamed by infection. All of these can trigger a neuropathic pain response. Allodynia is a common characteristic of neuropathic pain as the body becomes overly sensitive to sensory stimuli that is typically nonpainful. This type of pain may last months or years even when any injured tissue has apparently healed. The pain signaling is nonproductive and the alarm system itself is malfunctioning. Examples include post-shingle neuralgia, complex regional pain syndrome, nerve trauma, aspects of cancer pain, phantom limb pain, entrapment neuropathy such as thoracic outlet syndrome or carpal tunnel syndrome, and peripheral neuropathy (widespread nerve damage).

Diabetes is the most common peripheral neuropathy but the condition can also be caused by chronic alcohol use, exposure to other toxins including many chemotherapies, medication side effects, vitamin deficiencies, and medical conditions. It is not unusual for the cause of the condition to go undiagnosed. Neuropathic pain is frequently chronic, and does not respond well to opiate based medication, but may respond well to other drugs such as antiseizure and antidepressant medications. Usually, neuropathic problems are not fully reversible, but partial improvement is often possible with proper treatment.

A distinction can be made between central and peripheral neuropathic pain. Central neuropathic pain results from damage to the central nervous system. Peripheral pain originates in muscles, tendons, etc., or in the peripheral nerves themselves. Pain originating in the peripheral nerves, i.e. via trauma to the nerves, is called neurogenic pain.

In some conditions the pain appears to be caused by both nociceptive and neuropathic factors. An initial nervous system dysfunction or injury may trigger the neural release of inflammatory mediators and subsequent neurogenic inflammation (Cousins 1988). For example, migraine headaches probably represent a mixture of neuropathic and nociceptive pain. Myofascial pain is related to nociceptive input from the muscles and fascia, but the abnormal muscle activity may be the result of neuropathic conditions.

Acute and chronic

Pain can also be classified as acute and chronic. Acute pain is experienced for a short time and usually has a specific cause and purpose such as injury to body tissue. The inflammatory response is appropriately involved in an active healing process. Acute pain related to inflammation can be treated with anti-inflammatory medication such as aspirin or other method of pain relief such as ice. Acute pain also responds to opiate based medication.

Chronic pain has no time limit and can last for months or years, and serves no obvious biological purpose. Chronic pain can have a significant impact on the quality of person's life. It can trigger psychological as well as physical and emotional problems that lead to feelings of helplessness and hopelessness since chronic pain is resistant to treatment. Chronic pain is one of the most difficult conditions addressed by the health care system.

Chronic pain syndromes

Chronic pain syndromes share common characteristics of regional or generalized musculoskeletal pain, often associated with poor sleep, fatigue, sensory disturbances, headache, and visceral symptoms, and variously diagnosed in other settings as chronic widespread pain, fibromyalgia, and chronic fatigue syndrome.

Until recently the common conceptualization of these types of pain syndromes was within a psychosomatic framework ('all in their head'). We now understand that the problems of this type of pain occur in the signaling mechanism of the central nervous system rather than the absence of pathology in peripheral tissue structures and organs.

Interestingly there is a consistent relationship between certain beliefs, biases, and behaviors in individuals with these types of pain syndromes. There is a tendency for catastrophizing and fearful processing of internal and external information and avoidance of normal levels of activity. Deconditioning occurs and symptoms perpetuate. Symptoms of post traumatic stress disorder (PTSD) and chronic pain share some characteristics, particularly anxiety and increased sensitivity toward somatic cues, as well as avoidance behavior leading to isolation and increased distress.

It is likely that stress responses and pain modulation may be dysregulated in both conditions. Massage therapists need to be aware of the possibilities of interacting systems when they opt to focus only on pain and not on the total pain experience.

WHERE DOES PAIN COME FROM?

Pain basically results from a series of exchanges involving three major components: peripheral nerves, spinal cord, and brain. Pain is a neurological phenomenon involving the central nervous system (CNS), various types of sensory receptors, nerves, and neurotransmitters. Nociception is in the body but pain occurs in a group of interconnected brain regions known as the pain matrix. The cerebral cortex of the brain interprets location, quality, and intensity of the pain signals. The anterior cingulate cortex registers the unpleasant 'hurt' of pain. It connects the physical sensation of pain to feelings of danger, anxiety, and distress. Interestingly, the anterior cingulate cortex doesn't distinguish between psychological and bodily injury (Decety & Morigushi 2007). Body, mind, and spiritual pain are all the same to this aspect of the brain.

Peripheral nerves

As described by the Mayo Clinic (Swanson 1999) peripheral nerves encompass a network of nerve fibers that branch throughout the body. Attached to some of these fibers are special nerve endings (nociceptors) that can sense an unpleasant stimulus, such as a cut, burn, or painful pressure.

There are millions of nociceptors in the skin, bones, joints, and muscles and in the protective membranes around the internal organs. Nociceptors are concentrated in areas more prone to injury, such as the fingers and toes. There may be as many as 1300 nociceptors in just 1 square inch of skin. Skin stimulation during massage that is intense enough to stimulate the 'good hurt' response causes the nociceptors to fire. This is one of the mechanisms of counterirritation. This is also a major component of massage benefits for pain management.

Muscles, protected beneath the skin, have fewer nerve endings. Internal organs, protected by skin, muscle, and bone, have even less. Nociceptors sense pressure, temperature, and chemical changes determining injury potential. Nociceptors can also detect inflammation caused by illness and injury, disease, or infection.

Massage that addresses these receptors must have enough depth of pressure to elicit a response. When nociceptors detect a harmful stimulus, they relay their pain messages in the form of electrical impulses along a peripheral nerve to the spinal cord and brain. Severe pain sensations are transmitted almost instantaneously as the body protects itself from injury. Dull, aching pain – such as an upset stomach, toothache, or joint aching – is relayed on fibers that transmit at a slower speed.

Spinal cord pain

When pain messages reach the spinal cord, they meet up with specialized nerve cells that act as gatekeepers, which filter the pain messages on their way to the interpretive areas of the brain where the pain is felt, understood and coping strategies are developed. For severe pain that's linked to bodily harm, the 'gate' is wide open and the messages take an express route to the brain. Nerve cells in the spinal cord also respond to these urgent warnings by triggering other parts of the nervous system into action, especially the motor nerves to signal muscles to move away from harm, a process described as a reflex arc. However, if the pain signals are weak, such as from a scratch, they may be blocked by the gate.

Within the spinal cord, the messages can also change. Other sensations may overpower and diminish the pain signals. This is called counterirritation or hyperstimulation analgesia. Again, massage is an effective intervention to create counterirritation or hyperstimulation analgesia to suppress pain sensation.

Nerve cells in the spinal cord also release chemicals such as endorphins or substance P that amplify or diminish the strength of a pain signal that reaches the brain for interpretation. Massage can influence these chemical responses, although research has not yet identified the exact mechanism.

Pain in the brain

When pain messages reach the brain, they are first processed by the thalamus, which is a sorting and switching station. The thalamus quickly interprets the messages as pain and forwards them simultaneously to three specialized regions of the brain: the physical sensation region (somatosensory cortex), the emotional feeling region (limbic system), and the thinking (cognitive) region (frontal cortex). Awareness of pain is therefore a complex experience of sensing, feeling, and thinking. Pain tolerance comes from the interplay of these functions. Massage can influence all these areas, i.e. somatic sensation through nerve stimulation, limbic system by calming sympathetic dominance and nurturing, and the cognitive areas through education, reframing, and providing symptom relief.

The brain responds to pain by sending messages that trigger the healing process (see Box 1.3). Signals are sent to the autonomic nervous system, which then sends additional blood and nutrients to the illness and injury site. Pain suppressing chemicals send stop-pain messages.

Pain comes in many forms of physical sensations: sharp, jabbing, throbbing, burning, stinging, tingling, nagging, dull, and aching. Pain also varies from mild to severe. If you experience severe pain, it is realized very quickly and generally produces a greater physical and emotional response than mild pain. Severe

---

Box 1.3 Brain responses to pain

Brain responses to pain, assessed through positron emission tomography (PET) and functional magnetic resonance imaging (fMRI) are reviewed. Functional activation of brain regions are thought to be reflected by increases in the regional cerebral blood flow (rCBF) in PET studies, and in the blood oxygen level dependent (BOLD) signal in fMRI. rCBF increases to noxious stimuli are almost constantly observed in second somatic (SII) and insular regions, and in the anterior cingulate cortex (ACC), and with slightly less consistency in the contralateral thalamus and the primary somatic area (SI). Activation of the lateral thalamus, SI, SII and insula are thought to be related to the sensory-discriminative aspects of pain processing. SI is activated in roughly half of the studies, and the probability of obtaining SI activation appears related to the total amount of body surface stimulated (spatial summation) and probably also by temporal summation and attention to the stimulus. In a number of studies, the thalamic response was bilateral, probably reflecting generalized arousal in reaction to pain. ACC does not seem to be involved in coding stimulus intensity or location but appears to participate in both the affective and attentional concomitants of pain sensation, as well as in response selection. ACC subdivisions activated by painful stimuli partially overlap those activated in orienting and target detection tasks, but are distinct from those activated in tests involving sustained attention (Stroop, etc.). In addition to ACC, increased blood flow in the posterior parietal and prefrontal cortices is thought to reflect attentional and memory networks activated by noxious stimulation. Less noted but frequent activation concerns motor-related areas such as the striatum, cerebellum and supplementary motor area, as well as regions involved in pain control such as the periaqueductal grey. In patients, chronic spontaneous pain is associated with decreased resting rCBF in contralateral thalamus, which may be reverted by analgesic procedures. Abnormal pain evoked by innocuous stimuli (allodynia) has been associated with amplification of the thalamic, insular and SII responses, concomitant to a paradoxical CBF decrease in ACC. It is argued that imaging studies of allodynia should be encouraged in order to understand central reorganisations leading to abnormal cortical pain processing. A number of brain areas activated by acute pain, particularly the thalamus and anterior cingulate, also show increases in rCBF during analgesic procedures. Taken together, these data suggest that hemodynamic responses to pain reflect simultaneously the sensory, cognitive and affective dimensions of pain, and that the same structure may both respond to pain and participate in pain control. The precise biochemical nature of these mechanisms remains to be investigated.

Peyron R, Laurent B, García-Larrea L 2000 Functional imaging of brain responses to pain. A review and meta-analysis. Neurophysiol Clin 30(5):263–88.

---

pain can be incapacitating, making it difficult or impossible to function.

The location of pain can affect the response to it. A headache that interferes with the ability to focus or work may be more bothersome than, for example, arthritic pain in the ankle. Therefore the headache would receive a stronger pain response.

The emotional and psychological state, memories of past pain experiences, upbringing, and attitude also affect how people interpret pain messages and tolerate pain.

When pain persists beyond the time expected for healing, pain can become a chronic condition. No longer is the pain just the symptom of another disease, but a separate condition unto itself.

PAIN MODULATION

Descending neuronal pain control mechanisms

The CNS can control the pain response by transmitting impulses from the brain to the spinal cord signaling the periaqueductal gray area (PGA) to release enkephalins and the nucleus raphe magnus (NRM) to release serotonin. Stimulation of the PGA in the midbrain and NRM in the pons and medulla causes analgesia. The release of these neurotransmitters inhibits ascending neurons reducing the pain transition. Other neurotransmitters involved in pain modulation are the endogenous opioid peptides – endorphins and enkephalins that reduce pain perception by bonding to pain receptor sites (Nemmani & Mogil 2003).

Chemicals: endogenous and exogenous

The use of pain suppressing medication that mimics the body's own chemicals is controversial and may even slow healing. However, the stress of severe acute pain can slow the healing process and intractable chronic pain suppresses the immune system. In these cases, pain medication is appropriate.

The most potent painkillers detach us from our suffering. Opioids such as morphine and

OxyContin® (oxycodone), which mimic the brain's natural painkillers, not only dull the perception of pain but change our interpretation of it. In the cingulate, the drugs dampen emotional distress. Patients taking opioids often say that they still hurt, but it just doesn't bother them anymore. Chronic pain makes life hell for almost 30 million Americans. Cures are elusive, but in the meantime, emotions, expectations – and even sex – may help soothe the ache.

The pain experience is highly subjective and influenced by behavioral, physiological, sensory, emotional (e.g. attention, anxiety, fatigue, suggestion, prior conditioning), and cultural factors for a particular person under a certain set of circumstances. This accounts for the wide variation in individual responses to the sensation of pain. Pain medication can be addictive.

Incorporating massage into a substance abuse program is advantageous in all of the stages of quitting an addiction: withdrawal, detoxification, and abstinence. The physical, emotional, and spiritual components of recovery all can be directly benefited by the healing power of therapeutic touch. The nurturing contact of massage utilizes skin as the translator of the therapist's intent. Skin, the largest sensory organ in our body, is our primary sense for connecting information from our external surroundings to our internal environment.

The Touch Research Institute in Miami, Florida has performed scientific research documenting the physiological effects of massage on the body (see Box 1.4). Kosakoski (2003) reminds us of some of their findings on massage, such as decreased pain, diminished autoimmune response, enhanced immune response, and increased alertness and performance. These effects appear to be related to massage's ability to reduce cortisol, a stress hormone, as reported by the Touch Research Institute in 2003. Several of the Touch Research Institute's studies positively document the ability of massage to decrease anxiety, depression, agitation, and cravings.

In order to understand the connection between massage therapy and its benefit in addiction treatment, Kosakoski explains the neurological biochemistry of addiction:

Much attention has been directed to the mesolimbic reward system, the so-called 'pleasure pathway' of the brain. The area is activated in part by the release of the neurotransmitter dopamine, the chemical messenger responsible for making us feel good when we engage in any pleasurable activity. It is well known that dopamine is significantly involved in addiction and that dopamine levels are lower

---

Box 1.4 Pain transmission

The CNS is responsible for a conscious awareness of pain, integrates past experiences and emotions to determine the meaning of the pain, and reacts to stimulus. The afferent (ascending) nerves transmit impulses from the periphery to the CNS. The efferent (descending) nerves transmit impulses from the CNS to the periphery. Nerve types and the impulses they carry include:

Mylinated nerves
- A-alpha – non-pain impulses.
- A-beta – non-pain impulses.
- A-delta – pain impulses due to mechanical pressure.

Unmylinated nerves
- C – pain impulses due to chemicals or mechanical.

A nerve ending is the termination of a nerve fiber in a peripheral structure. Nerve endings may be sensory (receptor) or motor (effector).

Nerve endings related specifically to pain include:

- Free nerve endings – afferent: detects pain, touch, temperature, mechanical stimuli. Substance P is a peptide that functions as a neurotransmitter and neuromodulator thought to be responsible for the transmission of pain-producing impulses.
- Nociceptors – sensitive to repeated or prolonged stimulation.
- Mechanosensitive – excited by stress and tissue damage.
- Chemosensitive – excited by the release of chemical mediators.
- Bradykinin, histamine, prostaglandins, arachadonic acid.
- Primary hyperalgesia – due to injury.
- Secondary hyperalgesia – due to spreading of chemical mediators.

---

than average during the withdrawal process and into early recovery until brain chemistry normalizes.

In 1998, the Touch Research Institute published the findings that a regular massage regimen produced long-term results of increasing dopamine levels. The fact that massage naturally increases dopamine levels, and decreases cortisol levels, makes it a perfect addition to a standard detoxification program (Tiffany 2005).

Massage: the missing link in addiction treatment
People in the early stages of addiction recovery often experience an uncomfortable gap between their body and mind. Therapeutic massage can bridge that gap,

and is a powerful adjunct treatment in the addiction and recovery process.

Pain control theories

Pain and pain management remains somewhat mysterious. Theories to explain pain management attempt to describe why methods may work to control the experience of pain.

Gate control theory
The gate control theory states that nonpainful stimulus such as distraction competes with the painful impulse to reach the brain. This rivalry limits the number of impulses that can be transmitted in the brain by creating the hypothetical gate (see Fig 1.2).

The gate control takes into account the psychological factors of pain experiences. Experiences of pain are influenced by many physical and psychological factors such as beliefs, prior experience, motivation, emotional aspects, anxiety and depression, which can increase pain by affecting the central control system in the brain.

Melzack and Wall (2005) suggested that when pain signals first reach the nervous system, the pain messages are sent to the thalamus and the 'gate' opens to allow the pain messages to be sent to higher centers in the brain. However, the gate may remain closed if neurons come in contact with pain signals; the neurons have the ability to overpower the pain signals which results in the gate remaining closed. Pain signals can also be stopped if the hypothetical gate

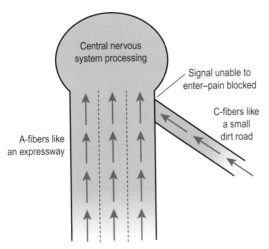

Touch, pressure, movement or moderate
acute pain purposefully applied = counterirritation
which may provide hyperstimulation analgesia

Figure 1.2 Gate-control theory of pain (based on Melzack and Wall's gate-control theory of pain). (From Fritz 2004.)

remains closed as our natural painkiller, endorphins, blocks the pain signals from getting to the brain.

Gate – located in the dorsal horn of the spinal cord.
Smaller, slower nerves carry pain impulses.
Larger, faster nerve fibers carry other sensations.
Impulses from faster fibers arriving at gate first inhibit pain impulses (acupuncture/pressure, cold, heat, chemical skin irritation).

Central biasing theory
Descending neurons are activated by the stimulation of A-delta and C neurons, cognitive processes, anxiety, depression, previous experiences, and so forth, causing the release of enkephalins (and serotonin which can block A-delta and C neuron firing).

Endogenous opiates theory
Least understood of all the theories. Stimulation of A-delta and C fibers causes the release of endorphins which can block ascending nerve impulses blocking pain signals.

PYSCHOSOCIAL CONTRIBUTIONS TO PAIN

Psychosocial risk factors, contributing to pain are:

Stress – feelings of being overwhelmed by the demands of life, time pressures, etc.
Distress – a combination of feelings of helplessness and unhappiness.
Anxiety – an exaggerated level of concern and fear. Usually catastrophizing is involved and almost always involved is altered (usually 'upper chest') breathing patterns, that contribute to lowered pain threshold and altered muscle tone (Nixon & Andrews 1996, Chaitow & Bradley 2002).
Depression – a profound unhappiness and sense of existence being pointless.
Cognitive dysfunction – misunderstanding and/or misinterpretation of facts.
Pain behavior – avoiding normal everyday activities that it is feared might aggravate the pain problem.
Job dissatisfaction – blaming the job for the problem, or simply unhappiness in the work situation.
Mental stress – inter-personal tensions, time (or other) pressures that make working and/or home environments difficult (Chaitow 2010).

Remedies for many of these psychosocial factors are to be found through patient education, stress management, counseling, and cognitive behavioral therapy.

Massage is one of the more effective interventions for managing chronic pain. Touch, vibration, and joint and muscle movement stimulate mechanoreceptors, causing a decrease in the pain information received by the brain. Massage stimulates the entire region of the body being worked on, along with localized pain areas. The large number of mechanoreceptors are stimulated, dramatically reducing the discomfort of working deep somatic tissues. This is why full body massage is better for pain management than localized spot work.

MANAGING PAIN

- Protect from further injury
- Encouraging progressive exercise
- Encourage motivation, positive thinking
- Practice relaxation methods
- Participate in breathing retraining
- Use hydrotherapy and thermotherapy methods
- Judicious use of medications
- Integrate appropriate massage therapy

KEY POINTS

- Pain is an unpleasant sensory emotional experience associated with actual or potential tissue damage composed of a variety of discomforts.
- Productive pain protects from continuous injury.
- Pain is a subjective sensation based on pain perceptions, expectations, past experience, anxiety, suggestions.
- Pain is multifaceted and the pain experience may have sensory, emotional, and cognitive aspects.

- Factors other than pain can affect the report of pain such as sleep disturbance, fatigue, depression, and anxiety.
- Physiological response is produced by activation of specific types of nerve fibers.
- There are cultural, environmental, and racial variations in pain experience and expression and in health care seeking and treatment.

References

Bond M: Pain: its nature analysis and treatment, ed 2, Edinburgh, 1984, Churchill Livingstone.

Chaitow L: Making sense of back pain. Online at from http://www.carenergy.com/articles-backpain1.php. Retrieved June 20, 2010.

Chaitow L, Bradley D, Gilbert C: Multidisciplinary approaches to breathing pattern disorders, Edinburgh, 2002, Churchill Livingstone.

Cousins MJ: Introduction to acute and chronic pain. In Cousins MJ, Bridenbaugh PO, editors: Neural blockade in clinical anesthesia and management of pain, Philadelphia, 1988, JB Lippincott.

Decety J, Moriguishi Y: The empathic brain and its dysfunction in psychiatric population: implications for intervention across different clinical conditions. Biopsychosoc Med, V1:22, 2007. http://www.ncbi.nlm.nih.gov/pmc/articles/pmc 22060360

Field T, Hernandez-Reif M, Diego M: Cortisol decreases and serotonin and dopamine increase following massage therapy, Intern J Neurosci 115:1397–1413, 2005, Taylor & Francis.

Fritz S: Mosby's essential sciences for therapeutic massage: anatomy, physiology, biomechanics, and pathology, ed 2, St Louis, 2004, Mosby.

Kauer J et al: Study raises caution on new painkillers. ScienceDaily 2008. Online at www.sciencedaily.com/releases/2008/03/080312141250.htm. Retrieved September 27, 2008.

Kosakoski J: Massage: hands down, a treatment for addiction. Counselor, The Magazine for Addiction Professionals 4(5): 26–38, Oct 2003.

Max MB: Pain. In Goldman L et al: Cecil medicine, ed 23, Philadelphia, 2007, Elsevier, p 151.

McMahon S, Koltzenburg M: Wall and Melzack's Textbook of pain, London, 2005, Churchill Livingstone.

Meldrum M: History of pain management, J Am Med Assoc 290:2470, 2003.

Merskey H, Bogduk N, editors: Part III: Pain terms, a current list with definitions and notes on usage. In Classification of chronic pain, ed 2, Seattle, 1994, IASP Press. IASP Task Force on Taxonomy, pp 209–214.

Moore J, Von Korff M, Cherkin D, et al: A randomized trial of a cognitive-behavioral program for enhancing back pain self-care in a primary care setting, Pain 88:45–153, 2000.

Nemmani KVS, Mogil JS: Serotonin–GABA interactions in the modulation of mu- and kappa-opiod analgesia, Neuropharmacology 44(3):304–310, 2003.

Nixon P, Andrews J: A study of anaerobic threshold in chronic fatigue syndrome (CFS), Biological Psychology 43(3):264, 1996.

Peyron R, Laurent B, García-Larrea L: Functional imaging of brain responses to pain. A review and meta-analysis, Neurophysiol Clin 30(5):263–288, 2000.

Swanson D: Mayo Clinic on chronic pain, New York, 1999, Kensington Publishing.

Szalavitz M: The pleasant truths about pain. Psychology Today, September 1, 2005. Online at http://www.psychologytoday.com/articles/200508/the-pleasant-truths-about-pain. Retrieved May 6, 2008.

CHAPTER TWO

Research supporting massage for pain management

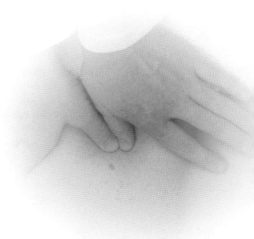

CHAPTER CONTENTS

INTRODUCTION

This chapter will focus on understanding and justifying massage as a treatment approach for pain management. Current research will be analyzed to support the premise that massage is a valuable intervention for pain management.

In review of Chapter 1, pain is usually described as acute or short term and as chronic or long term. Acute pain arises from sudden injury to the structures of the body (e.g. skin, muscles, viscera). The intensity of pain is usually proportional to the extent of tissue damage. The sympathetic nervous system is activated, resulting in an increase in the heart rate, pulse, respirations, and blood pressure. This also causes nausea, diaphoresis, dilated pupils, and elevated glucose. Continuing or persistent pain results from ongoing tissue damage or from chemicals released by the surrounding cells during the initial trauma (e.g. a crushing injury). The intensity diminishes as the stimulus is removed or tissue repair and healing take place. Acute pain serves an important protective physiologic purpose that warns of potential or actual tissue damage. Chronic pain has slower onset and lasts longer than 3 months beyond the healing process. Chronic pain does not relate to an injury or provide physiologic value. Depending upon the underlying etiology, it is often subdivided into malignant (cancer) or nonmalignant (causes other than cancer) pain. It may arise from visceral organs, muscular and connective tissue, or neurologic causes such as diabetic neuropathy, trigeminal neuralgia, or amputation. As chronic pain progresses, especially poorly treated pain, other physical and emotional factors come into play affecting almost every aspect of a patient's life – physical, mental, social, financial, and spiritual – causing additional stress, anger, chronic fatigue, and depression. Whereas pain has always been viewed as a symptom of a disease or a condition, chronic pain and its harmful physiologic effects are being looked upon as a disease itself.

As presented in Chapter 1, pain is caused by the stimulation of nociceptors. These receptors are usually stimulated by chemicals such as substance P, bradykinin, and histamine, which excite the nerve endings. Pain is elicited by three different classes of stimuli: mechanical, chemical, and thermal. Soft tissue pain is caused by the chemicals released from illness, injury, or from mechanical irritation caused by cumulative stress, microinflammation, or extreme heat or cold. Emotional or psychological stress, called autonomic disturbances, can cause pain by causing hypertonic muscles and shifts in fluid flow affecting oxygen and nutrient delivery and waste removal.

Within the spinal cord, the messages can also change. Other sensations may overpower and diminish the pain signals. This is called counterirritation or hyperstimulation analgesia. Again, massage is an effective intervention to create counterirritation or hyperstimulation analgesia to suppress pain sensation. The question becomes, is there sufficient research to support massage as evidence based and best practice intervention?

HOW DOES MASSAGE WORK?

We do not totally understand how massage therapy causes physiological change but researchers are beginning to uncover evidence that explains the value of the treatment. The focus of this text is massage therapy as an intervention for pain management. Much of the research has targeted pain reduction as an outcome. If massage can be considered a valid intervention then it must somehow influence pain production and perception. Additionally massage would work to reduce the source of the pain, such as to reduce nerve impingement, or modulate the transmission of pain signaling, or affect the pain tolerance, or activate or support the pain modulation neurochemical system of the body.

Treatment modalities in interdisciplinary pain management may include:

1. Education in pain mechanisms, physiology, and psychological aspects of pain.
2. Psychological interventions targeting cognitive and behavioral aspects of adaptation to pain and the relation between chronic pain and the effects of prolonged stress.

3. Physiotherapy with the principal goal of enhancing overall physical functioning and reducing musculoskeletal impairment caused by the pain experience. Pain mechanisms underlying chronic pain conditions include physical and emotional trauma, illness and deconditioning.
4. Pharmacological treatment to minimize symptoms and problems associated with pain. See: http://www.iasp-pain.org/AM/AMTemplate.cfm?Section=Home&TEMPLATE=/CM/ContentDisplay.cfm&CONTENTID=7626

Massage therapy needs to function to interface with one or more of these four points.

The most commonly used complementary modalities in the research are:

- chiropractic
- massage therapy
- acupuncture
- mind–body techniques.

If adaptation failure is the primary cause of pain then whatever treatment is offered should achieve one of three things:

- Removal or reduction in the stress load to which the local tissues (or the body as a whole) is adapting.
- Improvement in the way(s) the local tissues (or the body as whole) is coping and adapting.
- Symptomatic treatment to make the recovery period more comfortable – without adding to the adaptive load.
- Sometimes all three elements can be achieved, sometimes only one.

Since healing, or recovery, is a self-generated function (cuts heal, broken bones mend, etc.) the important element in any treatment choice is that it should be safe, should not add to the load, and should hopefully help recovery to be more rapidly achieved, and if not more rapidly, more comfortably.

Massage seems well able to offer a number of these features, with education and rehabilitation exercises doing the rest in most cases.

WHAT RESEARCH SHOWS US

Research is mixed for the efficacy of massage for pain. Generally massage for pain management was not found to be a definitive treatment on its own but was supportive of many other interventions either enhancing effects or managing side effects of other treatments. Massage was found to be generally safe. Some benefits of massage related to other conditions such as low back or neck pain can be logically applied to pain in general. Other researchers have looked at massage for pain in general and others delved into the general benefits of massage.

Based on a search using the terms massage, massage therapy and pain, the following is presented. Since research is an evolving process the studies and conclusions presented can be either confirmed or questioned and the massage professional needs to remain current with advances in the understanding of the benefits of massage. The search process for this text involved mainly Internet search using ScienceDirect, PubMed and Google Scholar. Representative studies, especially meta-analyses, were analyzed and the findings of some of these reports appear next.

MASSAGE BENEFITS AND SAFETY IN GENERAL

When looking at any treatment, safety is a primary concern, i.e. do no harm. If harm is possible, then the benefits of receiving massage must exceed the potential for harm. A summary of a review of massage safety by Ernst (2006) concludes that massage is generally safe (Box 2.1). Massage is not entirely risk free. However, serious adverse effects are rare. The majority of adverse effects from massage were associated with aggressive types of manual massage or massage delivered by untrained individuals. Serious adverse effects were associated mostly with massage techniques other than 'Swedish'(classic) massage.

Information provided by Moyer and others (2006) indicates that massage is effective as a treatment in some instances but they did not investigate why. The 'why massage works' remains elusive but there are reoccurring findings indicating possible physiologic mechanisms for massage benefit. One study by Field and her associates (2005) is particularly relevant for the topic of this text since it deals with serotonin, which is associated with the body pain modulation mechanisms. In the other studies (2004) Diego speaks of how massage needs to be applied with sufficient compressive force to stimulate antiarousal response and that massage that is considered light can be arousing (Moyer 2006).

Massage therapy appears to affect anxiety levels (Fig. 2.1). The therapeutic relationship established between massage therapist and client is similar to psychotherapy: a treatment that relies on communication and therapeutic relationship to provide effects. It is possible that massage effects related to the affective category are related to the therapeutic relationship (Fellowes 2004, Moyer 2006). As described it is common to find a correlation between stress, anxiety, depression, and pain. According to Hanley et al (2003) despite very strong patient preference for therapeutic massage, it did not show any benefits over either a relaxation tape used in the surgery or a relaxation tape used at home. This study indicates that massage is effective but no more effective than other relaxation interventions.

Box 2.1 Who is Edzard Ernst?

Professor Ernst qualified as a physician in Germany in 1978 where he also completed his MD and PhD theses. He has received training in acupuncture, autogenic training, herbalism, homoeopathy, massage therapy, and spinal manipulation. He was Professor in Physical Medicine and Rehabilitation (PMR) at Hannover Medical School and Head of the PMR Department at the University of Vienna. In 1993 he established the Chair in Complementary Medicine at the University of Exeter. He is founder/Editor-in-Chief of two medical journals (*Perfusion* and *FACT*). He has published more than 40 books and in excess of 1000 articles in the peer-reviewed medical literature and has been given visiting professorships in Canada and the USA. His work has been awarded with 13 scientific prizes. In 1999 he took British nationality. His unit's research is funded from two endowments by the late Sir Maurice Laing, by research grants and fellowships (not, however, by 'Big Pharma' as sometimes speculated). See: http://sites.pcmd.ac.uk/compmed/ernst.htm

Contact: Complementary Medicine, Peninsula Medical School, Universities of Exeter and Plymouth, Exeter, UK. Edzard.Ernst@pms.ac.uk

Edzard Ernst states:

My ultimate objective is to apply the principles of evidence-based medicine to the field of complementary medicine such that those treatments which demonstrably do generate more good than harm become part of conventional medicine and those which fail to meet this criterion become obsolete.

http://sites.pcmd.ac.uk/compmed/ErnstCV-extended.pdf. Retrieved December 14, 2009.

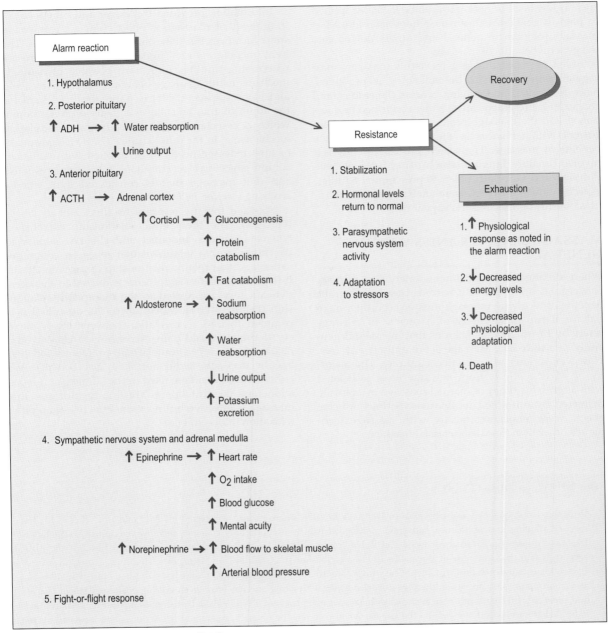

Figure 2.1 General adaptation syndrome (GAS).

A key is that people liked massage, which is important in compliance with treatment. Muller-Oerlinghausen et al (2004) concluded that slow-stroke massage is suitable for adjuvant intervention for depression and is readily accepted by very ill patients. Currin and Meister (2008) found that reduction in oncology patient distress was observed regardless of gender, age, ethnicity, or cancer type and therefore supported massage therapy for hospitalized oncology patients as a means of enhancing their course of treatment. Sturgeon et al (2009) found that therapeutic massage shows potential benefits for reducing breast cancer treatment side effects of chemotherapy and radiation and improving perceived quality of life and overall functioning.

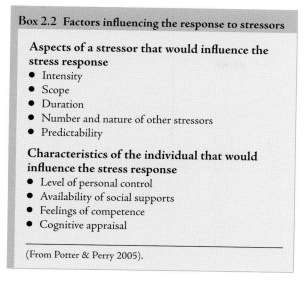

Mechanical effects related to massage benefits

Massage benefits appear to be related to mechanical forces applied to soft tissue which:

- alter pliability in connective tissue
- stimulate neuro signaling in fascia
- create changes in circulation
- stimulate changes in motor tone of muscles.

Let's look at each of these areas. As presented later in this text, massage methods apply mechanical forces to the soft tissue. According to Langevin and Sherman (2007) pain related fear leads to a cycle of decreased movement, connective tissue remodeling, inflammation and nervous system sensitization which combine into a cycle resulting in further decreased mobility. The mechanisms of a variety of treatments such as massage may reverse these abnormalities by applying mechanical forces to soft tissues. Based on a tensegrity principle, direct or indirect connections between fascia or muscles which stretch the aponeurosis or intermuscular septum may allow the transfer of tension over long distances. Massage applied in such a way to deform the soft tissue has an effect on electrical (EMG) and mechanical (MMG) activities of a muscle lying distant, but indirectly connected to, the massaged muscle. It was concluded that there was an electrical as well as a mechanical response of muscle connected indirectly by structural elements with the muscle being massaged, indicating an application for the tensegrity principle in massage therapy and influence on adverse muscle tension by massaging another distant muscle (Kassolik et al 2009).

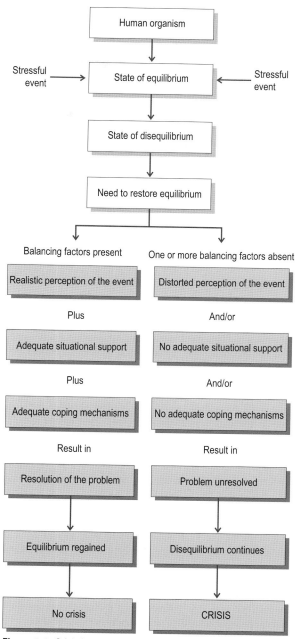

Figure 2.2 Crisis intervention model. (Redrawn from Aguilera 1998.)

Day et al (2009) found that deep muscular fascia design supports the premise that the myofascial system is a three-dimensional continuum, including the epimysium and the retinacula. Dr Carla Stecco and Dr Antonio Stecco have carried out extensive research into the anatomy and histology of the fascia via dissection of unembalmed cadavers. This technique presents a complete biomechanical model that assists in deciphering the role of fascia in musculoskeletal disorders.

The mainstay of this manual technique lies in the identification of a specific, localized area of the fascia in connection with a specific limited movement. Once a limited or painful movement is identified, then a specific point on the fascia is implicated and, through the appropriate manipulation of this precise part of the fascia, movement can be restored. These dissections have enhanced the pre-existing biomechanical model already elaborated by Luigi Stecco (2004, 2009) by providing new histological and anatomical data.

While part of the fascia is anchored to bone, part is also always free to slide.

Fascia is formed by undulated collagen fibers and elastic fibers arranged in distinct layers, and within each layer the fibers are aligned in a different direction. Due to its undulated collagen fibers, fascia can be stretched and, thanks to its elastic fibers, it can then return to its original resting state. Subcutaneous connective tissue forms a very elastic, sliding membrane essential for thermal regulation, metabolic exchanges, and the protection of vessels and nerves, whereas the deep fascia envelops the muscles, and surrounds a muscle's aponeurosis up to where it inserts into bone.

It is hypothesized that the richly innervated fascia could be maintained in a resting state of tension due to the different muscular fibers that insert into it. Due to this optimal resting state, or basal tension, of the fascia, the free nerve endings and receptors within the fascial tissue are primed to perceive any variation in tension and, therefore, any movement of the body, whenever it occurs (Stecco et al 2007).

Deep fascia is effectively an ideal structure for perceiving and, consequently, assisting in organizing movements. Whenever a body part moves in any given direction in space there is a myofascial, tensional rearrangement within the corresponding fascia. Afferents embedded within the fascia are stimulated, producing accurate directional information. Any impediment in the gliding of the fascia could alter afferent input resulting in incoherent movement.

It is hypothesized that fascia is involved in proprioception and peripheral motor control in strict collaboration with the CNS.

The method used in the Stecco studies involves a deep kneading of muscular fascia at specific points, termed centers of coordination (cc) and centers of fusion (cf), along myofascial sequences, diagonals, and spirals, and is called fascial manipulation technique. Visual analogue scale (VAS) measurement of pain administered prior to the first session and after

---

Box 2.3 Interview of Luigi Stecco

Fascial Manipulation© is a manual therapy that has been developed by Luigi Stecco, an Italian physiotherapist from the north of Italy. This method has evolved over the last 30 years through study and practice in the treatment of a vast caseload of musculoskeletal problems.

In the fascia, there are different Centres of Coordination that, incidentally, often coincide with acupuncture points. These centres are probably involved in the coordination of joint movements. When, or if, they become 'desensitized', pain results in the associated joint. In order to re-balance the various body structures the densifications need to be slowly dissolved. Not by chance, manipulation of the fascia can play a role in preventing dysfunction.

**http://www.fascialmanipulation.com/
Portals/0/Curingthefascia.pdf**

Curing the fascia. Interview of Luigi Stecco by Massimo Ilari. Published April 2003, Vita & Salute magazine. Translation: Julie Ann Day

---

the third session was compared with a follow-up evaluation at 3 months. Results suggested that the application of fascial manipulation technique may be effective in reducing pain in chronic situations (Pedrelli et al 2009).

Recent studies suggest that cyclic stretching of fibroblasts contributes to antifibrotic processes of wound healing by reducing connective tissue growth factor (CTGF) production (Kanazawa et al 2009). Robert Schleip (2003) indicates that fascia is imbedded with sensory mechanoreceptors, making fascia a sensory organ, and free nerve endings which respond to mechanical force stimulation. The intrafascial mechanoreceptors consist of four groups:

1. Golgi organs, which are found mostly in myotendinous junctions.
2. Large Pacini corpuscles, which respond to rapid changes in pressure.
3. Smaller and more longitudinal Ruffini organs, which do not adapt quickly to pressure.
4. Interstitial myofascial receptors.

Schleip (2006) indicates soft tissue strain involves a stimulation of intrafascial mechanoreceptors. This stimulation leads to an input to the central nervous system, altering the tone of motor units associated with the tissue. Combined with Ruffini organs and interstitial receptors, it can trigger changes in the autonomic nervous system.

The European Fascia Group (Schleip et al 2006) found that when fascia is stretched there are longitudinal relaxation changes in the collagen fibers and the water is squeezed out. Fascia seems to adapt with very complex and dynamic water changes to mechanical stimuli and the matrix reacts in smooth muscle-like contraction and relaxation responses of the whole tissue due to the sponge effect of fascia, like squeezing and refilling effects in the semiliquid ground substance.

Dr Leon Chaitow (2009) indicates that key fascia related topics are:

- The presence of contractile smooth muscle cells (SMCs/myofibroblasts) that are embedded in most connective tissues. For example, SMCs have been located widely in connective tissues including cartilage, ligaments, spinal discs, and lumbodorsal fascia (Ahluwalia 2001, Hastreite et al 2001). The extracellular matrix (ECM) plays a key role in the transmission of forces generated by the organism (e.g. muscle contraction) or externally applied (e.g. gravity, or by means of manually applied therapy).
- Cell-matrix adhesion sites appear to host a 'mechanosensory switch' as they transmit forces from the ECM to the cytoskeleton, and vice versa, triggering internal signals following mechanical stimulation, such as occurs in manual therapy (Chen & Ingber 1999). There appear to be forms of communication within the fascial matrix, for example caused by tugging in the mucopolysaccharides, created by twisting acupuncture needles (Langevin et al 2005).

German researchers, Robert Schleip et al (2005), note that:

> The ability of fascia to contract is further demonstrated by the widespread existence of pathological fascial contractures. Probably, the most well known example is Dupuytren disease (palmar fibromatosis), which is known to be mediated by the proliferation and contractile activity of myofibroblasts. Lesser known is the existence of similar contractures in other fascial tissues which are also driven by contractile myofibroblasts, e.g. plantar fibromatosis, Peyronies disease (induratio penis plastica), club foot, or – much more commonly – in the frozen shoulder with its documented connective tissue contractures. Given the widespread existence of such strong pathological chronic contractures, it seems likely that minor degrees of fascial contractures might exist among normal, healthy people and have some influence on biomechanical behavior.

The behavior of water that interacts with protein in the human body is becoming clearer. Professor Martin Gruebele of the University of Illinois explains:

> Water in our bodies has different physical properties from ordinary bulk water, because of the presence of proteins and other biomolecules. Proteins change the properties of water to perform particular tasks in different parts of our cells ... Water can be viewed as a 'designer fluid' in living cells.

http://www.biocompare.com/News/
NewsStory/239323/NewsStory.html
Retrieved December 17, 2009.

Sommer and Zhu (2008) note that interfascial water plays a key part in what is termed 'protein folding,' the process necessary for cells to form their characteristic shapes – and that nanocrystals are a part of this process – and that these are influenced by light:

> In the course of a systematic exploration of interfascial water layers on solids we discovered microtornadoes, found a complementary explanation to the surface conductivity on hydrogenated diamond, and arrived at a practical method to repair elastin degeneration, using light.

A leading researcher in this field, Pollack (2006), has shown that water can at times demonstrate a tendency to behave in a crystalline manner. He has discussed interfascial water in living cells known as vicinal water. Interfascial water exhibits structural organizations that differ from what is termed 'bulk' water. This vicinal water seems to be influenced by structural properties that make up the cell. In discussion of one example of this, in relation to the water in a temporomandibular joint, Pollack says:

> The combined data from three different methods lead to the conclusion that all or almost all of the water in the intact disc is bound water and does not have properties consistent with free or bulk water.

Pollack also says:

> If you want to understand what happens in any system – be it biological, or physical, or chemical, or oceanographic, or atmospheric, or whatever – it doesn't matter, anything involving water, you really have to know the behavior of this special kind of gel-like water, which dominates.

Several years ago Klingler and Schleip (2004) showed that the water content of fascia partially determines its stiffness, and that stretching, or compression, of fascia (as occurs during almost all manual therapies) causes water to be extruded (like a sponge) – making the tissues more pliable and supple. After a while the water is taken up again and stiffness returns, but in the meantime structures can be mobilized and stretched more effectively and comfortably than when were they still densely packed with water.

- Klingler et al measured wet and dry fresh human fascia, and found that during an isometric stretch, water is extruded, refilling during a subsequent rest period.
- As water extrudes during stretching, temporary relaxation occurs in the longitudinal arrangement of the collagen fibers.
- If the strain is moderate, and there are no micro-injuries, water soaks back into the tissue until it swells, becoming stiffer than before.

All this suggests that much manual therapy, and the tissue responses experienced, may relate to sponge-like squeezing and refilling effects in the semi-liquid ground substance, with its water binding glycosaminoglycans and proteoglycans.

Muscle energy technique-like contractions and stretches almost certainly have similar effects on the water content of connective tissue, as do myofascial release methods and the multiple force-loading elements of massage.

Most people nowadays are aware that acupuncture points in TCM are thought of as being linked along invisible lines (meridians) that apparently connect anatomical areas and organs, and along which energy (*chi*) is thought to travel. Obstructions to this flow, leading to areas of congestion or deficiency, are seen as contributing to health problems, and can be relieved by appropriate needle application (or manual treatment of the points – as in shiatsu). Please forgive this simplistic outline of what is in fact a far more complex theoretical construction, but it may help in my attempt to eventually get to the 'wow' moments from Vermont and outer space, below.

Apart from the hundreds of 'official' acupuncture points, lying on these meridian maps/lines, another class of acupuncture point has always fascinated me. This is the so-called Ah shi point. Ah shi points are areas that become spontaneously tender/painful in response to local problems (strain, draughts, etc.). They become 'eligible' for treatment in acupuncture (needles or acupressure) when they are sensitive. Now anyone who knows very much about Simons, Travell and Simons' (1999) work on trigger points might be forgiven for thinking that these points sound like those points ... if you see what I mean?

Since we already know that approximately 80% of the main trigger point sites lie on points located on the meridian maps (Wall & Melzack 1990), the conjunction of these two areas of study (TCM/acupuncture points and myofascial trigger points) should not come as a surprise. Indeed, many experts believe that trigger points and acupuncture points are the same phenomenon (Kawakita et al 2002). Whether this is so or not, it suggests that in trying to understand trigger points better, we need to pay attention to research that tries to explain the processes of acupuncture, and the structural aspects of these invisible points.

Dr Langevin and her research colleagues have helped to clarify the situation, having shown that acupuncture points, and many of the effects of acupuncture, seem to relate to the fact that most of these localized 'points' lie directly over areas where there is a fascial cleavage, where sheets of fascia diverge to separate, surround, and support different muscle bundles (Langevin et al 2001).

It seems that the meridians may, in fact, be fascial pathways. This is not too surprising, since we know the fascial network represents one continuum from the internal cranial reciprocal tension membranes to the plantar fascia of the feet. Now we know that acupuncture points (and it seems the majority of trigger points) are structurally situated in connective tissue, but how does application of a needle or pressure in one part of the fascia translate to distant sites? How does the fascia communicate with other parts of the body?

Well, the Vermont researchers have also shown that connective tissue is a sophisticated communication system, of as yet unknown potential:

'Loose' connective tissue forms a network extending throughout the body including subcutaneous and interstitial connective tissues. The existence of a cellular network of fibroblasts within loose connective tissue may have considerable significance as it may support yet unknown body-wide cellular signaling systems ...Our findings indicate that soft tissue fibroblasts form an extensively interconnected cellular network, suggesting they may have important, and so far unsuspected integrative functions at the level of the whole body. (Langevin et al 2004)

Author's note: Research information summarized in this article has been drawn from content in the 2nd edition of my book, *Clinical Applications of Neuromuscular Techniques: Volume 1* (Churchill Livingstone, 2001).

To understand how this signaling system works we need to be aware of the role of integrins – tiny projections emerging from each cell, that act like mini-transmitters and receivers. What Helene Langevin and her colleagues are now showing is that when deformation of cells and tissues occurs – such as that which happens to all of us when areas of the body are chronically shortened, crowded, compressed, stretched, or twisted due to age, disease, trauma, or progressive adaptation – the cells cannot function or communicate normally, or even demonstrate normal gene expression. And consider, from the bodyworker's point of view, the reverse of that scenario. When we normalize tissues that are tense/tight/deformed/compressed by means of massage, stretching, mobilizing, etc., we are not just normalizing the biomechanical aspects of the function of those tissues – so that, for example, the shoulder or elbow or neck or whatever 'feels' better – we are also improving internal cellular function, enhancing cellular communication and gene expression. If that's not a 'wow' I don't know what is!

The Amazing Fascial Web, Leon Chaitow

The observation of Langevin et al (2005) is:

> The dynamic, cytoskeleton-dependent responses of fibroblasts to changes in tissue length demonstrated in this study have important implications for our understanding of normal movement and posture, as well as therapies using mechanical stimulation of connective tissue including physical therapy, massage and acupuncture. (Langevin et al 2005)

Consider the connections I have attempted to put together in this brief communication regarding different elements of our understanding of how the body works:

1. The fascial cleavage planes seem to have a great deal to do with where acupuncture points (and many or most trigger points) are situated.
2. Cells communicate via (among other methods) mini-projections (integrins) that are capable of becoming deformed and distorted though age, overuse, misuse, abuse, and disuse (and loss of gravity!), with negative effects on cellular (and therefore tissue) function, including communication, nutrition, and reproduction (gene expression).
3. The function of tissues, down to the cellular level, can be enhanced by appropriate massage, bodywork, movement, and manipulation (and, it seems, by acupuncture).

Our work can really change the way the body works, and not just on the mechanical level. We influence emotion, the mind, the nervous system, immune function, and now we know that we also influence the way cells communicate and nourish themselves.

What type of methods influence fascia?
Any form of application that deforms the tissue and incorporates a stretching technique influences fascia. Fascia is a thin tissue that covers all the organs of the body. This tissue covers every muscle and every fiber within each muscle. All muscle stretching is, therefore, actually stretching of the fascia and the muscle, the myofascial unit. Injury to this tissue and subsequent healing can result in changes in the force distribution through the fascial network. Based on tensegrity structure, strain, shortening, and shape change in the tissue can cause pain and stiffness in areas of the body distant from the original injury site.

Fischer et al (2009) confirmed the interconnectedness of body areas with a study that suggests that temporomandibular joint dysfunction plays an important role in the restriction of hip motion experienced by patients with complex regional pain syndrome, which indicated a connectedness between these two regions of the body.

Various fascial techniques contain the same components. The therapist finds the area of tightness (better described as bind) and a light stretch (better called tension force) is applied to the tight area. The tension on the tissue is maintained for up to 30 seconds until softening occurs. Then the therapist moves to the next area of binding tissue and repeats constantly, sustaining bind and moving in multiple directions. The process is repeated until the area is fully softened. Then, the next area is addressed.

Circulation is also affected by massage. Castro-Sánchez et al (2009) found that connective tissue massage improves blood circulation in the lower limbs of type 2 diabetic patients at stage I or II-a and may be useful to slow the progression of peripheral artery disease. A different study lead by Castro-Sánchez indicated that a combined program of exercise and massage improves arterial blood pressure and ankle brachial index values in type 2 diabetics with peripheral arterial disease. Walton (2008) investigated efficacy of myofascial release techniques in the treatment of primary Raynaud's phenomenon and found that releasing restricted fascia using myofascial techniques may influence the duration and severity of the vasospastic episodes.

Arroyo-Morales et al (2008) found that massage reduces EMG amplitude and vigor when applied as a passive recovery technique after a high-intensity exercise protocol. Massage may induce a transient loss of muscle strength or a change in the muscle fiber tension–length relationship, influenced by alterations of muscle function and a psychological state of relaxation.

Research related to massage and pain

Existing research provides fairly robust support for the analgesic effects of massage for nonspecific low back pain, but only moderate support for such effects on shoulder pain and headache pain. There is only modest, preliminary support for massage in the treatment of fibromyalgia, mixed chronic pain conditions, neck pain, and carpal tunnel syndrome. Thus, research to date provides varying levels of evidence for the benefits of massage therapy (MT) for different chronic pain conditions (Tsao 2007).

Ho et al (2009) studied massage for adhesive capsulitis (AC), shoulder impingement syndrome (SIS) and nonspecific shoulder pain/dysfunction. For SIS, there was no clear evidence to suggest additional benefits of MT to other interventions. MT was not shown to be more effective than other conservative interventions for AC; however, massage and mobilizations-with-movement may be useful in comparison to no treatment for short-term outcomes for shoulder dysfunction. Massage is safe and may have clinical benefits for treating chronic neck pain at least in the short term (Sherman et al 2009). The application of a single session of manual therapy program produces an immediate increase of index heart rate variability (HRV) and a decrease in tension, anger status, and perceived pain in patients with chronic tension-type headache (CTTH), HRV, mood states, and pressure pain thresholds (PPTs) in patients with CTTH (Toro-Velasco et al 2009).

PAIN RELIEF BY TOPIC

Cancer pain

The value of massage therapy in cancer care
MT is increasingly available as a supportive therapy to patients in medical centers providing cancer treatment. This section provides an overview of the evidence base relevant to the use of massage with the intended goal of alleviating symptoms and side effects experienced by cancer patients. Collectively, the available data support the view that massage, modified appropriately, offers potential beneficial effects for cancer patients in terms of reducing anxiety and pain and other symptoms. Replication of preliminary studies with larger, more homogeneous patient samples and rigorous study designs will help to clarify which massage modalities have the most potential benefit for which patients before, during, and after specific types of cancer treatment.

Effects of a full-body massage on pain intensity, anxiety, and physiological relaxation in Taiwanese patients with metastatic bone pain: a pilot study

Sui-Whi Jane, Diana J. Wilkie, Betty B. Gallucci, Randal D. Beaton, Hsiu-Ying Huang Journal of Pain and Symptom Management, Volume 37, Issue 4, April 2009, Pages 754–763

Abstract
Bone involvement, a hallmark of advanced cancer, results in intolerable pain, substantial morbidity, and impaired quality of life in 34–45% of cancer patients. Despite the publication of 15 studies on MT in cancer patients, little is known about the longitudinal effects of MT and safety in cancer patients with bone metastasis. The purpose of this study was to describe the feasibility of MT and to examine the effects of MT on present pain intensity (PPI), anxiety, and physiological relaxation over a 16- to 18-hour period in 30 Taiwanese cancer patients with bone metastases. A quasi-experimental, one-group, pretest/post-test design with repeated measures was used to examine the time effects of MT using single-item scales for pain (PPI-visual analog scale [VAS]) and anxiety (anxiety-VAS), the modified Short-Form McGill Pain Questionnaire (MSF-MPQ), heart rate (HR), and mean arterial pressure (MAP). MT was shown to have effective immediate [$t(29) = 16.5$, $P = 0.000$; $t(29) = 8.9$, $P = 0.000$], short-term (20–30 minutes) [$t(29) = 9.3$, $P = 0.000$; $t(29) = 10.1$, $P = 0.000$], intermediate (1–2.5 hours) [$t(29) = 7.9$, $P = 0.000$; $t(29) = 8.9$, $P = 0.000$], and long-term benefits (16–18 hours) [$t(29) = 4.0$, $P = 0.000$; $t(29) = 5.7$, $P = 0.000$] on PPI and anxiety. The most significant impact occurred 15 [$F = 11.5(1,29)$, $P < 0.002$] or 20 [$F = 20.4(1,29)$, $P < 0.000$] minutes after the intervention. There were no significant time effects in decreasing or increasing HR and MAP. No patient reported any adverse effects as a result of MT. Clinically, the time effects of MT can assist health care providers in implementing MT along with pharmacological treatment, thereby enhancing cancer pain management. Randomized clinical trials are needed to validate the effectiveness of MT in this cancer population.

Effects of ice massage on neuropathic pain in persons with AIDS

Kristin Kane Ownby Journal of the Association of Nurses in AIDS Care, Volume 17, Issue 5, September–October 2006, Pages 15–22

Abstract

Peripheral neuropathic pain is a unique form of chronic pain that afflicts up to 50% of persons with AIDS. The purpose of this pilot study was to examine the effects of ice massage to reduce neuropathic pain and improve sleep quality, and to determine the feasibility of a larger study. A repeated measures design was used. The three treatments consisted of ice massage, dry-towel massage, and presence. Consecutive sampling was used to select 33 persons with AIDS who had neuropathic pain. Although the results of the study were negative, there was a decrease in pain intensity over time with both the ice massage and towel massage, suggesting that the intervention has some clinical benefit.

Massage therapy for symptom control: outcome study at a major cancer center

Barrie R. Cassileth, Andrew J. Vickers Journal of Pain and Symptom Management, Volume 28, Issue 3, September 2004, Pages 244–249

Abstract

Massage is increasingly applied to relieve symptoms in patients with cancer. This practice is supported by evidence from small randomized trials. No study has examined massage therapy outcome in a large group of patients. At Memorial Sloan-Kettering Cancer Center, patients report symptom severity pre- and post-massage therapy using 0–10 rating scales of pain, fatigue, stress/anxiety, nausea, depression and 'other'. Changes in symptom scores and the modifying effects of patient status (in- or outpatient) and type of massage were analyzed. Over a 3-year period, 1290 patients were treated. Symptom scores were reduced by approximately 50%, even for patients reporting high baseline scores. Outpatients improved about 10% more than inpatients. Benefits persisted, with outpatients experiencing no return toward baseline scores throughout the duration of 48-hour follow-up. These data indicate that massage therapy is associated with substantive improvement in cancer patients' symptom scores.

Chronic muscular skeletal pain

The effectiveness of manual therapy in the management of musculoskeletal disorders of the shoulder: A systematic review

Chung-Yee Cecilia Ho, Gisela Sole, Joanne Munn Manual Therapy, Volume 14, Issue 5, October 2009, Pages 463–474

Abstract

A systematic review of randomized controlled trials (RCTs) was conducted to determine the effectiveness of manual therapy (MT) techniques for the management of musculoskeletal disorders of the shoulder. Results were analyzed within diagnostic subgroups (adhesive capsulitis [AC], shoulder impingement syndrome [SIS], non-specific shoulder pain/dysfunction) and a qualitative analysis using levels of evidence to define treatment effectiveness was applied. For SIS, there was no clear evidence to suggest additional benefits of MT to other interventions. MT was not shown to be more effective than other conservative interventions for AC, however, massage and Mobilizations-with-Movement may be useful in comparison to no treatment for short-term outcomes for shoulder dysfunction.

Assessing the effect of sample size, methodological quality and statistical rigour on outcomes of randomised controlled trials on mobilisation, manipulation and massage for low back pain of at least 6 weeks duration

Dries M. Hettinga, Deirdre A. Hurley, Anne Jackson, Stephen May, Chris Mercer, Lisa Roberts Physiotherapy, Volume 94, Issue 2, June 2008, Pages 97–104

Abstract
Objectives
To assess the effect of sample size, methodological quality and statistical rigour on outcomes of randomised controlled trials (RCTs) on manual therapy (i.e. manipulation, mobilisation and/or massage) for non-specific low back pain (LBP) of at least 6 weeks duration, and to report results from RCTs with adequate sample size, methodological quality and statistical rigour.

Data sources
MedLine, EMBASE, CINAHL, AMED, Cochrane, PEDro and the library collection of the Chartered Society of Physiotherapy.

Review methods
RCTs were identified that compared manual therapy with a control or alternative intervention in adults with non-specific LBP of at least 6 weeks duration. The sample size, methodological quality (adapted 10-point van Tulder scale) and statistical rigour were then assessed. RCTs were regarded as higher quality if they fulfilled the following three criteria: (a) > 40 subjects in the manual therapy group; (b) scoring > 5/10 on the Van Tulder scale; and (c) reporting statistical tests that compared the change in the intervention group with the change in the control group.

Results
Ten RCTs were included in the review but only two qualified as higher quality RCTs. Results from smaller trials and lower quality RCTs showed more variation in differences between the intervention and control groups than larger or higher quality trials. Evidence from large, high-quality RCTs with adequate statistical analyses showed that, for improvement in pain and function, a mobilisation/manipulation package is an effective intervention [compared with general practitioner (GP) care], whilst manipulation used in isolation showed no real benefits over sham manipulation or an alternative intervention. No higher quality evidence considering massage was identified.

Conclusions
Many RCTs in the area of manual therapy for LBP have shortcomings in sample size, methodological quality and/or statistical rigour, but there remains evidence from higher quality RCTs to support the use of a manual therapy package, compared with GP care, for non-specific LBP of at least 6 weeks duration.

Massage therapy decreases frequency and intensity of symptoms related to temporomandibular joint syndrome in one case study

Lindsay Phipps Eisensmith Journal of Bodywork and Movement Therapies, Volume 11, Issue 3, July 2007, Pages 223–230

Summary
Objective
This study investigated the ability of massage therapy to mitigate the frequency and intensity of headaches, jaw clicking and masticatory pain associated with temporomandibular joint syndrome (TMJ).

Methods
The subject reported 3 years of masticatory pain, clicking, teeth grinding, reduced jaw opening and headaches prior to the study. A log was kept documenting frequency, intensity and type of pain. Pre- and post-treatment jaw opening was recorded. Western massage techniques combined with strain–counterstrain techniques targeted the upper torso, cervical region and oral cavity twice weekly for 30 min each over 3 weeks.

(Continued)

(Continued)

Results
TMJ-related pain decreased and maximal jaw opening increased by almost a third. Jaw clicking decreased fourfold to once monthly. Teeth grinding was unchanged.

Conclusion
The results suggest that western massage and strain–counterstrain techniques can improve jaw range of motion, alleviate the intensity and reduce the frequency of TMJ-related pain without surgical or pharmacological intervention.

Effects of traditional Thai massage versus joint mobilization on substance P and pain perception in patients with non-specific low back pain

Surussawadi Mackawan, Wichi Eungpinichpong, Rungthip Pantumethakul, Uraiwon Chatchawan, Tokamol Hunsawong, Pricha Arayawichanon Journal of Bodywork and Movement Therapies, Volume 11, Issue 1, January 2007, Pages 9–16

Summary
Although both Traditional Thai Massage (TTM) and joint mobilization have been practiced in Thailand to reduce musculoskeletal pain, a comparative study of these in relieving pain is not been found in the literature. The purpose of this study was to examine the immediate effects of TTM versus joint mobilization on substance P and pain perception in patients with non-specific low back pain. Sixty-seven adults with non-specific low back pain were randomly assigned to receive either TTM (35 people) or joint mobilization (32 people). The duration of each treatment was 10 min. The levels of substance P in saliva and a visual analog scale (VAS) were measured before and 5 min after each treatment. Both groups showed a decrease in the level of substance P after treatment when compared with levels pre-treatment. There was no significant difference in the substance P level after treatment between the two groups. However, the VAS pain score was slightly different between the groups after treatment. Both TTM and joint mobilization can relieve pain in patients with non-specific low back pain. However, TTM yields slightly more beneficial effects than joint mobilization.

The immediate effect of ischemic compression technique and transverse friction massage on tenderness of active and latent myofascial trigger points: a pilot study

César Fernández-de-las-Peñas, Cristina Alonso-Blanco, Josué Fernández-Carnero, Juan Carlos Miangolarra-Page Journal of Bodywork and Movement Therapies, Volume 10, Issue 1, January 2006, Pages 3–9

Summary
The aim of this pilot study was to compare the effects of a single treatment of the ischemic compression technique with transverse friction massage for myofascial trigger point (MTrP) tenderness. Forty subjects, 17 men and 23 women, aged 19–38 years old, presenting with mechanical neck pain and diagnosed with MTrPs in the upper trapezius muscle, according to the diagnostic criteria described by Simons and by Gerwin, participated in this pilot study. Subjects were divided randomly into two groups: group A which was treated with the ischemic compression technique, and group B which was treated with a transverse friction massage. The outcome measures were the pressure pain threshold (PPT) in the MTrP, and a visual analogue scale assessing local pain evoked by a second application of $2.5\,kg/cm^2$ of pressure on the MTrP. These outcomes were assessed pre-treatment and 2 min post-treatment by an assessor blinded to the treatment allocation of the subject. The results showed a significant improvement in the PPT ($P = 0.03$), and a significant decrease in the visual analogue scores ($P = 0.04$) within each group. No differences were found between the improvement in both groups ($P = 0.4$). Ischemic compression technique and transverse friction massage were equally effective in reducing tenderness in MTrPs.

The clinical effectiveness of therapeutic massage for musculoskeletal pain: a systematic review

Mark Lewis, Mark I. Johnson Physiotherapy, Volume 92, Issue 3, September 2006, Pages 146–158

Abstract
Objectives
To determine the effectiveness of therapeutic massage (TM) for the symptomatic relief of musculoskeletal pain, and to analyze TM intervention protocols used in studies.

Systematic review of randomized controlled clinical trials and experimental studies on healthy human participants.

Twenty studies (1341 participants) met the criteria for review. TM was superior to no treatment in five out of 10 comparisons, superior to sham (laser) treatment in one out of two comparisons, and superior to active treatment in seven out of 22 comparisons. TM was superior to comparison groups in six out of 11 studies using patients with musculoskeletal pain, and in three out of seven studies using patients with low back pain. TM was superior to comparison groups in four out of nine studies using healthy participants experiencing post-exercise pain and soreness. There were no relationships between study outcome and the TM regimen used. The available evidence is inconclusive. A combination of inadequate sample sizes, low methodological quality and insufficient TM dosing is likely to have contributed to the confused evidence base.

Effectiveness of traditional Thai massage versus Swedish massage among patients with back pain associated with myofascial trigger points

Uraiwon Chatchawan, Bandit Thinkhamrop, Samerduen Kharmwan, Jacqueline Knowles, Wichai Eungpinichpong Journal of Bodywork and Movement Therapies, Volume 9, Issue 4, October 2005, Pages 298–309

Abstract
The aim of this study was to verify the effectiveness of traditional Thai massage (TTM) among patients with back pain associated with myofascial trigger points (MTrPs). Swedish massage (SM) was selected as the treatment for the comparison group. One hundred and eighty patients were randomly allocated to receive either TTM or SM for 6 sessions during a 3–4 week period, with follow-up 1 month later. Results indicated that pain intensity, assessed using the visual analog scale (VAS), among patients in both groups was reduced by more than half after 3 weeks of treatment and for up to one month afterwards ($P < 0.05$) with no significant difference in VAS between the groups. Similar improvements were found for most other outcome measures. We conclude that TTM and SM are effective in reducing back pain among patients with MTrPs. We therefore suggest that massage therapy, and in particular Thai massage, be considered as an alternative primary health care treatment for this disorder.

Carpal tunnel syndrome symptoms are lessened following massage therapy

Tiffany Field, Miguel Diego, Christy Cullen, Kristin Hartshorn, Alan Gruskin, Maria Hernandez-Reif, William Sunshine Journal of Bodywork and Movement Therapies, Volume 8, Issue 1, January 2004, Pages 9–14

Abstract
Objective. To determine the effectiveness of massage therapy for relieving the symptoms of carpal tunnel syndrome (CTS).

Results. Participants in the massage therapy group improved on median peak latency and grip strength. They also experienced lower levels of perceived pain, anxiety, and depressed mood.

Conclusion. The results suggest that symptoms of CTS can be relieved by a daily regimen of massage therapy.

Hospice

Evaluating CAM treatment at the end of life: a review of clinical trials for massage and meditation

William E. Lafferty, Lois Downey, Rachelle L. McCarty, Leanna J. Standish, Donald L. Patrick Complementary Therapies in Medicine, Volume 14, Issue 2, June 2006, Pages 100–112

Background
There is a pressing need for improved end-of-life care. Use of complementary and alternative medicine (CAM) may improve the quality of care but few controlled trials have evaluated CAM at the end of life.

Objectives
To determine the strength of evidence for the benefits of touch and mind-body therapies in seriously ill patients.

Methods
Systematic review of randomized controlled trials of massage and mind-body therapies. A PubMed search of English language articles was used to identify the relevant studies.

Results
Of 27 clinical trials testing massage or mind-body interventions, 26 showed significant improvements in symptoms such as anxiety, emotional distress, comfort, nausea and pain. However, results were often inconsistent across studies and there were variations in methodology, so it was difficult to judge the clinical significance of the results.

Conclusions
Use of CAM at the end of life is warranted on a case-by-case basis. Limitations in study design and sample size of the trials analyzed mean that routine use of CAM cannot be supported. There are several challenges to be addressed in future research into the use of CAM in end-of-life patients.

Labor pain

Massage or music for pain relief in labour: a pilot randomised placebo controlled trial

L. Kimber, M. McNabb, C. McCourt, A. Haines, P. Brocklehurst European Journal of Pain, Volume 12, Issue 8, November 2008, Pages 961–969

Abstract
Research on massage therapy for maternal pain and anxiety in labour is currently limited to four small trials. Each used different massage techniques, at different frequencies and durations, and relaxation techniques were included in three trials. Given the need to investigate massage interventions that complement maternal neurophysiological adaptations to labour and birth pain(s), we designed a pilot randomised controlled trial (RCT) to test the effects of a massage programme practised during physiological changes in pain threshold, from late pregnancy to birth, on women's reported pain, measured by a visual analogue scale (VAS) at 90 min following birth. To control for the potential bias of the possible effects of support offered within preparation for the intervention group, the study included 3 arms – intervention (massage programme with relaxation techniques), placebo (music with relaxation techniques) and control (usual care). The placebo offered a non-pharmacological coping strategy, to ensure that use of massage was the only difference between intervention and placebo groups. There was a trend toward slightly lower mean pain scores in the intervention group but these differences were not statistically significant. No differences were found in use of pharmacological analgesia, need for augmentation or mode of delivery. There was a trend toward more positive views of labour preparedness and sense of control in the intervention and placebo groups, compared with the control group. These findings suggest that regular massage with relaxation techniques from late pregnancy to birth is an acceptable coping strategy that merits a large trial with sufficient power to detect differences in reported pain as a primary outcome measure.

Does regular massage from late pregnancy to birth decrease maternal pain perception during labor and birth? A feasibility study to investigate a program of massage, controlled breathing and visualization, from 36 weeks of pregnancy until birth

Mary T. McNabb, Linda Kimber, Anne Haines, Christine McCourt, Complementary Therapies in Clinical Practice, Volume 12, Issue 3, August 2006, Pages 222–231

Summary

The present study was undertaken to produce a detailed specification of a program of massage, controlled breathing and visualization performed regularly by birth partners, from 36 weeks gestation and assisted by a trained professional, following hospital admission during labour and birth. As current research on massage interventions for pain relief in labour is poorly characterized, we began by undertaking a feasibility study on an established massage program (Goldstone 2000). The intervention was designed in light of experimental findings that repeated massage sessions over 14 days increases pain threshold, by an interaction between oxytocin and opioid neurons (Lund I et al 2002). A 4 week time-frame was selected to coincide with a physiological increase in maternal pain threshold (Cogan R et al 1986, Gintzler, Komisaruk 1991, Gintzler, Liu 2001). The main objective was to measure the effects of the program on maternal pain perception during labour and birth. To detect any effect of massage during labour, on maternal cortisol and catecholamines, cord venous blood was taken to measure plasma concentrations following birth. Twenty-five nulliparous (N) and 10 multiparous (M) women participated in the study. Cortisol values were similar to published studies following labour without massage but pain scores on a Visual Analogue Scale (VAS), at 90 min following birth were significantly lower than scores recorded 2 days postpartum. The mean score was 6.6. Previous studies suggest that a reduction from 8.5 to 7.5 would significantly reduce pharmacological analgesia in labour (Capogna et al 1996).

Pain
_____

Quantitative application of transverse friction massage and its neurological effects on flexor carpi radialis

Hsin-Min Lee, Shyi-Kuen Wu, Jia-Yuan You Manual Therapy, Volume 14, Issue 5, October 2009, Pages 501–507

Abstract

The purpose of the study was to determine the effects of transverse friction massage (TFM) on flexor carpi radialis (FCR) motoneuron (MN) pool excitability.

Twenty-eight healthy subjects were randomly assigned into massage and control groups. Pre- vs post-TFM H-reflex data were collected. Controls received a rest period instead of massage. Massage dose was standardized by a novel electronic method which recorded the massage rate, momentary pressure and total cumulative pressure (energy). Two-way ANOVA of H/M ratios derived from maximal amplitudes of Hoffman reflexes (Hmax) and motor responses (Mmax) was used to analyze neurological effects and group differences.

Analysis of pressure/time curve data showed: mean massage rate was 0.501 ± 0.005 Hz; mean duration of massage sessions was 184.6 ± 26.4 s; mean peak pressure was 4.990 ± 1.006 psi. Hmax/Mmax ratios declined from 14.3% to 10.3% for massage ($P < 0.01$) but showed no change for controls ($P > 0.05$).

In conclusion a novel quantitative approach to the study of massage has been demonstrated while testing the effects of TFM on FCR MN pool excitability. TFM appears to reduce MN pool excitability. The novel method of quantifying massage permits more rigorous testing of client-centered massage in future research.

Effects of abdominal massage in management of constipation – A randomized controlled trial

Kristina Lämås, Lars Lindholm, Hans Stenlund, Birgitta Engström, Catrine Jacobsson, International Journal of Nursing Studies, Volume 46, Issue 6, June 2009, Pages 759–767

Abstract
Background
Associated with decreases in quality of life, constipation is a relatively common problem. Abdominal massage appears to increase bowel function, but unlike laxatives with no negative side effects. Because earlier studies have methodological flaws and cannot provide recommendations, more research is needed.

Objective
This study investigates the effects of abdominal massage on gastrointestinal functions and laxative intake in people who have constipation.

Participants and method
A sample of 60 people with constipation was included and randomized in two groups. The intervention group received abdominal massage in addition to an earlier prescribed laxative and the control group received only laxatives according to earlier prescriptions. Gastrointestinal function was assessed with Gastrointestinal Symptoms Rating Scale (GSRS) on three occasions; at baseline, week 4 and week 8. The statistical methods included linear regression, Wilcoxon sign rank test, and Mann–Whitney U-test.

Result
Abdominal massage significantly decreased severity of gastrointestinal symptoms assessed with GSRS according to total score ($p = .003$), constipation syndrome ($p = .013$), and abdominal pain syndrome ($p = .019$). The intervention group also had significant increase of bowel movements compared to the control group ($p = .016$). There was no significant difference in the change of the amount of laxative intake after 8 weeks.

Conclusions
Abdominal massage decreased severity of gastrointestinal symptoms, especially constipation and abdominal pain syndrome, and increased bowel movements. The massage did not lead to decrease in laxative intake, a result that indicates that abdominal massage could be a complement to laxatives rather than a substitute.

Massage reduces pain perception and hyperalgesia in experimental muscle pain: a randomized, controlled trial

Laura A. Frey Law, Stephanie Evans, Jill Knudtson, Steven Nus, Kerri Scholl, Kathleen A. Sluka The Journal of Pain, Volume 9, Issue 8, August 2008, Pages 714–721

Abstract
Massage is a common conservative intervention used to treat myalgia. Although subjective reports have supported the premise that massage decreases pain, few studies have systematically investigated the dose response characteristics of massage relative to a control group. The purpose of this study was to perform a double-blinded, randomized controlled trial of the effects of massage on mechanical hyperalgesia (pressure pain thresholds, PPT) and perceived pain using delayed onset muscle soreness (DOMS) as an endogenous model of myalgia. Participants were randomly assigned to a no-treatment control, superficial touch, or deep-tissue massage group. Eccentric wrist extension exercises were performed at visit 1 to induce DOMS 48 hours later at visit 2. Pain, assessed using visual analog scales (VAS), and PPTs were measured at baseline, after exercise, before treatment, and after treatment. Deep massage decreased pain (48.4% DOMS reversal) during muscle stretch. Mechanical hyperalgesia was reduced (27.5% reversal) after both the deep massage and superficial touch groups relative to control (increased hyperalgesia by 38.4%). Resting pain did not vary between treatment groups.

Perspective
This randomized, controlled trial suggests that massage is capable of reducing myalgia symptoms by approximately 25% to 50%, varying with assessment technique. Thus, potential analgesia may depend on the pain assessment used. This information may assist clinicians in determining conservative treatment options for patients with myalgia.

An experimental study on the effectiveness of massage with aromatic ginger and orange essential oil for moderate-to-severe knee pain among the elderly in Hong Kong

Yin Bing Yip, Ada Chung Ying Tam Complementary Therapies in Medicine, Volume 16, Issue 3, June 2008, Pages 131–138

Summary

Objectives
To assess the efficacy of an aromatic essential oil (1% *Zingiber officinale* and 0.5% *Citrus sinensis*) massage among the elderly with moderate-to-severe knee pain.

Method
Fifty-nine older persons were enrolled in a double-blind, placebo-controlled experimental study group from the Community Centre for Senior Citizens, Hong Kong. The intervention was six massage sessions with ginger and orange oil over a 3-week period. The placebo control group received the same massage intervention with olive oil only and the control group received no massage. Assessment was done at baseline, post 1-week and post 4 weeks after treatment. Changes from baseline to the end of treatment were assessed on knee pain intensity, stiffness level and physical functioning (by Western Ontario and McMaster Universities Osteoarthritis index) and quality of life (by SF-36).

Results
There were significant mean changes between the three time-points within the intervention group on three of the outcome measures: knee pain intensity ($p = 0.02$); stiffness level ($p = 0.03$); and enhancing physical function ($p = 0.04$) but these were not apparent with the between-groups comparison ($p = 0.48, 0.14$ and 0.45 respectively) 4 weeks after the massage. The improvement of physical function and pain were superior in the intervention group compared with both the placebo and the control group at post 1-week time (both $p = 0.03$) but not sustained at post 4 weeks ($p = 0.45$ and 0.29). The changes in quality of life were not statistically significant for all three groups.

Conclusion
The aroma-massage therapy seems to have potential as an alternative method for short-term knee pain relief.

A study to compare the effects of massage and static touch on experimentally induced pain in healthy volunteers

Jeff Kessler, Paul Marchant, Mark I. Johnson Physiotherapy, Volume 92, Issue 4, December 2006, Pages 225–232

Abstract

Objective
To investigate the hypoallergesic effects of massage on experimental pain.

Design
A cross-over intervention study separated by a 24-hour washout period. During each experiment, participants completed five cold-induced pain tests, two before the intervention and three during the intervention. During each test, participants immersed their hand in iced water and reported the first sensation of pain and pain intensity after a further 30 seconds.

A volunteer sample of 30 university staff and students without known pathology, recruited from notice board advertisements. Participants received massage in one experiment and static touch in the other experiment. Interventions were administered to the ipsilateral arm for 4 minutes immediately before the hand was immersed in iced water.

Main outcome measures
Time to pain threshold and the odds of a reduction in pain intensity and an increase in pain relief.

Results
A mixed model analysis was used to establish how measures varied, according to baseline, during static touch and during massage. Massage increased the pain threshold by a factor of 1.08 (95% confidence interval 0.99–1.17) compared with static

(Continued)

(Continued)

touch, but this failed to reach statistical significance (P = 0.088). Massage was more likely to result in a report of low pain intensity than static touch (odds ratio 0.26, 95% confidence interval 0.10–0.71, P = 0.007). Massage was more likely to result in a state of high pain relief than static touch (odds ratio 7.7, 95% confidence interval 3.0–19.8, P < 0.001).

Conclusion
Massage produced hypoallergenic effects on experimental pain in healthy volunteers.

Pain syndromes

Fascia: A missing link in our understanding of the pathology of fibromyalgia

G.L. Liptan Journal of Bodywork and Movement Therapies Volume 14, Issue 1, January 2010, Pages 3–12

Abstract

Significant evidence exists for central sensitization in fibromyalgia, however the cause of this process in fibromyalgia – and how it relates to other known abnormalities in fibromyalgia – remains unclear. Central sensitization occurs when persistent nociceptive input leads to increased excitability in the dorsal horn neurons of the spinal cord. In this hyperexcited state, spinal cord neurons produce an enhanced responsiveness to noxious stimulation, and even to formerly innocuous stimulation. No definite evidence of muscle pathology in fibromyalgia has been found. However, there is some evidence for dysfunction of the intramuscular connective tissue, or fascia, in fibromyalgia. This paper proposes that inflammation of the fascia is the source of peripheral nociceptive input that leads to central sensitization in fibromyalgia. The fascial dysfunction is proposed to be due to inadequate growth hormone production and HPA axis dysfunction in fibromyalgia. Fascia is richly innervated, and the major cell of the fascia, the fibroblast, has been shown to secrete pro-inflammatory cytokines, particularly IL-6, in response to strain. Recent biopsy studies using immuno-histochemical staining techniques have found increased levels of collagen and inflammatory mediators in the connective tissue surrounding the muscle cells in fibromyalgia patients. The inflammation of the fascia is similar to that described in conditions such as plantar fasciitis and lateral epicondylitis, and may be better described as a dysfunctional healing response. This may explain why NSAIDs and oral steroids have not been found effective in fibromyalgia. Inflammation and dysfunction of the fascia may lead to central sensitization in fibromyalgia. If this hypothesis is confirmed, it could significantly expand treatment options to include manual therapies directed at the fascia such as Rolfing and myofascial release, and direct further research on the peripheral pathology in fibromyalgia to the fascia.

Corticotropin releasing factor in urine – A possible biochemical marker of fibromyalgia: Responses to massage and guided relaxation

Irene Lund, Thomas Lundeberg, Joakim Carleson, Helene Sönnerfors, Björn Uhrlin, Elisabeth Svensson
Neuroscience Letters, Volume 403, Issues 1–2, 31 July 2006, Pages 166–171

Abstract

The purpose of this preliminary study was to evaluate the relationship between a possible biochemical marker of stress, 24-h urinary concentrations of Corticotropin Releasing Factor-Like Immunoreactivity (CRF-LI), and ratings of stress-related symptoms like depression and anxiety, as well as to evaluate pain and emotional reactions in patients with fibromyalgia (FM). Another purpose was to study the effects of massage and guided relaxation, with respect to change in the same variables. Urine sampling and ratings were performed before treatments, after and 1 month after completed treatments. Concentrations of CRF-LI was analyzed with radioimmunoassay technique. For the assessment of depression, anxiety and pain the CPRS-A questionnaire was used and for rated pain and emotional reactions the NHP questionnaire was used. The 24-h urinary concentration of the CRF-LI was found to be related to depression, mood and inability to take initiative. After treatment the urinary CRF-LI concentrations and the rated levels of pain and emotional reactions were found to have decreased. In conclusion, the 24-h urinary CRF-LI concentration may be used as a biochemical marker of stress-related symptoms such as depression in patients with FM and possibly also other conditions characterized by chronic pain. Therapies such as massage and guided relaxation may be tried for the amelioration of pain and stress but further studies are required.

Surgery related pain

A randomized trial of massage therapy after heart surgery

Nancy M. Albert, A. Marc Gillinov, Bruce W. Lytle, Jingyuan Feng, Roberta Cwynar, Eugene H. Blackstone Heart & Lung: The Journal of Acute and Critical Care, Volume 38, Issue 6, November–December 2009, Pages 480–490

Issues in cardiovascular nursing

Objectives

To determine whether massage therapy improves postoperative mood, pain, anxiety, and physiologic measurements; shortens hospital stay; and decreases occurrence of atrial fibrillation.

Conclusion

Massage therapy is feasible in cardiac surgical patients; however, it does not yield therapeutic benefit. Nevertheless, it should be a patient-selected and -paid option.

Effect of massage therapy on pain, anxiety, and tension in cardiac surgical patients: A pilot study

Susanne M. Cutshall, Laura J. Wentworth, Deborah Engen, Thoralf M. Sundt, Ryan F. Kelly, Brent A. Bauer Complementary Therapies in Clinical Practice, Volume 16, Issue 2, May 2010, Pages 92–95

Abstract

Objectives

To assess the role of massage therapy in the cardiac surgery postoperative period. Specific aims included determining the difference in pain, anxiety, tension, and satisfaction scores of patients before and after massage compared with patients who received standard care.

Interventions

Patients in the intervention group received a 20-minute session of massage therapy intervention between postoperative days 2 and 5. Patients in the control group received standard care and a 20-minute quiet time between postoperative days 2 and 5.

Results

Statistically and clinically significant decreases in pain, anxiety, and tension scores were observed for patients who received a 20-minute massage compared with those who received standard care. Patient feedback was markedly positive.

Conclusions

This pilot study showed that massage can be successfully incorporated into a busy cardiac surgical practice. These results suggest that massage may be an important therapy to consider for inclusion in the management of postoperative recovery of cardiovascular surgical patients.

Piloting tailored teaching on nonpharmacologic enhancements for postoperative pain management in older adults

Susanne M. Tracy Pain Management Nursing, Volume 11, Issue 3, September 2010, Pages 148–158

Abstract

Despite many advances in the pharmacologic treatment of pain, the issue of unresolved postoperative pain continues to plague patients and health care professionals. Little seems to be known about the reasons why nonpharmacologic methods are not more widely used, particularly as they are commonly low in cost, easy to use, and largely free of adverse side effects. A central

(Continued)

(Continued)

question has to do with what patients are taught about nonpharmacologic methods and how a novel mode of teaching can be embedded in practice. A seven-step pre-posttest teaching intervention pilot study was deployed with older joint replacement patients within the context of a translational research model. Results of the teaching pilot showed significant post-teaching changes in subjects' knowledge and attitudes about nonpharmacologic methods for pain management, high satisfaction with the nonpharmacologic methods they chose, and incrementally greater use of the nonpharmacologic methods over the course of the hospital stay. A randomized controlled trial of the study is now in the early planning stages in an effort to obtain generalizable results that will help solidify evidence of the impact of music, imagery, and slow-stroke massage on pain management and confirm the value of patient teaching as an important means of offering patients more options for managing their own pain.

Effect of massage therapy on pain, anxiety, and tension after cardiac surgery: A randomized study

Brent A. Bauer, Susanne M. Cutshall, Laura J. Wentworth, Deborah Engen, Penny K. Messner, Christina M. Wood, Karen M. Brekke, Ryan F. Kelly, Thoralf M. Sundt Complementary Therapies in Clinical Practice, Volume 16, Issue 2, May 2010, Pages 70–75

Abstract

Integrative therapies such as massage have gained support as interventions that improve the overall patient experience during hospitalization. Cardiac surgery patients undergo long procedures and commonly have postoperative back and shoulder pain, anxiety, and tension. Given the promising effects of massage therapy for alleviation of pain, tension, and anxiety, we studied the efficacy and feasibility of massage therapy delivered in the postoperative cardiovascular surgery setting. Patients were randomized to receive a massage or to have quiet relaxation time (control). In total, 113 patients completed the study (massage, n = 62; control, n = 51). Patients receiving massage therapy had significantly decreased pain, anxiety, and tension. Patients were highly satisfied with the intervention, and no major barriers to implementing massage therapy were identified. Massage therapy may be an important component of the healing experience for patients after cardiovascular surgery.

Foot and hand massage as an intervention for postoperative pain

Hsiao-Lan Wang, Juanita F. Keck, Pain Management Nursing, Volume 5, Issue 2, June 2004, Pages 59–65

Abstract

Physiological responses to pain create harmful effects that prolong the body's recovery after surgery. Patients routinely report mild to moderate pain even though pain medications have been administered. Complementary strategies based on sound research findings are needed to supplement postoperative pain relief using pharmacologic management. Foot and hand massage has the potential to assist in pain relief. Massaging the feet and hands stimulates the mechanoreceptors that activate the 'nonpainful' nerve fibers, preventing pain transmission from reaching consciousness. The purpose of this pretest-posttest design study was to investigate whether a 20-minute foot and hand massage (5 minutes to each extremity), which was provided 1 to 4 hours after a dose of pain medication, would reduce pain perception and sympathetic responses among postoperative patients. A convenience sample of 18 patients rated pain intensity and pain distress using a 0 to 10 numeric rating scale. They reported decreases in pain intensity from 4.65 to 2.35 (t = 8.154, p < .001) and in pain distress from 4.00 to 1.88 (t = 5.683, p < .001). Statistically significant decreases in sympathetic responses to pain (i.e., heart rate and respiratory rate) were observed although blood pressure remained unchanged. The changes in heart rate and respiratory rate were not clinically significant. The patients experienced moderate pain after they received pain medications. This pain was reduced by the intervention, thus supporting the effectiveness of massage in postoperative pain management. Foot and hand massage appears to be an effective, inexpensive, low-risk, flexible, and easily applied strategy for postoperative pain management.

Effectiveness of foot and hand massage in postcesarean pain control in a group of Turkish pregnant women

N. Degirmen, N. Ozerdogan, D. Sayiner, N. Kosgeroglu, U. Ayranci, Applied Nursing Research, Volume 23, Issue 3, August 2010, Pages 153–158

Abstract

The aim of this study was to determine the efficiency of foot and hand massage on reducing postoperative pain in patients who had cesarean operation. This pretest–posttest design study was planned as a randomized controlled experimental study. In the light of the results, it was reported that the reduction in pain intensity was significantly meaningful in both intervention groups when compared to the control group. It was also noted that vital findings were measured comparatively higher before the massage in the test groups, and they were found to be relatively lower in the measurements conducted right before and after the massage, which was considered to be statistically meaningful. Foot and hand massage proved useful as an effective nursing intervention in controlling postoperative pain.

Massage as adjuvant therapy in the management of acute postoperative pain: a preliminary study in men

Marcia M. Piotrowski, Cynthia Paterson, Allison Mitchinson, Hyungjin Myra Kim, Marvin Kirsh, Daniel B. Hinshaw Journal of the American College of Surgeons, Volume 197, Issue 6, December 2003, Pages 1037–1046

Abstract
Background

Opioid analgesia alone may not fully relieve all aspects of acute postoperative pain. Complementary medicine techniques used as adjuvant therapies have the potential to improve pain management and palliate postoperative distress.

Results

The rate of decline in the unpleasantness of postoperative pain was accelerated by massage ($p = 0.05$). Massage also accelerated the rate of decline in the intensity of postoperative pain but this effect was not statistically significant. Use of opioid analgesics was not altered significantly by the interventions.

Conclusions

Massage may be a useful adjuvant therapy for the management of acute postoperative pain. Its greatest effect appears to be on the affective component (i.e., unpleasantness) of the pain.

Symptom management

Pain after spinal cord injury: a review of classification, treatment approaches, and treatment assessment

Diana D. Cardenas, Elizabeth R. Felix PM&R, Volume 1, Issue 12, December 2009, Pages 1077–1090

Abstract

Pain is a prevalent consequence of spinal cord injury (SCI) that can persist for years after the injury and can have a significant impact on physical and emotional function and quality of life. There are a variety of types of pain that may develop after a SCI, including those of primarily nociceptive origin and those of primarily neuropathic origin. Recommendations for diagnostic and treatment strategies have been varied in part because of the lack of a universal classification system and in part because of the biopsychosocial nature of pain. The most recent taxonomy for pain after SCI is described herein. Pain-management strategies, including pharmacological, interventional, and psychological treatments, also are described. For neuropathic pains in

(Continued)

(Continued)

SCI anticonvulsant agents and tricyclic antidepressants often are tried, but these treatments have had limited success in many patients, and alternative interventions (e.g., massage therapy, acupuncture, meditation) often are just as successful. Treatment of nociceptive pain after SCI often includes nonsteroidal antiinflammatory agents and acetaminophen, but corrections of underlying etiologies and behavior adjustments also should be implemented if possible. An overview of self-report pain questionnaires and scales also is presented to provide the clinician and researcher with a set of tools to evaluate the efficacy of pain interventions.

A targeted search on Science Direct found 4,876 articles using search terms massage pain management intervention. The most current and representative of the topic of this text are listed chronologically by topic. In each category the researchers, title and summary of the abstract is provided.

Palliative care review

Interdisciplinary palliative care, including massage, in treatment of amyotrophic lateral sclerosis

Kendra Blatzheim, Journal of Bodywork and Movement Therapies, Volume 13, Issue 4, October 2009, Pages 328–335

Palliative care review
Interdisciplinary palliative care, including massage, in treatment of amyotrophic lateral sclerosis.

Summary
Amyotrophic lateral sclerosis (ALS) is a progressive fatal neurological disease that affects approximately 20,000 Americans. Symptoms include muscle weakness, fatigue, twitching, atrophy, spasticity, pain, oropharyngeal dysfunction, pseudobulbar affect, weight loss, and respiratory impairment. Death occurs within 3–5 yr after onset of symptoms, with diagnosis taking from 11 to 17.5 months. The only FDA-approved drug for ALS is Riluzole, which only increases the life expectancy by a few months. All other treatments for ALS provide symptom management to improve the patient's quality of life. An interdisciplinary palliative care team for the ALS patient helps to reduce the stress that the illness places on families. Massage can be a useful adjunctive treatment for spasticity and pain when medication side effects are unwanted. A holistic interdisciplinary palliative care team supports both the patient and the family improving their quality of life.

Symptom management with massage and acupuncture in postoperative cancer patients: a randomized controlled trial

Wolf E. Mehling, Bradly Jacobs, Michael Acree, Leslie Wilson, Alan Bostrom, Jeremy West, Joseph Acquah, Beverly Burns, Jnani Chapman, Frederick M. Hecht, Journal of Pain and Symptom Management, Volume 33, Issue 3, March 2007, Pages 258–266

Abstract
The level of evidence for the use of acupuncture and massage for the management of perioperative symptoms in cancer patients is encouraging but inconclusive. We conducted a randomized, controlled trial assessing the effect of massage and acupuncture added to usual care vs. usual care alone in postoperative cancer patients. Cancer patients undergoing surgery were randomly assigned to receive either massage and acupuncture on postoperative Days 1 and 2 in addition to usual care, or usual care alone, and were followed over three days. Patients' pain, nausea, vomiting, and mood were assessed at four time points. Providing massage and acupuncture in addition to usual care resulted in decreased pain and depressive mood among postoperative cancer patients when compared with usual care alone. These findings merit independent confirmation using larger sample sizes and attention control.

To assess the non-pharmacological treatments used and preferred by patients with spinal cord injury and pain.

(Continued)

(Continued)

Design
A cross-sectional descriptive study.

Interventions
One hundred and twenty three patients with spinal cord injury, matched for gender, age, level of lesion and completeness of injury were assessed in 1999 at the Spinalis SCI unit, Stockholm, Sweden and followed-up in a mailed survey 3 years later. In total, 82.1% of the questionnaires (n=101) were returned. Ninety of these patients still suffered pain and were thus included in the study.

Main outcome measures
Pain questionnaires, visual analogue scale (VAS), Hospital Anxiety and Depression Scale and Life Satisfaction instrument.

Results
63.3% of the patients had tried non-pharmacological treatments, where acupuncture, massage and transcutaneous electrical nerve stimulation (TENS) were the most commonly tried. Predictive for having tried non-pharmacological treatment were high ratings of pain intensity, presence of aching pain, and cutting/stabbing pain.

Conclusion
Massage, and heat were the non-pharmacological treatments reported to result in the best pain alleviation. Results from our study suggest that we need to (re)evaluate the treatments offered to patients with spinal cord injury and pain and combine non-pharmacological and pharmacological treatments.

Miscellaneous

Procedural pain heart rate responses in massaged preterm infants

Miguel A. Diego, Tiffany Field, Maria Hernandez-Reif, Infant Behavior and Development, Volume 32, Issue 2, April 2009, Pages 226–229

Abstract
Heart rate (HR) responses to the removal of a monitoring lead were assessed in 56 preterm infants who received moderate pressure, light pressure or no massage therapy. The infants who received moderate pressure massage therapy exhibited lower increases in HR suggesting an attenuated pain response. The heart rate of infants who received moderate pressure massage also returned to baseline faster than the heart rate of the other two groups, suggesting a faster recovery rate.

The culture of massage therapy: valued elements and the role of comfort, contact, connection and caring

Joanna M. Smith, S. John Sullivan, G. David Baxter, Complementary Therapies in Medicine, Volume 17, Issue 4, August 2009, Pages 181–189

Summary
Objective
To explore the attributes of the therapy encounter valued by repeat users of health-related massage therapy. A qualitative design with telephone focus group methodology was used. A total of 19 repeat users of massage therapy participated in three telephone focus groups where audiotaped semi-structured interviews were conducted.

(Continued)

(Continued)

Six valued elements of the massage encounter (time for care and personal attention, engaging and competent therapist, trust partnership, holism and empowerment, effective touch and enhancing relaxation); four modulators (comfort, contact, connection and caring); and two themes relating to adding experiential value (enjoyment, escapism) characterize the massage therapy culture. The culture of massage therapy care incorporates a number of characteristics that are congruent with the complementary and alternative medicine approach to health. In addition, massage specific factors were identified. The humanistic aspects of the therapy encounter valued by clients offer insight into the growing use of massage therapy and the success of massage therapy outcomes.

The effects of massage on delayed onset muscle soreness and physical performance in female collegiate athletes

Corrie A. Mancinelli, D. Scott Davis, Leila Aboulhosn, Misty Brady, Justin Eisenhofer, Stephanie Foutty, Physical Therapy in Sport, Volume 7, Issue 1, February 2006, Pages 5–13

Summary

The purpose of this study was to determine if post-exercise massage has an effect on delayed-onset muscle soreness (DOMS) and physical performance in women collegiate athletes. This study used a randomized pre-test post-test control group design. Twenty-two NCAA Division I women basketball and volleyball players participated. On the day of predicted peak soreness, the treatment group (n = 11) received a thigh massage using effleurage, petrissage and vibration while the control group (n = 11) rested.

Outcome measures

Paired t-tests were used to assess differences between pre and post massage measures ($\alpha = 0.05$) for vertical jump displacement, timed shuttle run, quadriceps length and pressure-pain threshold in the thigh.

Results

A significant increase (slowing) was found in shuttle run times for the control group (p = 0.0354). There were significant changes in vertical jump displacement (p = 0.0033), perceived soreness (p = 0.0011) and algometer readings (p = 0.0461) for the massage group.

Conclusions

This study supports the use of massage in women collegiate athletes for decreasing soreness and improving vertical jump.

Chair massage for carers in an acute cancer hospital

Peter Mackereth, Paola Sylt, Ashley Weinberg, Gwynneth Campbell, European Journal of Oncology Nursing, Volume 9, Issue 2, June 2005, Pages 167–179

Summary

The Chair Massage service considered in this evaluation study was provided to carers, visiting in-patients at a major cancer hospital in the UK. The two-stage evaluation comprised: firstly, a retrospective review of treatment records for the previous 12 months (n = 182), and secondly, a prospective study, gathering data by interview and a 'next-day' questionnaire from carers (n = 34), during 1 week of service delivery. The study at both stages sought to identify who used the service, post-treatment comments and changes in scores using a Feeling Good Thermometer (Field, T., 2000. Touch Therapy. Churchill Livingstone, London). During the second stage the carers were also asked about their concerns and worries, and to report changes in physical and emotional states using visual scales. Findings included significant improvements in physical and psychological scores; these were retained through to the next day. The next-day questionnaire also reported improved sleep for the majority of carers. A number of concerns and worries were raised at interview, notably anxieties about the patient and uncertainty about the future, family and financial worries. Overall, the service was well evaluated with parents and in particular female carers appearing to gain the most from the intervention.

KEY POINTS

- Pain is always a subjective experience.
- Pain has multiple components: intensity, unpleasantness, specific qualities (e.g. burning, allodynia), location, relief, and temporal aspects (e.g. onset of relief, duration of relief) (Backonja & Galer 1998).
- Factors other than pain can affect the report of pain. Common symptoms associated with the report of pain include sleep disturbance, fatigue, depression, and anxiety (http://www.iasp-pain.org/AM/Template.cfm?Section=Home&Template=/CM/ContentDisplay.cfm&ContentID=1961).
- Pain is a conscious, aversive aspect of somatic awareness, the product of complex, central, nociception induced processing, and not a primitive sensation.
- Nociception is never conscious and engages sensory, emotional, and cognitive processing areas of the brain.
- Pain is multidimensional AND the pain experience may have sensory, emotional, and cognitive aspects.
- Pain AFFECTS function, affective status, and quality of life (http://www.iasp-pain.org/AM/Template.cfm?Section=Home&Template=/CM/ContentDisplay.cfm&ContentID=1973).
- It is necessary to recognize concepts of catastrophizing and avoidance in relation to pain (Sullivan et al 2001, Turner and Aaron 2001, Rosenberger et al 2004, Severeijns et al 2004).
- An individual's motivation, coping style, social support, and responses to pain can influence pain and treatment outcome (Jensen et al 2001, Jensen et al 2002, Hanly et al 2004, Montoya et al 2004, Nielson and Jensen 2004).
- There are cultural, environmental, and racial variations in pain experience and expression and in health care seeking and treatment (Bonham 2001, Edwards et al 2001b, LeResche 2001, Green Davidhizar & Giger 2004).
- Pain behaviors and complaints are best understood in the context of social transactions among the individual, spouse, employers, and health professionals and in the context of community. (Charlton 2005).

References

Aguilera DC: Crisis intervention: theory and methodology, ed 8, St Louis, 1998, Mosby.

Ahluwalia S: Distribution of smooth muscle actin containing cells in the human meniscus, *J Orthop Res* 19(4):659–664, 2001.

Albert NM, Gillinov AM, Lytle BW, et al: A randomized trial of massage therapy after heart surgery, *Heart Lung* 38(6):480–490, 2009.

Arroyo-Morales M, Olea N, Martínez MM, et al: Psychophysiological effects of massage-myofascial release after exercise: a randomized sham-control study, *J Complement Altern Med* 14(10):1223–1229, 2008.

Bauer BA, Cutshall SM, Wentworth LJ, et al: Effect of massage therapy on pain, anxiety, and tension after cardiac surgery: a randomized study, *Compl Therap Clinl Practice* 16(2):70–75.

Beider S, Moyer CA: Randomized controlled trials of pediatric massage: a review, *Evid Based Complement Alternat Med* 4(1):23–34, 2007. PMCID: PMC1810360.

Blatzheim K: Meridians – palliative care review: interdisciplinary palliative care, including massage, in treatment of amyotrophic lateral sclerosis, *J Bodyw Mov Ther* 13(4):328–335, 2009.

Bonham VL: Race, ethnicity, and pain treatment: striving to understand the causes and solutions to the disparities in pain treatment, *J Law Med Ethics* 29:52–68, 2001.

Born B, Kim SJ, Ebbinghaus S, et al. The terahertz dance of water with the proteins: the effect of protein flexibility on the dynamical hydration shell of ubiquitin, Faraday Discussions, 141, pp 161–173, 2008.

Capogna G, Alahuhta S, Celleno D, et al: Maternal expectations and experiences of labour pain and analgesia: a multi-centre study of nulliparous women, *Int J Obstet Anaesth* 5:229–235, 1996.

Cardenas DD, Felix ER: Pain after spinal cord injury: a review of classification, treatment approaches, and treatment assessment, *PM&R* 1(12):1077–1090, 2009.

Cassileth BR, Vickers AJ: Massage therapy for symptom control: outcome study at a major cancer center, *J Pain Symptom Manage* 28(3):244–249, 2004.

Castro-Sánchez AM, Moreno-Lorenzo C, Matarán-Peñarrocha GA, et al: Connective tissue reflex massage for type 2 diabetic patients with peripheral arterial disease: randomized controlled trial, *Evid Based Complement and Alternat Med* Nov(23) PMID: 19933770.

Castro-Sánchez AM, Moreno-Lorenzo C, Matarán-Peñarrocha GA, et al: Efficacy of a massage and exercise programme on the ankle-brachial index and blood pressure in patients with diabetes mellitus type 2 and peripheral arterial disease: a randomized clinical trial, *Med Clin (Barc)* Oct(9) PMID: 19819486.

Chaitow L: Clinical applications of neuromuscular techniques (vol 1), Edinburgh, 2006, Elsevier.

Chaitow L: *Massage today the amazing fascial web* 5(5), 2005.

Charlton JE, editor: *Core curriculum for professional education in pain*, Seattle, 2005, IASP Press.

Chatchawan U, Thinkhamrop B, Kharmwan S, et al: Effectiveness of traditional Thai massage versus Swedish massage among patients with back pain associated with myofascial trigger points, *J Bodyw Mov Ther* 9(4):298–309, 2005.

Cogan R, Spinnato JA: Pain and discomfort thresholds in late pregnancy, *Pain* 27:63–68, 1986.

Currin J, Meister EA: A hospital-based intervention using massage to reduce distress among oncology patients, *Cancer Nurs* 31(3):214–221, 2008.

Cutshall AM, Wentworth LJ, Engen D, et al: Effect of massage therapy on pain, anxiety, and tension in cardiac surgical patients: a pilot study, *Complement Ther Clin Pract* 16(2):92–95.

Davidhizar R, Giger JN: A review of the literature on care of clients in pain who are culturally diverse, *Int Nurs Rev* 51:47–55, 2004.

Day JA, Stecco C, Stecco A: Application of Fascial Manipulation technique in chronic shoulder pain – anatomical basis and clinical implications, *J Bodyw Mov Ther* 13(2):128–135, 2009.

Degirmen N, Ozerdogan N, Sayiner D, et al: Effectiveness of foot and hand massage in postcesarean pain control in a group of Turkish pregnant women, *Appl Nurs Res* 23(3):153–158.

Diego MA, Field T, Hernandez-Reif M: Procedural pain heart rate responses in massaged preterm infants, *Infant Behavior and Development* 32(2):226–229, 2009.

Diego MA, Field T, Sanders C, et al: Massage therapy of moderate and light pressure and vibrator effects on EEG and heart rate, *Int J Neurosci* 114(1):31–44, 2004.

Edwards RR, Doleys DM, Fillingim RB, et al: Ethnic differences in pain tolerance: clinical implications in a chronic pain population, *Psychosom Med* 63:316–323, 2001.

Ernst E: The safety of massage therapy, *Rheumatology (Oxford)* 42(9):1101–1106, 2003.

Fellowes D, Barnes K, Wilkinson S: Aromatherapy and massage for symptom relief in patients with cancer, *Int J Neurosci* 106(3–4):131–145, 2004.

Fernández-de-las-Peñas C, Alonso-Blanco C, Fernández-Carnero J, et al: The immediate effect of ischemic compression technique and transverse friction massage on tenderness of active and latent myofascial trigger points: a pilot study, *J Bodyw Mov Ther* 10(1):3–9, 2006.

Field T, Diego M, Cullen C, et al: Carpal tunnel syndrome symptoms are lessened following massage therapy, *J Bodyw Mov Ther* 8(1):9–14, 2004.

Field T, Hernandez-Reif M, Diego M, et al: Cortisol decreases and serotonin and dopamine increase following massage therapy, *Int J Neurosci* 115(10):1397–1413, 2005.

Fischer MJ, Riedlinger K, Gutenbrunner C, et al: Influence of the temporomandibular joint on range of motion of the hip joint in patients with complex regional pain syndrome, *J Manipulative Physiol Ther* 32(5):364–371, 2009.

Frey Law LA, Evans S, Knudtson J, et al: Massage reduces pain perception and hyperalgesia in experimental muscle pain: a randomized, controlled trial, *J Pain* 9(8):714–721, 2008.

Gintzler AR, Komisaruk BR: Analgesia is produced by uterocervical mechano-stimulation in rats: roles of afferent nerves and implications for analgesia of pregnancy and parturition, *Brain Res* 566:299–302, 1991.

Gintzler AR, Liu N-J: The maternal spinal cord: biochemical and physiological correlates of steroid-activated antinociceptive processes. In Russell JA, Douglas AJ, Windle RJ, Ingram CD, editors: Progress in Brain Research. Volume 133. The maternal brain. Neurobiological and neuroendocrine adaptation and disorders in pregnancy and postpartum, Amsterdam, 2001, Elsevier, pp 83–97.

Goldstone LA: Massage as an orthodox medical treatment past and future, *Complement Ther Nurs Midwifery* 6:169–175, 2000.

Gruebele, M, Haverith M. Water as 'Designer Fluid' that helps proteins change shape. http://www.biocampare.com/News/NewsStory/239323/NewsStory.html. Retrieved Dec 17, 2009.

Hanley J, Stirling P, Brown C, Br J: Randomised controlled trial of therapeutic massage in the management of stress, *Gen Pract* 53(486):20–25, 2003.

Hanly MA, Jensen MP, Ehde DM, et al: Psychosocial predictors of long-term adjustment to lower-limb amputation and phantom limb pain, *Disabil Rehabil* 26:882–893, 2004.

Hastreite D, et al: Regional variations in cellular characteristics in human lumbar intervertebral discs, including the presence of alpha-smooth muscle actin, *J Orthop Res* 19(4):597–604, 2001.

Hettinga DM, Hurley DA, Jackson A, et al: Assessing the effect of sample size, methodological quality and statistical rigour on outcomes of randomised controlled trials on mobilisation, manipulation and massage for low back pain of at least 6 weeks duration, *Physiotherapy* 94(2):97–104, 2008.

Ho CY, Sole G, Munn J: The effectiveness of manual therapy in the management of musculoskeletal disorders of the shoulder: a systematic review, *Man Ther* 14(5):463–474, 2009.

Ilari M: Curing the fascia, Interview of Luigi Stecco, *Vita & Salute magazine*, April 2003.

Ingber DE: Cellular tensegrity: defining new rules of biological design that govern the cytoskeleton, *J Cell Sci* 104:613–627, 1993.

Ingber DE, Folkman J: Tension and compression as basic determinants of cell form and function: utilization of a cellular tensegrity mechanism. In Stein W, Bronner F, editors: Cell shape: determinants, regulation and regulatory role, San Diego, 1989, Academic Press, pp 1–32.

Jane S-W, Wilkie DJ, Gallucci BB, et al: Effects of a full-body massage on pain intensity, anxiety, and physiological relaxation in Taiwanese patients with metastatic bone pain: a pilot study, *Journal of Pain* 37(4):754–763, 2009.

Jensen MP: Enhancing motivation to change in pain treatment. In Turk DC, Gatchel R, editors: Psychological approaches to pain management: a practitioner's handbook, New York, 2002, Guildford Press, pp 71–93.

Jensen MP, Turner JA, Romano JM: Changes in beliefs, catastrophizing, and coping are associated with improvement in multidisciplinary pain treatment, *J Consult Clin Psychol* 69:655–662, 2001.

Kanazawa Y, Nomura J, Yoshimoto S, et al: Cyclical cell stretching of skin-derived fibroblasts downregulates connective tissue growth factor (CTGF) production, *Connect Tissue Res* 50(5):323–329, 2009.

Kassolik K, Jaskólska A, Kisiel-Sajewicz K, et al: Tensegrity principle in massage demonstrated by electro- and mechanomyography, *J Bodyw Mov Ther* 13(2):164–170, 2009.

Kawakita K, Itoh K, Okada K: The polymodal receptor hypothesis of acupuncture and moxibustion, and its rational explanation of acupuncture points, *Int Congr Ser: Acupuncture – is there a physiological basis?* 1238:63–68, 2002.

Kessler J, Marchant P, Johnson MI: A study to compare the effects of massage and static touch on experimentally induced pain in healthy volunteers, *Physiotherapy* 92(4):225–232, 2006.

Kimber L, McNabb M, McCourt C, Massage or music for pain relief in labour: a pilot randomised placebo controlled trial, *Eur J Pain* 12(8):961–969, 2008.

Klingler W, Schleip R, Zorn A: European Fascia Research Project Report. 5th World Congress Low Back and Pelvic Pain, Melbourne, 2004.

Kuan TS: Current studies on myofascial pain syndrome, *Curr Pain Headache Rep* 13(5):365–369, 2009. PMID: 19728962.

Lämås K, Lindholm L, Stenlund H, et al: Effects of abdominal massage in management of constipation – a randomized controlled trial, *Int J Nurs Stud* 46(6):759–767, 2009.

Langevin HM, Bouffard NA, Badger GJ, et al: Dynamic fibroblast cytoskeletal response to subcutaneous tissue stretch ex vivo and in vivo, *Am J Physiol Cell Physiol* 288:C747–C756, 2005.

Langevin H, Churchill D, Cipolla M: Mechanical signaling through connective tissue: a mechanism for the therapeutic effect of acupuncture, *FASEB J* 15:2275–2280, 2001.

Langevin H, Cornbrooks C, Taatjes D, et al: Fibroblasts form a body-wide cellular network, *Histochem Cell Biol* 122(1):7–15, 2004.

Langevin HM, Sherman KJ: Pathophysiological model for chronic low back pain integrating connective tissue and nervous system mechanisms, *Med Hypotheses* 68(1):74–80, 2007.

Langevin HM, Yandow JA: Relationship of acupuncture points and meridians to connective tissue planes, *Anat Rec* 269:257–265, 2002.

Lee HM, Wu SK, You JY: Quantitative application of transverse friction massage and its neurological effects on flexor carpi radialis, *Man Ther* 14(5):501–550, 2009.

LeResche L: Gender, cultural, and environmental aspects of pain. In Loeser JD, Butler SH, Chapman CR, Turk DC,

editors: *Bonica's Management of pain*, Philadelphia, 2001, Lippincott Williams & Wilkins, pp 191–195.

Lewis M, Johnson M: The clinical effectiveness of therapeutic massage for musculoskeletal pain: a systematic review, *Physiotherapy* 92(3):146–158, 2006.

Liptan GL: Fascia: A missing link in our understanding of the pathology of fibromyalgia, *J Bodyw Movem Ther* 14(1):3–12, 2010.

Lund I, Yu L-C, Uvnas-Moberg K, Wang J, et al: Repeated massage-like stimulation induces long-term effects on nociception: contribution of oxytocinergic mechanisms, *Eur J Neurosci* 16:330–338, 2002.

Mackawan S, Eungpinichpong W, Pantumethakul R, et al: Effects of traditional Thai massage versus joint mobilization on substance P and pain perception in patients with non-specific low back pain, *J Bodyw Mov Ther* 11(1):9–16, 2007.

Mackereth P, Sylt P, Weinberg A, et al: Chair massage for carers in an acute cancer hospital, *Europ J Oncology Nurs* 9(2):167–179, 2005.

Mancinelli CA, Davis DS, Aboulhosn L, et al: The effects of massage on delayed onset muscle soreness and physical performance in female collegiate athletes, *Phys Ther Sport* 7(1):5–13, 2006.

McNabb MT, Kimber L, Haines A, et al: Does regular massage from late pregnancy to birth decrease maternal pain perception during labor and birth? A feasibility study to investigate a program of massage, controlled breathing and visualization, from 36 weeks of pregnancy until birth, *Compl Ther Clin Prac* 12(3):222–231, 2006.

Mehling WE, Jacobs B, Acree M, et al: Symptom management with massage and acupuncture in postoperative cancer patients: a randomized controlled trial, *J Pain Symp Manage* 33(3):258–266, 2007.

Meiss RA: Persistent mechanical effects of decreasing length during isometric contraction of ovarian ligament smooth muscle, *J Muscle Res Cell Motil* 14(2):205–218, 1993.

Montoya P, Larbig W, Braun C, et al: Influence of social support and emotional context on pain processing and magnetic brain responses in fibromyalgia, *Arthritis Rheum* 50:4035–4044, 2004.

Moyer CA, Rounds J, Hannum JW: A meta-analysis of massage therapy research, *Psychol Bull* 130(1):3–18, 2004.

Moyer CA, Rounds J, Hannum JW: A meta-analysis of massage therapy research, Belmont, 2006, Thomson Wadsworth.

Muller-Oerlinghausen B, Berg C, Scherer P, et al: Effects of slow-stroke massage as complementary treatment of depressed hospitalized patients, *Dtsch Med Wochenschr 11* 129(24):1363–1368, 2004.

Murray M, Spector M: Fibroblast distribution in the anteromedial bundle of the human anterior cruciate ligament: the presence of alpha-smooth muscle actin-positive cells, *J Orthop Res* 17(1):18–27, 1999.

Nielson WR, Jensen MP: Relationship between changes in coping and treatment outcome in patients with fibromyalgia syndrome, *Pain* 109:233–241, 2004.

Ownby KK: Effects of ice massage on neuropathic pain in persons with AIDS, *J Assoc Nurses AIDS Care* 17(5):15–22, 2006.

Pedrelli A, Stecco C, Day JA: Treating patellar tendinopathy with Fascial Manipulation, *J Bodyw Mov Ther* 13(1):73–80, 2009. Epub 2008 Jul 26 PMID: 19118795.

Phipps Eisensmith L: Massage therapy decreases frequency and intensity of symptoms related to temporomandibular joint syndrome in one case study, *J Bodyw Mov Ther* 11(3):223–230, 2007.

Piotrowski MM, Paterson C, Mitchinson A, et al: Massage as adjuvant therapy in the management of acute postoperative pain: a preliminary study in men, *J Amer Coll Surg* 197(6):1037–1046, 2003.

Potter PA, Perry AG: *Fundamentals of nursing* (ed 6), St Louis, 2005, Mosby.

Rosenberger PH, Ickovics JR, Epel ES, et al: Physical recovery in arthroscopic knee surgery: unique contributions of coping behaviors to clinical outcomes and stress reactivity, *Psychology & Health* 19:307–320, 2004.

Schleip R: Fascial plasticity – a new neurobiological explanation, *J Bodyw Mov Ther* 7:11–19, 2003.

Schleip R, Klingler W, Lehmann-Horn F: Active fascial contractility: fascia may be able to contract in a smooth muscle-like manner and thereby influence musculoskeletal dynamics, *Med Hypotheses* 65:273–277, 2005.

Schleip, R, Zorn, A, Else MJ, et al: The European Fascia Research Project Report 2006. Online at www.somatics.de/FasciaResearch/ReportIASIyearbook06.htm

Severeijns R, Vlaeyen JWS, van den Hout MA, et al: Pain catastrophizing is associated with health indices in musculoskeletal pain: a cross-sectional study in the Dutch community, *Health Psychol* 23:49–57, 2004.

Sherman KJ, Cherkin DC, Hawkes RJ, et al: Randomized trial of therapeutic massage for chronic neck pain, *Clin J Pain* 25(3):233–238, 2009.

Smith JM, Sullivan SJ, Baxter GD: The culture of massage therapy: valued elements and the role of comfort, contact, connection and caring, *Compl Therap Med* 17(4):181–189, 2009.

Stecco C, Gagey O, Belloni A, et al: Anatomy of the deep fascia of the upper limb. Second part: study of innervation, *J Pain* 20:433–439, 2004.

Stecco L: Fascial Manipulation for musculoskeletal pain, Padua, 2004, Piccin.

Stecco L, Stecco C: Fascial Manipulation: practical part, Padua, 2009, Piccin.

Sturgeon M, Wetta-Hall R, Hart T, et al: Effects of therapeutic massage on the quality of life among patients with breast cancer during treatment, *J Altern Complement Med* 15(4):373–380, 2009.

Sullivan MJ, Thorn B, Haythornthwaite JA, et al: Theoretical perspectives on the relation between catastrophizing and pain, *Clin J Pain* 17:52–64, 2001.

Toro-Velasco C, Arroyo-Morales M, Fernández-de-Las-Peñas C, et al: Short-term effects of manual therapy on heart rate variability, mood state, and pressure pain sensitivity in patients with chronic tension-type headache: a pilot study, *J Manipulative Physiol Ther* 32(7):527–535, 2009.

Tracy SM: Piloting tailored teaching on nonpharmacologic enhancements for postoperative pain management in older adults, *Pain Manage Nurs* 11(3):148–158, 2010.

Tsao JC: Effectiveness of massage therapy for chronic, non-malignant pain: a review, *Evid Based Complement Alternat Med* 4(2):165–179, 2007.

Turner JA, Aaron LA: Pain-related catastrophizing: what is it? *Clin J Pain* 17:65–71, 2001.

Wall P, Melzack R: Textbook of pain, ed 2, Edinburgh, 1990, Churchill Livingstone.

Walton A: Efficacy of myofascial release techniques in the treatment of primary Raynaud's phenomenon, *J Bodyw Mov Ther* 12(3):274–280, 2008. Epub 2008 Mar 5. PMID: 19083682.

Wang HL, Keck JF: Foot and hand massage as an intervention for postoperative pain, *Pain Mgmt Nurs* 5(2):59–65, 2004.

Whipple B, Josimovich JB, Komisaruk BR: Sensory thresholds during the antepartum, intrapartum, and postpartum periods, *Inter J of Nurs Stud* 27(3):213–221, 1990.

Yahia L, Pigeon P, et al: Viscoelastic properties of the human lumbodorsal fascia, *J Biomed Eng* 15:425–429, 1993.

Yip Yin Bing, Ying Tam Ada Chung: An experimental study on the effectiveness of massage with aromatic ginger and orange essential oil for moderate-to-severe knee pain among the elderly in Hong Kong, *Complement Ther Med* 16(3):131–138, 2008.

CHAPTER THREE
The pain experience

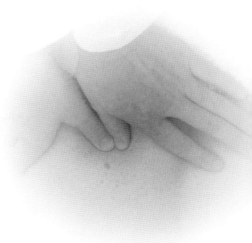

INTRODUCTION

Pain can be described using a variety of terms and concepts. Pain is a noxious stimulus resulting from an actual or potential tissue damaging event that stimulates nociceptors. Nociceptors are receptors sensitive to a noxious stimulus or to a stimulus which would become noxious if prolonged (Seaman 1997). The experience of pain begins with the pain threshold, which is the smallest pain producing stimulus a person can perceive as painful, and pain tolerance, which is the maximum intensity of a stimulus that evokes pain and that a subject is willing to tolerate. An individual can modify pain tolerance and to a lesser extent pain threshold based on their perception of the pain sensation. There are also physiological mechanisms that can occur that modify pain threshold and pain tolerance. The pain experience can be altered by using changes in perception and activating physiological pain control mechanisms. These methods will be described in future chapters.

Some individuals experience pain due to hyperalgesia and/or sensitization. Hyperalgesia is an increased response to a stimulus which is normally painful. In other words the body overreacts to a pain producing stimulus. Hyperalgesia may include a decrease in both pain threshold and pain tolerance. Sensitization, a neurophysiological process resulting, is an increased responsiveness of neurons to their normal input or recruitment of a response to normally subthreshold inputs. In other words the body is interpreting nonpainful stimuli as pain. Like hyperalgesia, sensitization includes a drop in pain threshold and an increased sensitivity of neuroresponse. The nervous system may generate pain signals without any

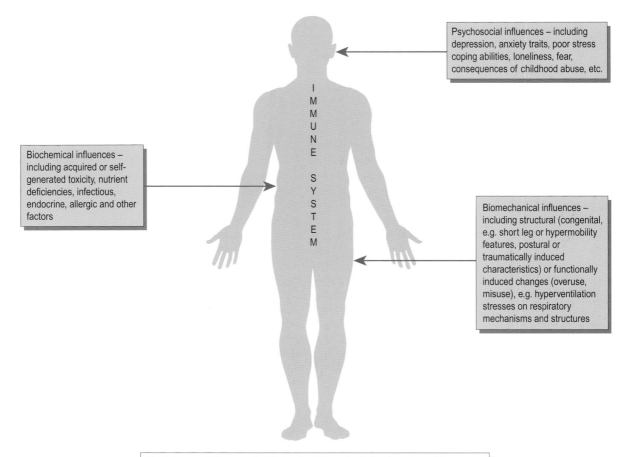

Psychosocial influences – including depression, anxiety traits, poor stress coping abilities, loneliness, fear, consequences of childhood abuse, etc.

Biochemical influences – including acquired or self-generated toxicity, nutrient deficiencies, infectious, endocrine, allergic and other factors

Biomechanical influences – including structural (congenital, e.g. short leg or hypermobility features, postural or traumatically induced characteristics) or functionally induced changes (overuse, misuse), e.g. hyperventilation stresses on respiratory mechanisms and structures

The interacting influences of a biochemical, biomechanical and psychosocial nature do not produce single changes. For example:
- A negative emotional state (e.g. depression) produces specific biochemical changes, impairs immune function and leads to altered muscle tone.
- Hyperventilation modifies blood acidity, alters neural reporting (initially hyper and then hypo), creates feelings of anxiety/apprehension and directly impacts on the structural components of the thoracic and cervical region – muscles and joints.
- Altered chemistry affects mood; altered mood changes blood chemistry; altered structure (posture for example) modifies function and therefore impacts on chemistry (e.g. liver function) and potentially on mood.
Within these categories – biochemical, biomechanical and psychosocial – are to be found most major influences on health.

Figure 3.1 Biochemical, biomechanical, and psychosocial influences on health. (Adapted from Chaitow & DeLany 2000.)

stimulus and increase the receptive field size. Pain tolerance is usually affected as well. Peripheral sensitization is an increased responsiveness and reduced threshold of nociceptors to stimulation of their receptive fields. Central sensitization is an increased responsiveness of nociceptive neurons in the central nervous system to their normal or subthreshold afferent input, which may be due to dysfunction of the endogenous pain control system.

In simple terms hyperalgesia is like the saying making mountains out of mole hills, and sensitization is making something out of nothing. Knowing this terminology is all well and good in our task of understanding pain and being able to communicate with multidisciplinary heath care professions. However, these terms and descriptions do not describe what it is like to be in pain and to live the pain experience. Massage therapists must appreciate the mechanisms

Box 3.1 A pain experience

Even though every individual's experience of pain is unique to them there is a level of shared understanding. Following is author Sandy Fritz's pain experience story.

I have had babies and experienced the productive process of labor except with my third child. He was stuck full-face presentation. The labor pain was not productive, I could not push him out, and I was afraid. It was the only time I recall begging for help. I finally did push him out resulting in structural damage to my pelvis that continues to produce a level of chronic pain over 20 years later but my youngest son is a constant reminder to me that in the whole scheme of life, an aching and stiff sacral iliac joint is not horrible even if it is aggravating.

At age 54 I had open heart surgery (coronary artery triple bypass) – a big surprise, sort of. The post surgery experience was very painful. I am forever grateful for morphine and Demerol. Recovery was acutely painful. When the chest cavity and ribs have been injured everything is painful but currently there is not another way to correct the blockage I had. I could be dead instead. If pain exists you are alive and I feel blessed to have been sawed open, replumbed, and sewn and wired closed. Currently my chest and mid back will ache and I get stiff. There are a couple of spots that remain painful but every time I stretch to relieve the sensations I am thankful I am alive.

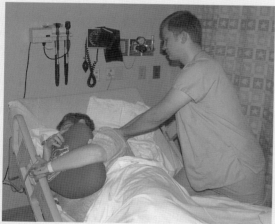

Figure 3.2 Massage for medical purposes. (Photograph courtesy Laura Cochran.)

When I was 55 my eldest child was tragically killed when hit by a car. I cannot imagine an experience more horrible than the gut wrenching experience of pain. I felt as if I stood by his side as he died. Not only do I continue to experience physical, emotional, and spiritual pain but I also suffer. His first and only child was born four months later. I was the labor coach for my daughter-in-law and she commented that the real honest productive pain of giving birth actually felt right and good in contrast to her pain and suffering of a broken heart. My granddaughter heals us all and yes, when I carry her around it makes my back and chest stiff and painful, but she alleviates my suffering and supports my hope and joy. I am a massage therapist and have been for many, many years. I know that when I massage someone in pain that hurts I help them for a while. I am much more tolerant, understanding, and compassionate of others because of my own pain experiences.

causing, enhancing, and creating the pain experience to competently use massage to help those experiencing pain. It hurts to be in pain whether that pain is acute or chronic, physical, emotional or spiritual, helpful or harmful. There are differences between harm and hurt. Pain hurts whether there is harm or not. Hurting is disempowering, fatiguing, miserable, and the foundation of suffering (Box 3.1).

SUFFERING

Massage can help reduce pain and suffering for a short period but the complex process of suffering requires multilevel intervention. The connection between physical and mental pain has been studied extensively by Matthew Lieberman, Naomi Eisenberger, and associates at the Social, Cognitive Neuroscience Lab at UCLA, Department of Psychology. Their research has shown that the pain and suffering that occurs when social relationships are damaged or lost and the pain experienced from physical injury share parts of the same underlying physiological processing system (Eisenberger & Lieberman 2004). Since physical and social pain rely on similar neural systems, factors that increase tolerance of the experience of social pain, such as social support, should also increase the tolerance to physical pain.

Grieving over the death of a loved one and being treated unfairly also activate these regions. Grief is one of life's most painful experiences (Eisenberger & Lieberman 2005). In 1998, researchers suggested that the social attachment system uses opiate substrates of the physical pain system. This overlap in function results in pleasure when with those we care about and elicits distress when we are separated from the social attachment system. This pleasure/pain experience of connectiveness and separation piggyback onto the pre-existing pain system, borrowing the pain signal to signify and prevent the danger of social separation (Nelson & Panksepp 1998, Panksepp 1998). Ongoing studies by Lieberman and Eisenberger (Eisenberger, Lieberman & Williams 2003, Eisenberger et al 2004, 2006, 2007, Eisenberger & Lieberman 2005, Lieberman & Eisenberger 2005) continue to support that pain distress and social distress share neurocognitive function and increased social distress will increase sensitivity to physical pain and vice versa. Understanding this overlap in the neural systems underlying pain distress and social distress supports alternative ways to treat and manage chronic pain conditions. For example, rather than treating pain symptoms directly, it may be possible to reduce physical pain symptoms by addressing the social stressors that may go along with them.

Massage therapists need to realize the importance of multidisciplinary care in the treatment of pain and appreciate the importance of nurturance and compassion as aspects of the massage application.

This relationship may also help to explain why massage and the therapeutic relationship are effective in pain management systems.

NEUROANATOMY OF PAIN AND PLEASURE

Pain is the individual or subjective experience to a stimulus, not only the perception of the noxious stimulus but also the interpretation of that sensation as an unpleasant one. Without this psychological component, the noxious stimulus would not constitute a painful stimulus, and the individual could not be said to be in pain (Seaman 1997).

To appreciate how the experiences of pain occurs it is necessary to understand the neuroanatomy.

The pain network consists of the dorsal anterior cingulate cortex, insula, somatosensory cortex, thalamus, and periaqueductal gray area. The somatosensory cortex is associated with sensory aspects of cutaneous physical pain (e.g. its location on the body); the dorsal anterior cingulate cortex is associated with the distressing aspect of pain (suffering).

The reward or pleasure network consists of the ventral tegmental, ventral striatum, ventromedial prefrontal cortex, and the amygdala. The brain's reward circuitry consists of neural structures receiving the neurotransmitter dopamine. Major dopaminergic

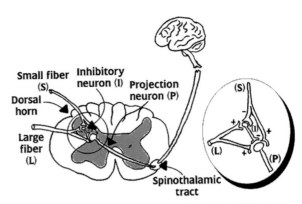

Figure 3.3 Gate-control theory of pain (based on Melzack and Wall's gate-control theory of pain). (From Fritz 2004.)

targets in the brain have been implicated in reward/pleasure processes (Lieberman & Eisenberger 2009).

According to pain experts Melzack and Wall (McMahon & Koltzenburg 2010), pain has three dimensions:

1. Sensory discriminative – thalamus and somatosensory cortex.
2. Motivational-affective – brain stem reticular formation, limbic system.
3. Cognitive-evaluative – frontal cortex.

In other words, the pain experience results in the perception of tissue damage and the interpretation of the unpleasantness, and the aversive nature of the experience motivates responses to avoid further injury or promote healing (voluntarily or involuntarily). All pain experiences are a normal response to what your brain perceives as a threat. And the amount of pain you experience does not necessarily relate to the amount of damage to tissue.

If massage therapy is going to be beneficial in pain management it must interact with the pain/pleasure anatomy and physiology. One of the greatest benefits of massage is that it feels good. Massage is pleasurable. The pain/pleasure system is like so many processes in the body. One dominates the other and then vice versa. When the agonist muscle is activated the antagonist muscle is inhibited. When the pain network dominates it is difficult to feel pleasure and also if the pleasure network is activated it is hard to experience pain (Fig. 3.3).

PAIN TYPES AND PAIN DYSFUNCTION

I hurt
I am tired
I hurt and I am tired.

Box 3.2 The pain experience

Pain is a subjective experience influenced by:
- Arousal
- Alarm phase
- Adaptation phase
- Age
- Sex
- Cultural background
- Level of anxiety
- Level of understanding
- Expectation
- Motivation

(From http://www.womenshealthapta.org/csm04/6412. pdf).

The pain experience is influenced by anxiety and depression.

Physical symptoms associated with anxiety or depression
- Changes in sleep patterns
- Shortness of breath
- Constipation
- Nausea
- Weight loss or gain
- Persistent fatigue
- Decreased sexual drive
- Palpitations
- Dizziness
- Unexpected crying
- Menstrual changes

Emotional symptoms associated with depression
- Feelings of guilt
- Hopelessness
- Unworthiness
- Fear of mental or physical disease or death
- Poor concentration, little ambition, no interest in life, indecisiveness, or poor memory
- Job conflicts
- Personal relationships conflicts

The acute pain experience

Acute and chronic pain are both physically and emotionally different.

Acute pain is triggered by tissue damage. It's the type of pain that generally accompanies illness, illness and injury, or surgery, and is location specific (see: http://www.changingstates.co.uk/issues/pain_control.html).

Acute pain may be mild and last just a moment, such as from an insect sting, or it can be severe and last for weeks or months, such as from a burn, pulled muscle, or broken bone. In a fairly predictable period, and with treatment of the underlying cause, acute pain generally fades away. Massage targets acute pain with symptom management and healing support. It is fairly easy to treat. The experience of acute pain is intense and tasking on the individual but typically it is easier to endure because it can be specifically related to events that are tangible. Acute pain is usually effectively managed by medication used in the short term, therefore it is possible to remain in control of the experience. This is the case when acute pain is related to an event that has a definite beginning and end. The classic example is surgery pain. When there is a reason for the surgery and the outcome adds to the quality of one's life then the pain experience can be framed as productive.

There are acute pain experiences that are not related to life enhancement intervention. Abuse, torture, and trauma fall into this experience of acute pain. Many times the individual is helpless in the situation and powerless to control or prevent or protect themselves. It is the sacrifice of the self that is an underlying aspect of this type of pain experience and the victimization often leads to an ongoing chronic pain, anxiety, and depression pain experience. Individuals with this type of pain experience can truly be said to suffer. UCLA and University of North Carolina researchers have found that women with irritable bowel syndrome (IBS) who have experienced sexual and/or physical abuse may have a heightened brain response to pain that makes them more sensitive to abdominal discomfort. IBS is a condition that affects 10–15% of the population and causes gastrointestinal discomfort along with diarrhea, constipation or both (Mayer et al 2008).

Acute stress and pain can actually increase pain threshold and tolerance. Stress induced analgesia occurs when the stress hormone noradrenaline floods the bloodstream during stressful events affecting the brain's pain processing pathway to produce analgesia. The amygdala is the brain's emotion processing region known to mediate the emotional and stress related aspects of pain, and the amygdala based processes are controlled by neurons that originated in the brainstem regulated by noradrenaline (adapted from materials provided by Brown University 2008).

Early exposure to acute pain is associated with changes in stress hormone receptors in certain regions of the brain. Premature infants exposed to multiple noxious stimuli such as experienced in the neonatal intensive care unit are less sensitive and responsive to everyday pain at 18 months of age. Full-term circumcised boys reacted more strongly than uncircumcised boys to the pain of a routine vaccination at 4–6 months. Infants and young children may not clearly remember painful experiences as actual events but there is evidence that memory for pain occurs. Even at 6 months of age, most infants appear capable of remembering and displaying fear in anticipation of a previously experienced painful procedure (Center For The Advancement Of Health 1999).

Undertreated pain leads to other problems, including reduced quality of life, decreased socialization, depression, sleep disturbances, cognitive impairment, and malnutrition. When considering the opposite of the infant, the elderly population is already vulnerable to the detrimental effects of the pain experience because of social isolation, financial strain from reduced income and the costs incurred by frequent physician visits, hospitalizations, and long term care. Older people are also more likely to be living with multiple chronic diseases and medications, increasing the risk of negative drug–disease and drug–drug interactions. Older patients often show atypical presentations of pain. Depression can also play a role in the assessment and treatment of pain. For a number of reasons, many older people choose not to report their pain. Often they are afraid that they will be involuntarily hospitalized or subjected to invasive procedures if they report pain. Another important barrier to successful pain management is the fact that older people and their social support system are often misinformed about the aging process, analgesics, pain management, and opioid addiction.

Health professionals have a moral imperative to help elderly people in pain and massage therapy can play an important part. The management of pain in geriatric clients can be complicated by the changing physiology that occurs with aging (Robinson 2007).

What are the implications of early pain experiences and the changes that occur in the pain/pleasure pathways? What can be the process of acute stress and pain as a pain control measure? How do these factors interface with the chronic pain experience? What is the impact of the pain experience throughout the life span? As this chapter and future chapters unfold, we may be able to respond to some of these questions.

The chronic pain experience

Chronic pain is different. It lingers after the illness and injury is healed. The pain may remain constant, or it can come and go. At times the pain will linger even though the injury or illness shows no other symptoms – and the pain may become more intense than before. Chronic pain caused by damage to the central nervous system (i.e. brain, brainstem, or spinal cord) or peripheral nervous system is called neurogenic pain. Central pain syndrome, trigeminal neuralgia, and phantom pain are types of neurogenic pain (see: http://www.neurologychannel.com/chronicpain/causes.shtml).

Chronic pain can also occur without any indication of illness or injury. The cause of chronic pain is not well understood and there may be no evidence of disease or damage to the body tissues that doctors can directly link to the pain. This is extremely frustrating for the medical team and client. Chronic pain that is not related to physical disease or injury, or to other physical cause, is called psychogenic pain. This type of pain is also referred to as pain disorder with psychological factors. Mental and emotional disorders may cause, increase, or prolong pain. Headache, muscle pain, back pain, and stomach pain are the most common types of psychogenic pain. Physicians and mental health specialists work together to treat patients with this disorder. Massage therapy as part of the multidisciplinary intervention is justified (see Chapter 2 and http://www.neurologychannel.com/chronicpain/causes.html).

Pain types and pain dysfunction

Pain and fatigue typically occur together. Sleep supports the healing process accompanying acute pain. Unfortunately pain interferes with restorative sleep. Many people with chronic, widespread musculoskeletal pain report having fatigue and most people with chronic fatigue syndromes report muscle pain. Women make up the majority of patients with these conditions.

Chronic pain causes underlying biological changes affecting physical and psychosocial factors caused by the bombardment of the central nervous system (CNS) with nociceptive impulses, which causes changes in the neural response (sensation). The pain experience can include changes in the behavior and as a result, the individual may also become physically deconditioned. For example, fibromyalgia is a chronic pain condition that causes widespread pain and tenderness throughout the body. A University of Michigan study, published in the journal *Current Pain and Headache Reports*, shows that fibromyalgia is associated with central nervous system abnormalities evidenced by patients' elevated sensitivity to auditory and pressure sensations. Noise and pressure are interpreted as somatic pain. This suggests that a mismatch between sensory and motor neurons could be a contributing factor in fibromyalgia (Eazella 2006 materials provided by American Pain Society, via Newswise. American Pain Society 2008).

Avoidance behavior occurs leading to physical deconditioning which spirals into more sensitivity

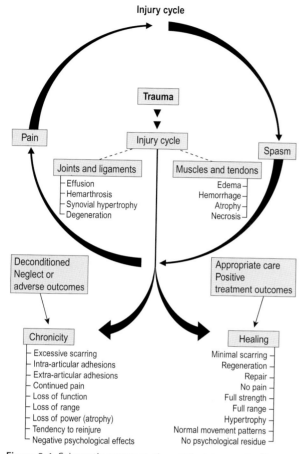

Figure 3.4 Schematic representation of the injury cycle. (From Chaitow & DeLany 2000.)

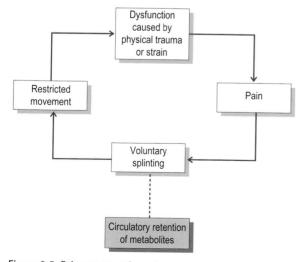

Figure 3.5 Pain–spasm–pain cycle.

to normal activity leading to even more avoidances and deconditioning. A biological link between pain and fatigue does exist. A study performed by the University of Iowa revealed a link between chronic pain and fibromyalgia, which is found in more women due to the lack of the male hormone testosterone, which protects against muscle fatigue (adapted from materials provided by University of Iowa 2008).

It may seem counterintuitive to exercise when suffering with pain, but physical activity is actually a natural pain reliever and mood modulator for most people suffering from pain. For example, The Arthritis Foundation Exercise Program is effective for improving and managing arthritis pain. Participants report a decrease in pain and fatigue, an increase in upper and lower extremity function, and an increase in strength after participating in the basic, 8-week exercise program. Also, participants who continued the exercise program beyond 8 weeks sustained improvement in reduced stiffness. The basic 8-week Arthritis Foundation Exercise Program consists of low impact routines with gentle range of motion movements that can be done while sitting or standing. This type of program would be appropriate for most experiencing reconditioning and fatigue from chronic pain (adapted from materials provided by Arthritis Foundation 2008).

IS THERE A COMMON LINK IN THE PAIN EXPERIENCE?

Maybe. Breathing pattern disorders (BPDs) can cause, aggravate, and perpetuate pain. Disordered breathing can decrease both pain threshold and pain tolerance resulting in increased pain awareness exacerbating the pain experience. Breathing pattern disorder can be simply defined as breathing in excess of need based on activity. The extreme of a BPD is hyperventilation (HVS), which is defined as breathing in excess of metabolic requirements.

BPD is a functional issue. There is no specific pathology but normal functions are occurring at abnormal times leading to physiologic changes causing the symptoms. Those with disordered breathing are breathing too much. Therapeutic massage intervention coupled with breathing retraining is effective in breaking the cycle of pain, stiffness and aching. About 10% of all patients attending general internal medicine practice in the USA are estimated to be suffering from chronic hyperventilation (Lum 1987). The authors' clinical experience with this sort of problem suggests that a large patient population exists with BPDs who don't meet the criteria for hyperventilation, but whose breathing patterns contribute greatly to their symptom picture. The vast majority of people who chronically overbreathe experience symptoms such as fatigue, widespread pain (e.g. fibromyalgia), irritable bowel symptoms, chronic bladder problems, anxiety, allergies, chemical sensitivities, headaches, premenstrual syndromes, photophobia, and increased sensitivity to noise. In many such conditions, BPDs rarely are causal (except perhaps if anxiety is a major feature), but they almost always are contributory, and sometimes become a major obstacle to recovery. The effects of BPDs are body wide, affecting all systems, having profound neurological, psychological, digestive, and circulatory influences. Disordered breathing is typically habitual. The good news is that massage therapy can support more effective breathing action, and breathing retraining and education can normalize the response with an outcome of improvement in the individual experience of pain by creating new breathing habits.

What happens during overbreathing?

Breathing too much results in an increase in oxygen beyond need and too much loss of carbon dioxide. Excessive carbon dioxide loss during overbreathing causes blood pH to rise, creating respiratory alkalosis causing sympathetic arousal and altering nerve function (including motor control). Calcium and magnesium ions are lost as the kidneys attempt to restore pH balance by excreting bicarbonate. This enhances neural sensitization, encouraging spasm and reducing pain threshold. Smooth muscle cells constrict, leading to vasoconstriction and possibly altering fascial tone causing connective tissue to shorten. Smooth muscle constriction can lead to colon spasm and pseudo-angina. Breathing pattern disorders automatically increase levels of anxiety and apprehension.

Due to alkalinity, the so-called Bohr effect reduces oxygen release to the cells, because hemoglobin retains oxygen more effectively in an alkaline environment. This reduction in oxygen availability affects tissues and the brain, encouraging ischemia, fatigue, and pain. Ischemia encourages the development of myofascial trigger points.

Overbreathing creates biomechanical overuse stresses, particularly on the accessory breathing muscles (scalenes, sternomastoid, upper trapezius, etc.),

There is evidence that the effects of breathing pattern disorders interfere with motor control, a key component in spinal (and all joint) injury prevention. Loss of motor control involves failure to control joints, commonly because of poor coordination of the agonist–antagonist muscle coactivation and trigger point development (Wheeler 2004).

Blood sugar and BPD

Feelings of faintness, cold sweats, weakness, and disturbed consciousness are common to BPD, HVS, and low blood sugar, and symptoms are far worse when both situations are present at the same time. During overbreathing, both EEG and cortical function deteriorate when glucose values are below 100 mg (Brostoff 1992).

Three minutes of hyperventilation presents mild effects when blood sugar is in the 85–90 mg range, but with blood sugar at 70–75 mg (still within normal range), gross EEG disturbances are noted (Lum 1994). It also has been found that fluctuating blood glucose levels, even when these stay within normal limits, can trigger HVS/BPD symptoms. People affected in this way are recommended to eat breakfast (including protein) and to avoid going without food for more than 3 hours or to follow a little-and-often or grazing pattern of eating. This is particularly important to those who experience panic attacks or seizures (Timmons & Ley 1994).

HVS/BPD is female dominated, ranging from a ratio of 2:1 to 7:1 (peak ages 15–55 years). Women are more at risk, possibly because progesterone is a respiratory accelerator. This also can have implications for women on hormone replacement therapy. During the postovulation phase, carbon dioxide levels drop about 25% and additional stress then 'increases ventilation at a time when CO_2 levels are already low' (Damas-Mora 1980).

In future chapters we will describe how massage and various bodywork methods can be use to support normal breathing as well as activate other pain modulating processes and help ease the pain and suffering of the pain experience.

KEY POINTS

- Pain is a noxious stimulus resulting from an actual or potential tissue damaging event that stimulates nociceptors.
- The experience of pain begins with the pain threshold, which is the smallest pain producing stimulus a person can perceive as painful, and

pain tolerance, which is the maximum intensity of a stimulus that evokes pain and that a subject is willing to tolerate.
- The pain experience can be altered by using changes in perception and activating physiological pain control mechanisms.

- In simple terms hyperalgesia is like the saying 'making mountains out of mole hills' and sensitization is making something out of nothing.
- Pain hurts whether there is harm or not. Hurting is disempowering, fatiguing, miserable, and the foundation of suffering.
- Since physical and social pain rely on similar neural systems, factors, such as social support, that increase tolerance of the experience of social pain should also increase the tolerance to physical pain.
- If massage therapy is going to be beneficial in pain management it must interact with the pain/pleasure anatomy and physiology. One of the greatest benefits of massage is that is feels good. Massage is pleasurable.
- Acute and chronic pain are both physically and emotionally different.
- Early exposure to acute pain is associated with changes in stress hormone receptors in certain regions of the brain.

- Undertreated pain leads to other problems, including reduced quality of life, decreased socialization, depression, sleep disturbances, cognitive impairment, and malnutrition.
- Pain and fatigue typically occur together.
- The pain experience can include changes in the behavior and as a result, the individual may also become physically deconditioned.
- Participants report a decrease in pain and fatigue, an increase in upper and lower extremity function, and an increase in strength after participating in the basic, 8-week exercise program.
- Breathing pattern disorders can cause, aggravate, and perpetuate pain. Disordered breathing can decrease both pain threshold and pain tolerance resulting in increased pain awareness which exacerbates the pain experience.
- Therapeutic massage intervention coupled with breathing retraining is effective in helping break the cycle of pain, stiffness, and aching.

References

Arthritis Foundation: Physical activity is natural pain reliever for arthritis, *ScienceDaily*, April 17, 2008. Online at http://www.sciencedaily.com/releases/2008/04/080408173045.htm. Retrieved September 27, 2008.

Brostoff J: Complete guide to food allergy, London, 1992, Bloomsbury.

Brown University: Pain receptor in brain may be linked to learning and memory, *ScienceDaily*, March 14, 2008. Online at http://www.sciencedaily.com/releases/2008/03/080313125347.htm. Retrieved September 27, 2008.

Center For The Advancement Of Health: Infant pain may have long-term effects, *ScienceDaily*, August 16, 1999. Online at http://www.sciencedaily.comreleases/1999/08/990816065623.htm. Retrieved September 27, 2008.

Chaitow L, DeLany J: Clinical application of neuromuscular techniques, vol 1. The upper body, Edinburgh, 2000, Churchill Livingstone.

Damas-Mora J: Menstrual respiratory changes and symptoms, *Br J Psychiatry* 136:492–497, 1980.

Eisenberger NI, Jarcho JM, Lieberman MD, et al: An experimental study of shared sensitivity to physical pain and social rejection, *Pain* 126:132–138, 2006.

Eisenberger NI, Lieberman MD: Why rejection hurts: a common neural alarm system for physical and social pain, *Trends in Cognitive Sciences* 8:294–300, 2004.

Eisenberger NI, Lieberman MD: Broken hearts and broken bones: the neurocognitive overlap between social pain and physical pain. In Williams KD, Forgas JP, von Hippel W, editors: The social outcast: ostracism, social exclusion rejection, and bullying, New York, 2005, Cambridge University Press, pp 109–127.

Eisenberger NI, Lieberman MD, Williams KD: Does rejection hurt: an fMRI study of social exclusion, *Science* 302:290–292, 2003.

Eisenberger NI, Taylor SE, Gable SL, et al: Neural pathways link social support to attenuated neuroendocrine stress response, *NeuroImage* 35:1601–1612, 2007.

Fibromyalgia pain caused by neuron mismatch, suggests study, *ScienceDaily*, November 2, 2007. Online at http://www.sciencedaily.com/releases/2007/10/071030220054.htm. Retrieved September 27, 2008.

Fritz S: Mosby's essential sciences for therapeutic massage: anatomy, physiology, biomechanics, and pathology, ed 2, St Louis, 2004, Mosby.

Gazella K: The pain from Fibromyalgia is real, reasearchers say, *Curr Pain Headache Rep*: 403–407, Dec 2006.

Lieberman MD, Eisenberger NI: A pain by any other name (rejection, exclusion, ostracism), still hurts the same: the role of dorsal anterior cingulate in social and physical pain. In Cacioppo JT, Visser P, Pickett C, editors: Social neuroscience: people thinking about people, Cambridge, MA, 2005, MIT Press, pp 167–187.

Lieberman M, Eisenberger N: Pains and pleasures of social life, *Science* 323:890–891, 2009.

Lum L: Hyperventilation syndromes in medicine and psychiatry, *Journal of the Royal Society of Medicine* 80: 229–231, 1987.

Lum L: HVS: Physiological considerations. In Timmons B, Ley R, editors: Behavioural and psychological approaches to breathing disorder, New York, 1994, Plenum Press.

Mayer E, Drossman D, Ringel Y: Adapted from materials provided by University of California, Los Angeles (February 3, 2008). Abuse history affects pain regulation in women with irritable bowel syndrome, *ScienceDaily*, February 3, 2008. Online at http://www.sciencedaily.com/releases/2008/02/080201085752.htm. Retrieved September 27, 2008.

McMahon S, Koltzenburg M, editors: Wall and Melzack's Textbook of pain, ed 5, St Louis, 2010, Elsevier.

Nelson EE, Panksepp J: Brain substrates of infant–mother attachment: contributions of opioids, oxytocin, and norepinephrine, *Neurosci Biobehav Rev* 22:437–452, 1998.

O'Connor M-F, Wellisch DK, Annette L, et al: Craving love? Enduring grief activates brain's reward center, *Neuroimage* 42:969–972, 2008.

Panksepp J: A critical analysis of ADHD, psychostimulants, and intolerance of childhood playfulness: a tragedy in the making? *Curr Dir Psychol Sci* 7:91–97, 1998.

Panksepp J: Affective neuroscience: the foundations of human and animal emotions (series in affective science), New York, 1998, Oxford University Press.

Panksepp J: The quest for long-term health and happiness: to play or not to play, that is the question, *Psychol Inq* 9:56–65, 1998.

Panksepp J: The periconscious substrates of consciousness: affective states and the evolutionary origins of the SELF, *J Consciousness Stud* 5:566–582, 1998.

Robinson CL: Relieving pain in the elderly, *Health Prog* 88(1): 48-53, 70, 2007.

Seaman D: The catastrophic effects of pain and the nature of tissue healing are not a focus in chiropractic practice, *Dynam Chiropr* 28(4). Online at http://www.chiroweb.com/mpacms/dc/article.php?id=38010.

Timmons B, Ley R, editors: Behavioural and psychological approaches to breathing disorders, New York, 1994, Plenum Press.

University of Iowa: Biological link between pain and fatigue discovered, *ScienceDaily*, April 9, 2008. Online at http://www.sciencedaily.com/releases/2008/04/080407153037.htm. Retrieved September 27, 2008.

Wheeler AH: Myofascial pain disorders: theory to therapy, *Drugs* 64(1):45–62, 2004.

Websites

Changing States: www.changingstates.co.uk/issues/pain_control.html

Neurology Channel: www.neurologychannel.com/chronicpain/causes.shtml

American Physical Therapy Association: www.womenshealthapta.org/csm04/6412.pdf

CHAPTER FOUR

Medical treatment for pain and implications for massage application

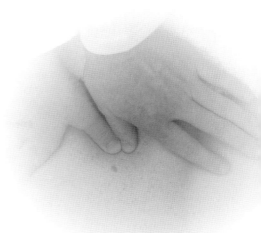

CHAPTER CONTENTS

INTRODUCTION

Those experiencing pain usually seek help from a family medical practitioner. If the problem is not relieved by standard treatments, the patient may then be referred to a specialist such as an internist or neurologist. Additional referrals may be made to psychologists.

The massage therapist needs to understand the diagnostic process and target of various treatments so that the massage application can support specific medical treatment. When therapeutic massage is used in conjunction with typical medical treatments such as medication, supplements or herbs, surgery, manipulation, physical therapy, etc. it is necessary to evaluate the massage application so that it is supportive of medical intervention as well as taking into account potential risks for massage associated with treatment.

THE DIAGNOSTIC PROCESS

The process of identifying the cause of the symptoms related to pain includes typical assessment procedures such as history taking, physical assessment, specific assessment (X-ray, blood tests, strength and stability testing, etc.), and interpretation of the information gathered.

History taking

A physician's detailed question and answer session with a patient can often produce enough information for a diagnosis. Many types of pain have clearcut symptoms which fall into an easily recognizable pattern. Most physicians will also obtain a full medical history from the patient, inquiring about past trauma or surgery, occupation related strain, lifestyle behaviors, sleep habits, levels of emotional and physical stress, and the use of medications, both prescribed and over the counter. Typical health history questions used to diagnose pain include:

- Were you injured and, if yes, what was the nature of the injury?
- Do you experience radiating pain and the presence of any symptoms that suggest nerve problems such as:
  - weakness
  - numbness
  - tingling or loss of function
  - difficulty breathing
  - dizziness, nausea, or vomiting
- How often do you experience pain?
- Where is the pain?
- How long does the pain last?
- When did you first develop pain?
- What factors make you feel better (relieving) or worse (exacerbating)?

Physical examination

- Observation includes: posture, gait, facial expression, willingness to move for examination, and ease of movement.
- Physical tests and palpation:
  - Neuromuscular testing to determine whether there are any injuries to the pain area. These tests typically involve moving the body both passively and actively, to assess for strength, range of motion, and any loss of sensation.
  - Assessment of the blood vessels, feeling the pulses to assess for briskness of upstroke and fullness, and the presence of any abnormal sounds.
  - Soft tissue will be palpated for tender area, signs of inflammation (heat and edema), tissue texture changes, differences in temperature and dryness or excessive moisture, tremor (shaking) and muscle twitches, and changes in muscle and motor tone.

Diagnostic imaging

Plain film radiography (X-rays)
Plain X-rays are still the primary means of looking for trauma to bones involving the cervical spine. They have the advantages of low cost, wide availability, and good anatomic resolution. X-rays do not give a good image of soft tissue structures (muscles and ligaments).

Computed tomography (CT scan)
This painless, noninvasive technique produces cross-sectional images of tissues. CT scans offer far better tissue contrast resolution when compared with plain X-rays and are excellent for displaying bony architecture, although soft tissues are seen less well.

They are useful in assessing for complex fractures and dislocations, disk protrusions and disease of the joints of the vertebrae, and spinal stenosis (a narrowing of the space containing the spinal cord). CT scans produce X-ray images of the brain that show structures or variations in the density of different types of tissue.

Magnetic resonating imaging (MRI)
MRI is a noninvasive, painless imaging technique used to obtain images of bone and soft tissue. It uses magnetic fields and is based on detecting the effect of a strong magnetic field on hydrogen atoms contained in water. MRI scans use magnetic fields and radio waves to produce an image that provides information about the structure and biochemistry of the brain.

MRI cannot be used for people with implanted or other metallic foreign bodies not firmly fixed to bone but is reportedly safe with prosthetic joints and internal fixation devices. It is often preferred over myelography for the assessment of disk disease because it is noninvasive. Its principal disadvantages include cost and lack of availability.

Myelography (spinal cord imaging)
A water soluble contrast dye is injected into the epidural space via lumbar puncture and allowed to flow to different levels of the spinal cord. Plain X-rays, or more commonly CT scan, are then performed, to indirectly visualize structures outlined by the dye.

This technique is very sensitive at detecting disk disease, disk herniation, nerve entrapment, spinal stenosis, and tumors of the spinal cord. Side effects of the procedure include headache, dizziness, nausea, vomiting, and seizures.

Diskography
This involves the injection of radio-opaque dye into the center of an intervertebral disk (nucleus pulposus), using radiographic guidance, and may be used to determine disk disruptions.

Blood tests
Blood tests may be ordered to screen for thyroid disease, anemia, or infections which might cause pain.

Hopefully the diagnostic process will identify the cause of the pain and guide the treatment process. The massage therapist would utilize the information gathered during diagnosis as well as gather similar information themselves as they develop and implement an appropriate massage intervention. There are a variety of pain conditions. However, pain does not always neatly fit into a specific diagnosis and sometimes there is no identifiable reason at all making the pain experience so difficult to treat with traditional health care measures.

THE A TO Z OF PAIN

Hundreds of pain syndromes or disorders make up the spectrum of pain. There are the most benign, fleeting sensations of pain, such as a pin prick. There is the pain of childbirth, the pain of a heart attack, and the pain that sometimes follows amputation of a limb. There is also pain accompanying cancer and the pain that follows severe trauma, such as that associated with head and spinal cord injuries. A sampling of common pain syndromes follows, listed alphabetically.

Amputation refers to loss of a body part. Care includes managing wound, postoperative, and phantom limb sensation or pain. Abnormal sensations can be felt from the amputated body part which is no longer part of the body. These unusual 'phantom limb' sensations can vary from feelings of size, position, movement to actual feelings of heat, cold, itching and, or touch. Stump pain is specific to its location: at or near the amputation site. Unlike phantom pain, it occurs in the body part that actually exists, in the stump that remains. Stump pain has been commonly described as sharp, burning, shock-like, or super-sensitive to the skin region. Stump pain results from nerve damage in the stump region. As nerves heal from injury or surgery they may form abnormally sensitive regions, called neuromas, which fire abnormally, resulting in pain and skin sensitivity.

Arachnoiditis is a condition in which one of the three membranes covering the brain and spinal cord, called the arachnoid membrane, becomes inflamed. A number of causes, including infection or trauma, can result in inflammation of this membrane. Arachnoiditis can produce disabling, progressive, and even permanent pain.

Arthritis affects millions who suffer from arthritic conditions such as osteoarthritis, rheumatoid arthritis, ankylosing spondylitis, and gout. These disorders are characterized by joint pain in the extremities.

Many other inflammatory diseases affect the body's soft tissues, including tendonitis and bursitis.

Back pain has become the high price paid by our modern lifestyle and is a startlingly common cause of disability for many Americans, including both active and inactive people. Back pain that spreads to the leg is called sciatica and is a very common condition (see below). Another common type of back pain is associated with the discs of the spine, the soft, spongy padding between the vertebrae (bones) that form the spine. Discs protect the spine by absorbing shock, but they tend to degenerate over time and may sometimes rupture. Spondylolisthesis is a back condition that occurs when one vertebra extends over another, causing pressure on nerves and therefore pain. Also, damage to nerve roots is a serious condition – called radiculopathy – that can be extremely painful. Treatment for a damaged disc includes drugs such as painkillers, muscle relaxants, and steroids; exercise or rest, depending on the patient's condition; adequate support, such as a brace or better mattress; and physical therapy. In some cases, surgery may be required to remove the damaged portion of the disc and return it to its previous condition, especially when it is pressing a nerve root. Surgical procedures include discectomy, laminectomy, or spinal fusion.

Burn pain can be profound and poses an extreme challenge to the medical community. First-degree burns are the least severe; with third-degree burns, the skin is lost. Depending on the injury, pain accompanying burns can be excruciating, and even after the wound has healed patients may have chronic pain at the burn site. For more on central pain syndrome, see 'Trauma' below.

Cancer pain can accompany the growth of a tumor, the treatment of cancer, or chronic problems related to cancer's permanent effects on the body. Fortunately, most cancer pain can be treated to help minimize discomfort and stress to the patient.

Headaches affect millions of Americans. The three most common types of chronic headache are migraines, cluster headaches, and tension headaches. Each comes with its own telltale brand of pain:

- Migraines are characterized by throbbing pain and sometimes by other symptoms, such as nausea and visual disturbances. Migraines are more frequent in women than men. Stress can trigger a migraine headache, and migraines can also put the sufferer at risk for stroke.
- Cluster headaches are characterized by excruciating, piercing pain on one side of the head; they occur more frequently in men than women.
- Tension headaches are often described as a tight band around the head.

Head and facial pain can be agonizing, whether it results from dental problems or from disorders such as cranial neuralgia, in which one of the nerves in the face, head, or neck is inflamed. Another condition, trigeminal neuralgia (also called tic douloureux), affects the largest of the cranial nerves, and is characterized by a stabbing, shooting pain.

Lyme disease can cause severe neurological problems and pain if untreated. Those with chronic pain syndromes associated with Lyme disease may develop a heightened activation of the pain pathways, sensitizing them not just to one type of pain, but to multiple types of pain. This means that otherwise mild symptoms might be perceived as abnormally intense, problematic, or distressing for a patient with a history of Lyme disease, or for those with other pre-existing pain conditions like fibromyalgia.

Muscle pain can range from an aching muscle, spasm, or strain to the severe spasticity that accompanies paralysis. Another disabling syndrome is fibromyalgia, a disorder characterized by fatigue, stiffness, joint tenderness, and widespread muscle pain. Polymyositis, dermatomyositis, and inclusion body myositis are painful disorders characterized by muscle inflammation. They may be caused by infection or autoimmune dysfunction and are sometimes associated with connective tissue disorders, such as lupus and rheumatoid arthritis.

Myofascial pain syndromes affect sensitive areas known as trigger points, located within the body's muscles. Myofascial pain syndromes are sometimes misdiagnosed and can be debilitating. Fibromyalgia is a type of myofascial pain syndrome.

Neuropathic pain is a type of pain that can result from injury to nerves, either in the peripheral or central nervous system. Neuropathic pain can occur in any part of the body and is frequently described as a hot, burning sensation, which can be devastating to the affected individual. It can result from diseases that affect nerves (such as diabetes) or from trauma, or, because chemotherapy drugs can affect nerves, it can be a consequence of cancer treatment. Among the many neuropathic pain conditions are diabetic neuropathy (which results from nerve damage secondary to vascular problems that occur with diabetes); reflex sympathetic dystrophy syndrome, which can follow injury; phantom limb and post amputation pain, which can result from the surgical removal of a limb; postherpetic neuralgia, which can occur after an outbreak of shingles; and central pain syndrome, which can result from trauma to the brain or spinal cord.

Pelvic pain or chronic pelvic pain refers to pain in the pelvic region (located between the navel and hips), lasting 6 months or longer. Chronic pelvic pain can be a symptom of another disease, or it can be designated as a condition in its own right. Spasms or tension of the pelvic floor muscles can lead to recurring pelvic pain as can long-term infection and **pelvic congestion** caused by enlarged, varicose-type veins. The condition is more common in females but does occur in males.

Reflex sympathetic dystrophy syndrome, or RSDS, is accompanied by burning pain and hypersensitivity to temperature. Often triggered by trauma or nerve damage, RSDS causes the skin of the affected area to become characteristically shiny. In recent years, RSDS has come to be called complex regional pain syndrome (CRPS); in the past it was often called causalgia.

Repetitive stress injuries are muscular conditions that result from repeated motions performed in the course of normal work or other daily activities. They include:

- writer's cramp, which affects musicians, writers, and others
- compression or entrapment neuropathies, including carpal tunnel syndrome, caused by chronic overextension of the wrist
- tendonitis or tenosynovitis, affecting one or more tendons.

Sciatica is a painful condition caused by pressure on the sciatic nerve, the main nerve that branches off the spinal cord and continues down into the thighs, legs, ankles, and feet. Sciatica is characterized by pain in the buttocks and can be caused by a number of factors. Exertion, obesity, and poor posture can all cause pressure on the sciatic nerve. One common cause of sciatica is a herniated disc.

Shingles and other painful disorders affect the skin. Pain is a common symptom of many skin disorders, even the most common rashes. One of the most vexing neurological disorders is shingles or herpes zoster, an infection that often causes agonizing pain resistant to treatment. Prompt treatment with antiviral agents is important to arrest the infection, which, if prolonged, can result in an associated condition known as postherpetic neuralgia. Other painful disorders affecting the skin include:

- vasculitis, or inflammation of blood vessels
- other infections, including herpes simplex
- skin tumors and cysts
- tumors associated with neurofibromatosis, a neurogenetic disorder.

Spinal stenosis refers to a narrowing of the canal surrounding the spinal cord. The condition occurs naturally with aging. Spinal stenosis causes weakness in the legs and leg pain usually felt while the person is standing up and often relieved by sitting down.

Sports injuries are common. Sprains, strains, bruises, dislocations, and fractures are all well known words in the language of sports. Pain is another. In extreme cases, sports injuries can take the form of costly and painful spinal cord and head injuries, which cause severe suffering and disability.

Surgical pain may require regional or general anesthesia during the procedure and medications to control discomfort following the operation. Control of pain associated with surgery includes presurgical preparation and careful monitoring of the patient during and after the procedure.

Temporomandibular disorders are conditions in which the temporomandibular joint (the jaw) is damaged and/or the muscles used for chewing and talking become stressed, causing pain. The condition may be the result of a number of factors, such as an injury to the jaw or joint misalignment, and may give rise to a variety of symptoms, most commonly pain in the jaw, face, and/or neck muscles. Physicians reach a diagnosis by listening to the patient's description of the symptoms and by performing a simple examination of the facial muscles and the temporomandibular joint.

Trauma can occur after injuries in the home, at the workplace, during sports activities, or on the road. Any of these injuries can result in severe disability and pain. Some patients who have had an injury to the spinal cord experience intense pain ranging from tingling to burning and, commonly, both. Such patients are sensitive to hot and cold temperatures and touch. For these individuals, a touch can be perceived as intense burning, indicating abnormal signals relayed to and from the brain. This condition is called central pain syndrome or, if the damage is in the thalamus (the brain's center for processing bodily sensations), thalamic pain syndrome. It affects as many as 100000 Americans with multiple sclerosis, Parkinson's disease, amputated limbs, spinal cord injuries, and stroke. Their pain is severe and is extremely difficult to treat effectively. A variety of medications, including analgesics, antidepressants, and anticonvulsants, and electrical stimulation, are options available to central pain patients.

Vascular disease or injuries – such as vasculitis or inflammation of blood vessels, coronary artery disease, and circulatory problems – all have the potential to cause pain. Vascular pain affects millions of Americans and occurs when communication between blood vessels and nerves is interrupted. Ruptures, spasms, constriction, or obstruction of blood vessels, as well as a condition called ischemia in which blood supply to organs, tissues, or limbs is cut off, can also result in pain.

Vulvodynia is chronic pain of the vulva – the external female genital organs. Women living with this condition report burning, stinging, irritation, and rawness in the vulva area that lasts for at least 3 months or more with no evidence of other possible causes such as infection, including sexually transmitted diseases, or skin problems. The pain associated with vulvodynia can occur all the time or just once in a while. It may or may not be promoted by touch. For many women, the pain is often triggered when pressure is applied to the vulva area, either when inserting a tampon, engaging in sexual activity, undergoing pelvic examination, wearing tight-fitting pants, or during exercise, especially bicycling or horseback riding.

NINDS health-related material is provided for information purposes only and does not necessarily represent endorsement by, or an official position of, the National Institute of Neurological Disorders and Stroke or any other Federal agency. Advice on the treatment or care of an individual patient should be obtained through consultation with a physician who has examined that patient or is familiar with that patient's medical history.

All NINDS-prepared information is in the public domain and may be freely copied. Credit to the NINDS or the NIH is appreciated.

See: http://www.ninds.nih.gov/disorders/chronic_pain/detail_chronic_pain.htm#102993084Pain

MEDICAL TREATMENT

The primary therapeutic outcomes from appropriate pain management therapy are as follows:

1. Relief of pain intensity and duration of pain complaint.
2. Prevention of the conversion of persistent pain to chronic pain.
3. Prevention of suffering and disability associated with pain.
4. Prevention of psychological and socioeconomic consequences associated with inadequate pain management.
5. Control of side effects associated with pain management.
6. Optimization of the ability to perform activities of daily living.

Acceptable outcomes include:

- pain at rest <3 on pain scale
- pain with movement <5 on pain scale
- ability to have at least 6 hours of sleep uninterrupted by pain
- ability to work at a hobby (e.g. crafts, play cards, gardening) for 1 hour.

Optimal outcomes include:

- minimizing physical and emotional suffering
- decreasing the disability caused by pain
- eliminating excessive reliance on medication or inappropriate medical resources
- accelerating return to a wide array of normal activities, including personal, family, and work.

Treatment for pain depends on the cause and on the individual needs of the person. Complete pain relief is not always possible; it is important for patients, physicians and other health professionals including massage therapists to work together to find the best treatment plan. Understanding the mechanisms of action of medical treatment, especially medication, helps the massage therapist make logical decisions about when massage may either support the outcome of treatment, and therefore reduce the medication dosage, or in some cases replace the medication. The health care system needs to take the treatment of pain seriously and be proactive and encompassing in pain management methods, conventional as well as alternative, within an integrated health care delivery system. The conventional health care practitioners need to learn about and respect the beneficial application of massage, and massage therapists need to learn about and integrate into the traditional (conventional) health care system. The management of pain is not an either/or process but instead a cooperative partnership among all (Box 4.2).

Medical procedures to treat pain

Surgery (e.g. joint replacement, tumor excision, discectomy) may eliminate some types of chronic pain. Cordotomy may be used in severe cases of lower body pain when other treatments are ineffective. This procedure involves severing the nerve fibers on one or both sides of the spinal cord, eliminating the sensations of pain and temperature.

Brain stimulation may be used to treat widespread, severe pain. This invasive procedure involves surgically implanting electrodes in the brain, which the patient controls by means of an external transmitter.

Transcutaneous electrical nerve stimulation (TENS; brief pulses of electricity) is applied to nerve endings to block pain transmission. This procedure has proven effective for many different types of chronic pain, and is safe and noninvasive. The feeling is described as a buzzing, tingling, or tapping feeling. The small electric impulses seem to interfere with pain sensations. The current can be adjusted so that the sensation is pleasant and relieves pain. Pain relief lasts beyond the time that the current is applied.

Nerve blocks are an injection of an anesthetic around a nerve's fiber to prevent pain messages that are traveling along that nerve pathway from reaching the brain. Nerve blocks are most often used to relieve pain for a short period, such as during surgery. If there is inflammation around a nerve, an injection of corticosteroid in conjunction with the nerve block may provide longer pain relief. There are three main types of nerve block:

1. *Peripheral.* For localized pain, an anesthetic is injected around a nerve that is away from the spine, such as in an ankle. The result is reduced feeling and less pain in that area.
2. *Spinal.* For pain that affects a broader area, such as the lower back or a leg, an anesthetic is injected in or near the spinal column. An injection directly into the spinal fluid is called an intrathecal injection. This type of injection is often used during surgery on the abdomen or legs.
3. If the injection is not into the spinal fluid, it is called an *epidural* injection. Epidurals are often used to relieve the pain of childbirth and sometimes to relieve some types of back pain, such as sciatica.

MEDICATIONS FOR PAIN MANAGEMENT

Over-the-counter (OTC) analgesics (e.g. aspirin, ibuprofen, acetaminophen) may be used to treat chronic pain. These medications should not be used to relieve pain for longer than 10 days without consulting a physician. Side effects of nonsteroidal anti-inflammatory drugs (NSAIDs) include nausea, abdominal pain, dizziness, and rash. When OTC medications are ineffective, stronger prescription medications may be used. The World Health Organization (http://www.who.int/cancer/palliative/painladder/en/) (Box 4.3) recommends a stepwise approach to pain management. Mild, acute pain is effectively treated with analgesics such as NSAIDs or acetaminophen. NSAIDs include aspirin, naproxen, and ibuprofen. Pain associated with inflammation responds well to NSAIDs. Acetaminophen is another type of OTC pain medication. Unrelieved or moderate pain is generally treated with a moderate potency opiate such as codeine or oxycodone, which are often used in combination with acetaminophen or aspirin (e.g. Empirin 3, Tylenol with Codeine No. 3, Percodan®). Severe, acute pain is treated with opiate agonists (e.g. morphine, hydromorphone, levorphanol). Morphine sulfate is usually the drug of choice for the treatment of severe, chronic pain. Other medication may be used as adjunctive therapy with analgesics such as antidepressants or anticonvulsants, depending on the cause of the pain.

Box 4.2 Australian and New Zealand College of Anaesthetists ABN 82 055 042 852. Faculty of Pain Medicine: Statement on patients' rights to pain management and associated responsibilities

1. Introduction

Since the time of Hippocrates, the treatment of pain has been an important priority of the physician. As knowledge of disease processes has advanced, the emphasis in medicine moved to diagnosis and treatment of the underlying causes of pain. However, there has been a renewed focus on the management of pain itself, arising out of the complex nature of the experience of pain, humanitarian aspects, and better methods and tools for symptom control. Enhanced pain management has been associated with improved outcomes after surgery and trauma, more successful rehabilitation in patients with persistent pain and potentially improved survival of patients with cancer pain. Standards and practice guidelines have been developed for the management of all forms of pain (Merskey & Bogduk 1994, Macintyre et al 2010, Brennan & Cousins 2004). Effective pain management requires assessment of physical, psychological, social and environmental factors in each patient, to facilitate strategies to improve physical, mental and emotional functioning, and to improve quality of life as rapidly and completely as possible given each individual's circumstances.

ANZCA recognises that unrelieved pain can have severe adverse physical and psychological effects on patients, with emotional, social and spiritual consequences causing suffering in patients, their families and those close to them (Macintyre et al 2010). *At times severe pain can be difficult to treat and management must be subject to the availability in each health care setting of appropriate, safe and effective methods.*

2. Rights

ANZCA recognizes that patients with pain, whether it is acute pain, pain related to cancer or persistent noncancer pain, have the following rights:

2.1 To have their complaint of pain respected and taken seriously, recognizing that pain is a personal experience and that individuals vary greatly in their responses to painful predicaments (Merskey & Bogduk 1994).

2.2 To be cared for in a timely manner by health professionals who have training and experience in assessment and management of pain, and who maintain such competencies through professional development consistent with their discipline. Where such competencies are unavailable, patients should have access to appropriate referral.

2.3 To participate actively, or have their families, carers or guardians participate, in education regarding pain and in the development of realistic goals for their pain management plan.

2.4 To expect that their 'pain history', current assessment and management plan and responses to therapies will be recorded regularly and in a way that promotes optimal and ongoing pain relief.

2.5 To have access to best practice care, including appropriate assessment and effective pain management strategies, and access to suitably qualified interdisciplinary pain management teams or individuals who should be able to address physical and psychological aspects of management. These must be supported by appropriate policies and procedures.

2.6 To be informed of the evidence for the efficacy of a pain treatment, of the likelihood and duration of a successful outcome of an intervention, of other possible consequences and of alternative treatments.

2.7 To have appropriate planning for pain management after discharge from immediate care.

3. Responsibilities

In addition, ANZCA recognises that patients or their carers and families have responsibilities that include:

3.1 To engage openly with their health care providers

3.2 To become informed about pain and its management

3.3 To participate actively in their own care and in decisions about their care

3.4 To consider bestpractice advice

3.5 To advocate for better pain management.

4. Footnotes

4.1 Use of the words 'rights' and 'appropriate'
   A 'right to pain relief' does not imply that all pain can or will be treated successfully, that all patients will be free from pain, or that any analgesic treatment will necessarily be provided on demand, including the prescription of opioids (Brennan & Cousins 2004, Rich 2007). That right requires that the professional response be reasonable and

(Continued)

Box 4.2 (Continued)

proportionate to the level and character of the pain experience and that the assessment and management of a patient's pain be appropriate to that patient' (Brennan & Cousins 2004).

4.2   International Association for the Study of Pain (IASP) Definition of Pain

An unpleasant sensory and emotional experience, associated with actual or potential tissue damage, or described in terms of such damage (Merskey & Bogduk 1994)

4.3   Particular patient groups

The rights outlined above apply to all patients, including neonates, preverbal children and patients with cognitive impairment, whether due to developmental delay, dementia or other causes. These patients have a right to age-appropriate, development-appropriate and other suitable pain assessment tools and management (Australian Pain Society 2005). In such cases, a parent, carer or other guardian must be recognised as the agent for the rights and responsibilities of the patient.

Related documents

Particular note should be taken of the following College and Faculty Documents:

PS3 Guidelines for the Management of Major Regional Analgesia
PS20 Recommendations on the Responsibilities of the Anaesthetist in the Post-Anaesthesia Period
PS38 Statement Relating to Relief of Pain and Suffering and End of Life Decisions
PS41 Guidelines on Acute Pain Management
PM2 Guidelines for Units Offering Training in Multidisciplinary Pain Medicine

The following document of the College of Intensive Care Medicine of Australia and New Zealand is also relevant:

IC-9 Statement on the Ethical Practice of Intensive Care Medicine, available at www.cicm.org.au

College professional documents

College professional documents are progressively being coded as follows:

TE Training and educational
EX Examinations
PS Professional standards
T Technical.
Policy – defined as 'a course of action adopted and pursued by the College'. These are matters coming within the authority and control of the College.
Recommendations – defined as 'advisable courses of action'.
Guidelines – defined as 'a document offering advice'. These may be clinical (in which case they will eventually be evidence-based), or non-clinical.
Statements – defined as 'a communication setting out information'.

This document has been prepared having regard to general circumstances, and it is the responsibility of the practitioner to have express regard to the particular circumstances of each case, and the application of this document in each case.

Professional documents are reviewed from time to time, and it is the responsibility of the practitioner to ensure that the practitioner has obtained the current version. Professional documents have been prepared having regard to the information available at the time of their preparation, and the practitioner should therefore have regard to any information, research or material which may have been published or become available subsequently.

Whilst the College endeavours to ensure that professional documents are as current as possible at the time of their preparation, it takes no responsibility for matters arising from changed circumstances or information or material which may have become available subsequently.

Promulgated: 2001. Reviewed: 2008. Date of current document: Oct 2008. Republished: Feb 2010; April 2010
PS45 (2010) © This document is copyright and has been reproduced with permission from WHO.
ANZCA website: http://www.anzca.edu.au/
FPM website: http://www.anzca.edu.au/fpm/

Box 4.3 The World Health Organization (WHO)

'WHO is the directing and coordinating authority for health within the United Nations system. It is responsible for providing leadership on global health matters, shaping the health research agenda, setting norms and standards, articulating evidence-based policy options, providing technical support to countries and monitoring and assessing health trends.'

According to WHO, pain management and palliative care include:

- An initial assessment of the patient includes believing the patient's complaint and establishing the severity of the pain and restriction it causes.
- Relief obtained from previous treatment.
- A physical examination that includes a psychological assessment.
- Rule out any treatable causes of the pain.
- If examination and investigations reveal treatable conditions then these are treated accordingly with appropriate pain relief.
- If there is no treatable cause of pain then symptomatic relief can be given with the three step ladder approach.
- Appropriate counseling, to help the patient cope, and other forms of palliation should be considered.
- If adequate pain relief is achieved an appropriate schedule for review or follow up should be arranged.
- Should the pain persist then a decision should be taken about how care can be provided in the home or hospital. This may involve the relatives of the patient or other supportive services in the community.
- The type of drug to relieve pain and duration of use needs to be agreed upon including consideration of psychological support for the family and the patient.
- It should be recognized that if death is an inevitable outcome of the condition then spiritual preparation may be requested by the patient.

This approach to care works best when there is a team of care givers working to meet the various needs of the patient. From http://www.searo.who.int/LinkFiles/Publications_ch11.pdf (Clinical Management of HIV and AIDS at District Level).

Pain management

It is important to recognize that pain is a problem in its own right, not 'just' an indicator of an underlying disease or damage process, but one which extracts a great toll on individuals and society. Alleviation of pain itself, as a symptom, should be a therapeutic target. In order to improve the quality of life, the objective should be to avoid any unpleasant perception with an approach based on the right communication between the care giver and the patient. Initial evaluation and ongoing reassessment are necessary. It is important to assess not only the intensity and frequency of physical pain but also the presence and intensity of other suffering called total pain. In total pain, we consider not only the physical suffering but also the social, emotional, and spiritual suffering. There is no amount of morphine that can alleviate such a suffering. This is an important message to send to nurses, physicians, and other caregivers. Otherwise there is only an increase in the doses of opioids administered, which results in adverse effects and no response to the real suffering of the patients.

The correct diagnosis and proper treatment of pain is an important public health concern. Millions of people in the world with severe acute and chronic pain suffer because the lack of a standardized scientific approach to pain management. Most experts agreed that WHO needs to develop guidelines (keeping broad distinction in acute and chronic and specific clinical situations) on the following three categories of pain:

1. Acute pain (including pre- and postoperative pain, post traumatic pain, burns pain, acute pain during childbirth, spinal cord injury, acute headache, HIV/AIDS, sickle cell crisis, pain in trigeminal neuralgia (tic douloureux), interventional pain (diagnostic and therapeutic procedures), pancreatitis and other colic pain, myocardial infarction and other major cardiac events, acute or chronic pain).
2. Chronic malignant pain (including pain in patients with cancer, HIV/AIDS, amyotrophic lateral sclerosis (ALS), multiple sclerosis, end stage organ failure, advanced chronic obstructive pulmonary disease, advanced congestive heart failure, Parkinsonism).
3. Chronic nonmalignant pain including:
   i) chronic musculoskeletal pain such as spinal pain or low back pain, chronic degenerative arthritis, osteoarthritis, rheumatoid arthritis, myofascial and rheumatic pain, chronic headache, migraine, bone pain

(Continued)

Box 4.3 (Continued)

 ii) neuropathic pain (including nerve compression pain, post nerve injury and postamputation pain), diabetic neuropathy, complex regional pain syndromes (type I and type II), skeletal muscle spasm, postherpetic neuralgia, chronic postsurgical pain

 iii) visceral pain (like distension of hollow viscera and colic pain), and

 iv) chronic pain in sickle cell anemia.

WHO guidelines on the treatment of all types of pain provide guidance to governments, institutions, and health care professionals for policy, legislation, and practice.

At present many physicians from different specialties (e.g. neurosurgery, neurology, surgery, anesthesiology, psychiatry, and physiotherapy) are involved in the care of pain patients. There is a bias for surgeons to operate, anesthesiologists to do pain procedures, physiotherapists to emphasize function improvement, and psychiatrists and physiologists to prescribe medication and behavior modification techniques. This reflects a particular physician's education and training. The medical curriculum does not have a common plan of pain management and uniform nomenclature of various pain states. Therefore there is a strong need for WHO to develop guidelines using a multidisciplinary approach. WHO published extensive guidelines on the relief of pain related to cancer in adults in 1986, which was updated in 1996, followed by guidelines on cancer related pain relief and palliative care in children in 1998.

However, there is a need to look at the problem of pain in a comprehensive manner as there are many cross-cutting issues across the sectors managing pain that can only be addressed by a comprehensive approach.

Low back pain is the most common musculoskeletal pain in the hospital, as well as in the clinics not dedicated to pain treatment alone. Chronic nonmalignant pain is invalidating and less researched than cancer related pain. Over the past 15–20 years there has been a great amount of effort to improve the management of cancer related pain, but the need for the optimal management of nonmalignant pain remains largely unrecognized. Pain in about 70% of older patients is chronic nonmalignant pain. There are no established procedures and as a result, chronic nonmalignant pain often goes untreated. Patients with chronic nonmalignant pain need separate guidelines using a multimodality approach. Thus, the greatest need for guidelines is in the area of chronic nonmalignant pain as these patients are at the highest risk of having inadequately managed pain. Measurement is being standardized now using scales. Newer diagnostic tests are being developed for precise measurement of pain, including quantitative sensory testing and functional brain imaging.

According to some experts, in previous WHO guidelines, the use of drugs is overprescribed and overemphasized, ignoring nonpharmacological methods of pain control. In both acute and chronic phase, for adequate pain relief and prevention of the side effects of the oral morphine, the use of interventional procedures, surgical procedures, physiotherapy, and other alternative treatments (including acupuncture, herbal therapy, meditation, and faith based treatments) should be recommended. For example, in the acute phase, pharmacological management is vital and very efficient. On the other hand, in the chronic phase, pharmacological management is inefficient and may require a rehabilitative approach. Nondrug interventions need to be considered when there is no change in the pain state or when the patient has severe side effects due to the medications.

Pain management is moving towards a mechanism based approach and molecular targeted pharmacological therapy. Treatment guidelines should consider the acute and chronic phase of the pain state, and recommend the appropriate treatment considering the recent advances and evidence base. They should also indicate when a single modality of treatment is appropriate and when multiple modalities are essential.

(Source: http://www.who.int/about/en/.

Modified and annotated from WHO Normative Guidelines on Pain Management. Report of a Delphi Study to determine the need for guidelines and to identify the number and topics of guidelines that should be developed by WHO, Geneva, June 2007. Online at http://www.who.int/medicines/areas/quality_safety/delphi_study_pain_guidelines.pdf.)

Analgesics

Analgesics are drugs that relieve pain without producing loss of consciousness or reflex activity. All OTC and prescription pain medications can have side effects. Overusing medications, beyond the labeling instructions and doctor's prescription, can lead to dependency and side effects that outweigh the benefits. Since medications have an increased potential for side effects it is advisable to treat pain with conservative care such as massage and other noninvasive methods if possible. The search for an ideal analgesic continues, but it is difficult to find one that meets this definition. It should be potent so that it will afford maximum relief of pain; it should not cause dependence; it should exhibit a minimum of side effects such as constipation, hallucinations, respiratory depression, nausea, and vomiting; it should not cause tolerance; it should act promptly and over a long period with a minimum amount of sedation so that the patient is able to remain conscious and responsive; and it should be relatively inexpensive. Researchers have not yet found such a medication.

It is important to maintain a relatively steady blood level of analgesic to gain the best control of pain. However, drug absorption, metabolism, and excretion are affected by age. Dosages and frequency of administration of analgesics may have to be increased in children, especially teenagers, because many medicines are more rapidly metabolized and excreted in this age group. Conversely, an older adult may need a somewhat smaller dose of an analgesic less frequently because of slower metabolism and excretion.

Pain medication works best if used on a regular basis before the pain escalates and becomes severe. Although the smallest dose possible to control the pain is the goal of treatment, it is also important that the dose be sufficient to provide adequate relief. However, in the case of chronic pain or intractable pain, it has been found that giving analgesics to people on a scheduled basis every 3–4 hours will maintain a more constant plasma level of the drug, providing more effective analgesia. This approach can result in better control of the pain while using less of the medication. Patient controlled analgesia (PCA) has gained acceptance and allows the patient to control an interventions dose of medication, usually morphine. When initiating the PCA pump procedure, a loading dose is often given to gain rapid blood levels necessary for analgesia. The patient then receives a slow, continuous infusion from the syringe pump. Depending on the activity level and the level of analgesia needed, the patient may push a button, self-administering a small bolus of analgesic to meet the immediate need. A timing device on the pump limits the amount and frequency of the dose that can be self-administered per hour. Transdermal (patch) opioid analgesia uses fentanyl (Duragesic®) for relief of chronic pain. With long-term use of analgesics the major issues are obtaining sufficient pain control to ensure comfort, ensuring that the patient has ample rest, and enhancing the quality of life.

It is also important to implement multiple measures to manage pain in chronic conditions to keep medication use at a minimum over long periods of time. There are different types of chronic pain that will influence the medication used:

- **Intermittent pain** is episodic. Mild to moderate intermittent pain is often treated with NSAIDs, adjuvant medicines, and nondrug therapies. Moderate to severe intermittent pain may be treated with short acting opioids.
- **Persistent pain** lasts 12 or more hours every day for more than 3 months. It is usually treated with medication taken at specific times daily. Moderate to severe pain maybe treated with opioids.
- **Breakthrough pain** comes on quickly or 'breaks through' the medicine taken to control persistent pain. This type of pain can be treated with short acting medication used as needed for quick pain relief.
- **Pain flares** are short-term increases in level of pain that suddenly erupts or emerges with or without an aggravating event or activity. As with breakthrough pain this type of pain can be treated with short acting medication used as needed for quick pain relief.

Medications commonly used to treat chronic pain include the following:

Opiates

The term opiate was once used to refer to drugs derived from opium, such as heroin and morphine. It has been found that many other analgesics not related to morphine act at the same sites within the brain. It is now understood that opiate agonists or opiate antagonists are drugs that act at the same site as morphine either to stimulate analgesic effects (opiate agonists) or block the effects of opiate agonists (opiate antagonists). Another outdated term is narcotic. Originally it referred to medications that induced a stupor or sleep. With the development in recent years of analgesics that are as potent as morphine but do not have its sedative or addictive properties, the word narcotic should be abandoned in exchange for opiate agonists and opiate partial agonists.

Opiates are a group of naturally occurring semisynthetic and synthetic medications that have the capability to relieve severe pain without the loss of consciousness. Opiate analgesics are used to relieve acute or chronic, moderate to severe pain such as that associated with acute injury, postoperative pain, myocardial infarction (MI), or cancer. Opiate medications act by stimulation of the opiate receptors in the CNS resulting in analgesia, suppression of the cough reflex, respiratory depression, drowsiness, sedation, mental clouding, euphoria, nausea, and vomiting. There may also be significant effects on the cardiovascular system, and gastrointestinal (GI) and urinary tracts. Opiates make the respiratory centers less sensitive to carbon dioxide, causing respiratory depression. Opiates may produce spasms of the ureters and bladder, causing urinary retention. Continued use may cause constipation.

Opiates have the ability to produce physical dependence and are thus considered controlled substances. With continued, prolonged use opiate agonists may produce tolerance or psychological and physical dependence (addiction). Drug tolerance occurs when a patient requires increases in dosing to receive the same analgesic relief. Patients who are physically dependent on opiate agonists remain asymptomatic as long as they are able to maintain their daily opiate agonist requirement. Addiction may develop after 3–6 weeks of continual use. Addiction following the use of opiates for acute pain management is infrequent. Signs of withdrawal are restlessness, perspiration, gooseflesh, runny nose, muscular spasm and pain, hot and cold flushes, insomnia, nausea, vomiting, diarrhea, and severe sneezing; and increases in body temperature, blood pressure, and respiratory and heart rate. These symptoms reach a peak at 36–72 hours after discontinuation of the medication and disappear over the next 5–14 days. Patients do not have to undergo the symptoms of withdrawal to be treated for addiction. Patients may be treated by gradual reduction of daily opiate agonist doses. If withdrawal symptoms become severe, the patient may receive methadone. Temporary administration of tranquilizers and sedatives may aid in reducing patient anxiety and craving for the opiate agonist.

Salicylates

The salicylates are the most common analgesics used for the relief of slight to moderate pain. The most common salicylate is aspirin. The primary therapeutic outcomes expected from salicylates are reduced pain, reduced inflammation, and elimination of fever. Salicylates are the drugs of choice for symptomatic relief of discomfort, pain, inflammation, or fever associated with bacterial and viral infections, headache, muscle aches, and rheumatoid arthritis. Caution is necessary for children and adolescents using aspirin because of the potential for developing Reye's syndrome. Salicylates can be taken to relieve pain on a long-term basis without causing drug dependence. Although the mechanisms of action are not fully known, most of the activity of the salicylates comes from inhibition of prostaglandin synthesis. They inhibit the formation of prostaglandins that sensitize pain receptors to stimulation causing pain (analgesia); they inhibit the prostaglandins that produce the signs and symptoms of inflammation (e.g. redness, swelling, warmth); and they inhibit the synthesis and release of prostaglandins in the brain that cause the elevation of body temperature (antipyresis). A major benefit of salicylates is that they do not cause mental sluggishness, memory disturbances, hallucinations, euphoria, or sedation.

A unique property of aspirin, compared with other salicylates, is inhibition of platelet aggregation and enhancement of bleeding time. Because of its antiplatelet activity, aspirin is also indicated for reducing the risk of recurrent transient ischemic attacks (TIAs). Aspirin is also used to reduce the risk of MI in patients with previous MI or unstable angina pectoris.

In normal therapeutic doses, salicylates may produce GI irritation, occasional nausea, and gastric bleeding. If gastric irritation occurs, taking medication with food, milk, or large amounts of water may help. Aspirin is available in enteric coated form to reduce gastric irritation.

Salicylism is a condition that occurs with overdose. Symptoms include tinnitus (ringing in the ears), impaired hearing, dimming of vision, sweating, fever, lethargy, dizziness, mental confusion, nausea, and vomiting. This condition is reversible if medication is discontinued or dose reduced.

NSAIDs

The primary therapeutic outcomes expected from NSAIDs are reduced pain, reduced inflammation, and elimination of fever. NSAIDs are used for those who do not tolerate aspirin. The cost of NSAIDs is much higher than aspirin and there is little difference between them in effectiveness or tolerance. They are chemically unrelated to the salicylates but are prostaglandin inhibitors and share many of the same therapeutic actions and side effects of aspirin. NSAIDs act by blocking cyclooxygenase (COX-1 and COX-2). Other NSAIDS are ibuprofen, ketoprofen, and naproxen, which are available OTC to be used for the temporary relief of minor aches and pains associated with the common cold, headache, toothache, muscle aches, backaches, arthritis, and menstrual cramps, as well as to reduce fever. Side effects include gastric irritation, constipation, dizziness, and drowsiness.

In April 2005, the US Food and Drug Administration (FDA) issued a new warning about an increased risk of potentially fatal cardiovascular adverse effects (heart attack, stroke) that may be a class effect of NSAIDs. The FDA also reiterated the well described risk of serious and potentially life-threatening GI bleeding associated with NSAIDs.

If a decision is made to prescribe an NSAID for chronic use, the lowest effective dose for the shortest duration should be used. NSAIDs should not be used in patients who are immediately postoperative from coronary artery bypass graft surgery.

Miscellaneous analgesics

Acetaminophen is a synthetic nonopiate analgesic. This drug has no anti-inflammatory activity and is therefore ineffective (other than as an analgesic) in the relief of symptoms of rheumatoid arthritis or other inflammatory conditions. Brand names include Tylenol, Datril, and Tempra. The primary therapeutic outcomes expected from acetaminophen are reduced pain and fever. The mechanism of action for acetaminophen is unknown. Acetaminophen is an effective analgesic-antipyretic for fever and discomfort associated with bacterial and viral infections, headache, and conditions involving musculoskeletal pain. It can be used as a substitute if aspirin is contraindicated.

Liver toxicity and failure Overdose due to acute and chronic ingestion has risen dramatically in the past few years. Severe life-threatening hepatotoxicity has been reported in patients who either ingest 5–8 g daily for several weeks or attempt suicide by consuming large quantities at one time.

Darvon® (propoxyphene) is an effective, well tolerated synthetic opiate analgesic structurally related to methadone. It is one-third to one-half as potent as codeine. The primary therapeutic outcome expected is reduced pain. It is similar to aspirin in potency and duration of analgesic effect and used for the relief of mild to moderate pain associated with muscular spasms, premenstrual cramps, bursitis, minor surgery and trauma, headache, and labor and delivery. Greater pain relief may be attained when used in combination with aspirin or acetaminophen.

Antiseizure medications

Antiseizure medications are primarily used to reduce or control epileptic seizures, but they also help control stabbing or shooting pain from nerve damage. These drugs seem to work by quieting damaged nerves to slow or prevent uncontrolled pain signals.

Adjuvant medication

Adjuvant medication (used to increase or support) may be used to treat chronic pain that does not respond to other pain relievers and to reduce the side effects of other medications. Adjuvant drugs include muscle relaxants, antidepressants, anticonvulsants, and corticosteroids.

Individuals using analgesic medication should eat a well balanced diet high in B-complex vitamins; limit or eliminate sugar, nicotine, caffeine, and alcoholic intake; and drink 8–10, 8-ounce (250 ml) glasses of water per day to maintain normal elimination patterns. To minimize or avoid the constipating effects of opiates, increase intake of fiber and fluids. If long-term use of opiates is planned, stool softeners may be necessary.

Massage implications when medication is used

Analgesics interfere with normal feedback mechanisms and the individual may not be able to monitor when pressure and intensity levels during massage application are inappropriate. Analgesics will also interfere with assessment by reducing pain sensation.

Aspirin and similar medication are anticoagulants and anti-inflammatories as well as analgesics and present many cautions for massage application. There may be an increased tendency for tissue damage and bruising. Feedback on pain sensation is altered and massage pressure and intensity need to be carefully monitored.

Specific massage application that relies on creating mild inflammation (friction) is ineffective if the individual is taking anti-inflammatory medication. Since the application of massage methods create an inflammatory response intense and uncomfortable massage should be avoided.

Medication that affects various mood regulating neuron chemicals can be either facilitated or inhibited by massage to a small degree and can result in a typical response to the medication. Massage appears to influence the action of serotonin and dopamine, therefore careful observation of the individual's response to massage is necessary to make sure that massage is supporting and not interfering with the medication actions.

Since massage typically increases serotonin blood levels and acts as a vasodilator, the interaction of massage with medication can become a concern. Massage can also stimulate histamine release that may decrease pain threshold.

Muscle relaxant medication interferes with the neuron chemical control of muscle contractions. The normal response to massage is going to be altered since the motor tone function of muscle is affected by the medication. Caution is required to avoid overstretching tissue since protective mechanisms are inhibited.

Massage can result in lower blood pressure and combined with medication that can also lower blood pressure can result in hypotensive symptoms of dizziness, fatigue, and weakness.

If cortisone is injected to reduce inflammation in soft tissue such as bursitis do not massage in the injection site area. Massage could spread the medication and reduce effectiveness on localized tissue.

Massage may be a beneficial treatment for constipation which is a common side effect of pain medication.

TREATMENT NOT USING SURGERY OR MEDICATION

There are methods that can alter the pain experience that do not rely on invasive methods such as surgery and medication but can stimulate similar physiological pathways. The main advantage of nonmedication methods is significant reduction of side effects. These methods can be used alone but are often used as adjunctive methods so that medication use can be reduced. Many of these methods combine well with massage and will be expanded upon in future chapters. These pain reduction methods can be very empowering to the individual experiencing pain since they provide a sense of control that is initiated by the person.

Psychosocial interventions should be introduced early as part of a multimodal approach to pain management. Because of the many misconceptions regarding pain and its treatment, education about the ability to control pain effectively and correction of myths about pain should be included as part of the treatment plan.

Pain relief may result from the power of suggestion, distraction, or optimism, or from a neurochemical reaction in the brain. Similar mechanisms are activated by relaxation and behavior modification therapy, meditation, hypnosis, and biofeedback. Typically called placebo, these types of responses are valuable in pain management programs. Based on research findings described in Chapter 2, massage benefits also affect these pain control processes in the body. Let's look at these methods in a bit more depth.

Psychosocial interventions

Biofeedback
With the help of special machines, people can learn to control certain body functions such as heart rate, blood pressure, and muscle tension. Biofeedback is sometimes used to help people learn to relax.

Imagery
Imagery is using imagination to create mental pictures or situations. The way imagery relieves pain is not completely understood. Imagery can be thought of as a deliberate daydream that uses all senses – sight, touch, hearing, smell, and taste. Some people believe that imagery is a form of self-hypnosis.

Distraction
Distraction means turning attention to something other than the pain. People use this method without realizing it when they watch television or listen to the radio to 'take their minds off' a worry or their pain. Distraction may be used alone to manage mild pain or used with medicine to manage brief episodes of severe pain, such as pain related to procedures. Any activity that occupies attention can be used for distraction. Distractions can be internal, for example, such as counting, singing, praying, or repeating statements such as 'I can cope.' Distractions can be external, for example, doing crafts such as needlework, model building, or painting. Reading, going to a movie, watching television, or listening to music are also good distraction methods. Slow, rhythmic breathing can be used as distraction as well as relaxation.

Hypnosis
Hypnosis is a trance-like state of high concentration between sleeping and waking. In this relaxed state, a person becomes more receptive or open to suggestion. Hypnosis can be used to block the awareness of pain, to substitute another feeling for the pain, and to change the sensation to one that is not painful. This can be brought on by a person trained in hypnosis, often a psychologist or psychiatrist. People can easily be taught, by a hypnotherapist, to place themselves in a hypnotic state, make positive suggestions to themselves, and to leave the hypnotic state.

Exercise
Proper exercise can strengthen muscles throughout the body, improve bone strength, reduce the risk for injuries, and enhance feelings of wellbeing. Physical therapy and massage therapy can reduce pain, improve function, and prevent recurrences.

Spinal manipulation
Spinal manipulation (adjustment) can be used to relieve chronic pain caused by musculoskeletal conditions (e.g. osteoarthritis).

Acupuncture
Acupuncture, which involves inserting and manipulating fine needles under the skin at selected points in the body, may be used to relieve chronic pain. Each point controls the pain sensation of a different part of the body. When the needle is inserted, a slight ache, dull pain, tingling, or electrical sensation is felt for a few seconds. Once the needles are in place, no further discomfort should be experienced. The needles are usually left in place for between 15 and 30 minutes, depending on the condition treated. No discomfort is felt when the needles are removed. Acupuncture is now a widely accepted and proven method of pain relief. Acupuncture should be performed by a licensed acupuncturist. Patients who choose to have acupuncture for pain management should be encouraged to

report new pain problems to their health care team before seeking palliation through acupuncture.

Heat and cold

Locally applied thermal treatments (ice and heat packs) and more general applications such as baths and showers are commonly used in painful conditions and can be easily applied by the individual at home.

Heat often relieves sore muscles and is comforting. Heat produces many responses including increase in blood flow, increased pliability of collagen tissues, and increased capillary permeability supporting local circulation. Superficial heating of skin produces muscle relaxation due to decreased gamma fiber activity and results in decreased spindle excitability, thus decreasing pain and spasm.

Cold lessens pain sensations by numbing the painful area and reducing inflammation. Heat and cold can raise pain threshold significantly; ice therapy is more effective than heat. Many people with prolonged pain use only heat and have never tried cold. Some people find that cold relieves pain faster, and relief may last longer. Alternate heat and cold for added relief.

Precautions:
- Heating modalities should not be used for persons with impaired consciousness, over anesthetized areas, or where circulation is decreased.
- Do not use a heating pad on bare skin. Do not go to sleep with the heating pad turned on.

- Do not use heat over a new injury because heat can increase bleeding – wait at least 24 hours.
- Heat is contraindicated in acute rheumatoid arthritis and in acute trauma, as it may increase bleeding tendency and edema.
- Deep heating modalities (extended sauna, hot bath, extended local heat application) should not be used over active malignancies, over gonads, or over a developing fetus.
- Avoid heat or cold over skin that is fragile.
- Do not use heat or cold over any area where circulation or sensation is poor.
- Do not use heat or cold application for more than 10–15 minutes before allowing temperature to return to normal and then repeat.

Menthol and/or capsicum based rubs

Many preparations are available for pain relief. There are creams, lotions, liniments, or gels that contain menthol or capsicum. When they are rubbed into the skin, they increase blood circulation to the affected area and produce a warm (sometimes cool) soothing feeling that lasts for several hours to produce counter-irritation. The essential oil peppermint is often used for headaches and is rubbed on the temples and back of the neck.

Precautions Do not rub product near eyes, over broken skin, a skin rash, or mucous membranes (such as inside mouth, or around genitals and rectum).

KEY POINTS

Medical management of pain is an important and often necessary part of a comprehensive approach to treating pain. Pain management has made significant progress in recent years, primarily because of better understanding of the pain experience; however, there is still a great deal to do in educating patients, family, and some health care providers about appropriate pain management and the implementation of an integrated intervention approach. Pain management is part of a broader therapeutic process known as palliative care. Palliative care provides a model for control of pain and symptoms, maintenance of function, psychosocial and spiritual support for the patient, family, and health care providers. Palliative care involves a variety of health care professionals and the well trained massage therapist can be an important part of the health care team.

- Appropriate diagnosis is necessary to determine an effective treatment process. The diagnostic process includes a history, physical assessment, and special tests.

- Physician monitored or delivered treatment includes medication, surgery, manipulation, and rehabilitative exercise.
- Analgesics are drugs that relieve pain without producing loss of consciousness or reflex activity. All over-the-counter and prescription pain medications can have side effects. Overusing medications, beyond the labeling instructions and doctor's prescription, can lead to dependence and side effects that outweigh the benefits.
- While there are very effective medications available for many types of pain, there are also other treatments available that can be used instead of or in combination with drug therapies. Many of these treatments are considered to be 'complementary' in that they work with other medical care and treatment.
- The massage therapist needs to understand the types of intervention, benefits, and side effects and apply massage to support treatment.

References

Australian Pain Society 2005 Pain in residential aged care facilities: management strategies. Online at http://www.apsoc.org.au/news.php?scode=9e2c2n.

Brennan F, Cousins MJ: Pain relief as a human right, *IASP Pain Clinical Updates* XII(5) 1–4, September 2004. Online at http://www.iasp-pain.org/AM/AMTemplate.cfm?Section=Home&CONTENTID=7636&TEMPLATE=/CM/ContentDisplay.cfm.

Macintyre PE, Scott DA, Schug SA, et al: ANZCA and FPM. Acute pain management: scientific evidence, ed 3, Melbourne, 2010, ANZCA and FPM. Online at http://www.anzca.edu.au/resources/books-and-publications/Acute%20pain%20management%20-%20scientific%20evidence%20-%20third%20edition.pdf.

Merskey H, Bogduk N: IASP Task Force on Taxonomy Classification of Chronic Pain, ed 2, Seattle, 1994, IASP Press. Online at http://www.iasp-pain.org/AM/Template.cfm?Section=Pain_Definitions&Template=/CM/HTMLDisplay.cfm&ContentID=1728.

Rich BA: Ethics of opioid analgesia for chronic non-malignant pain, *IASP Pain Clinical Updates* XV(9) 1–4 December 2007. Online at http://www.iasp-pain.org/AM/Template.cfm?Section=Home&CONTENTID=7624&TEMPLATE=/CM/ContentDisplay.cfm.

Further reading

Kumar N 2007 *WHO normative guidelines on pain management, report of a Delphi study to determine the need for guidelines and to identify the number and topics of guidelines that should be developed by WHO*, Geneva. June 2007. http://www.who.int/medicines/areas/quality_safety/delphi_study_pain_guidelines.pdf

Lynch ME, Watson PCN: The pharmacotherapy of chronic pain, a review, *Pain Res Manag* 11(1):11–38, 2006.

Websites

National Institute of Neurological Disorders and Strokes: www.ninds.nih.gov/disorders/chronic_pain/detail_chronic_pain.htm#Phantom

Mayo Clinic: www.mayoclinic.com/health/chronic-pelvic-pain/ds00571/dsection=causes

Mayo Clinic: www.mayoclinic.com/health/DiseasesIndex/DiseasesIndex

American Pain Foundation: www.painfoundation.org/learn/publications/pcn/PCN09Spring.pdf

CHAPTER FIVE
Massage based outcomes and assessment

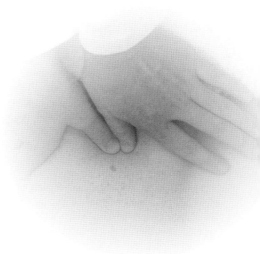

CHAPTER CONTENTS

INTRODUCTION

Assessment is a process of asking relevant questions and performing activities and then testing to answer those questions. Once a person has been able to obtain an accurate diagnosis of the pain condition and massage is recommended, then the massage therapist needs to perform assessment to determine the dysfunctional aspects that best respond to massage as well as to determine how massage will be delivered to support other treatments. Since massage has been shown through both clinical experience and scientific research to have beneficial outcomes for those with pain, it is important to be able to assess accurately for the factors that can be addressed by massage and to know when to refer the person for necessary medical treatment.

CLINICAL REASONING

Clinical reasoning is a process of decision making. It is like solving a puzzle. Using an outcome based process for massage application means that we know where we want to end up. Does the client want to relax, or is stress management the goal? Often managing general aches and pains is what the client desires. Sometimes we as massage therapists are involved in very complex care, such as sports medicine rehabilitation or cancer treatment. To solve these types of puzzles, we need to know the final outcome and we need to know where to start.

We start with a health history and physical assessment. These procedures provide a great deal of information, but information alone does not solve the puzzle; it is just one of the pieces of the puzzle. We have to use our logic and intuition to sort and categorize the pieces of information to determine both the beginning and ending points. This sorting is the beginning of a clinical reasoning process.

The middle steps in a clinical reasoning process help brainstorm and sort patterns, meanings, possible causes and interventions, as well as indications, contraindications, anticipation of unexpected results, research, and logical planning.

Finally, a treatment or care plan is developed in a clear and concise format using health care language. Implementation of this plan over a period of time should result in the predetermined outcome. Details of the implementation and what happens along the way are written down – like a journal but much more formal and precise – following the rules of health care charting.

So a clinical reason process starts with the end point – the goals. Then it returns to the beginning – data collection. The middle is when it is all sorted out, resulting in a plan or map. Implementing the plan should bring us to the destination, and along the way the process is documented.

Clinical reasoning is both a process and a set of skills. Using the clinical reasoning process teaches us how to be critical thinkers. A critical thinker considers what is important in a situation, imagines, and explores alternatives, considers ethical principles, and makes informed decisions.

Even though there is a series of steps in the various systems, there are many ways that the process can be used creatively and intuitively. Regardless of the system or the name, we need to use an active, organized, cognitive process to carefully examine our thinking and the thinking of others in the professional setting. This process involves:

- Recognizing the nature of the client's reason for massage by clearly defining the outcome. Define the problem.
- Collecting and analyzing information related to the client and their outcome for massage. Collect the facts and do research.
- Evaluating information relative to the specifics of the client and brainstorming potential interventions. Generate possibilities.
- Drawing conclusions and making decisions. Develop an intervention plan.

This process is then written down so others understand what you are doing and why you are doing it. Thinking and communicating are closely related processes. Critical thinkers use language precisely and clearly. When language is unclear and inaccurate, it reflects sloppy thinking, and that is why this content is in this chapter of the textbook.

Begin at the end – what is the outcome?

For a massage care plan to be effective it is necessary to identify the outcome of the intervention. That may seem obvious – reduce pain – but let's take a closer look.

Many things can occur when pain is modulated. Massage can be applied to support a specific outcome. Below are a few examples:

An individual may remain in pain but tolerance increases so they are able to perform daily work activities more effectively.
 Typical outcomes – increase restorative sleep, reduce pain perception with methods that create counter irritation and hyperstimulation analgesia, override pain sensation using pleasurable sensation, identify and alter impediments to normal breathing.
The cause of the pain condition – trigger point activity or myofascial shortening for example – can be altered resulting in pain reduction.
 Typical outcomes – identify and inactivate trigger points related to pain symptoms, and identify and lengthen shortened myofascial structures.
The individual's pain threshold and tolerance remain unaltered but palliative measures mask sensation temporarily or reduce the suffering.
 Typical outcomes – implement massage methods that support pain modulation such as counterirritation, hyperstimulation analgesia, override pain sensation with pleasure sensation, increase parasympathetic dominance, increase levels of pain modulating neurochemicals, and provide compassionate support.
The painful condition remains but the individual is better able to cope because they are less anxious or depressed.
 Typical outcomes – reduce sympathetic dominance and identify and alter impediments to normal breathing.

These few examples illustrate how important it is to know the desired outcome so one can alter the type of massage application. Two main categories of massage care can be identified:

1. **General full body massage.** Outcomes – support autonomic nervous system balance (Box 5.1), normalize breathing, support production and utilization of neurochemicals that alter pain (i.e. endorphins, serotonin), support restorative sleep though relaxation and overriding painful sensation with pleasurable sensation, and develop a supportive therapeutic relationship.

Box 5.1　Autonomic nervous system (ANS)

The ANS serves as the vast network of bridges between the central nervous system including cognition and emotions, the external environment, and the rest of our body. Its primary function is to maintain homeostasis. If a new stimulation (including pain) is maintained for a sufficiently long time, it becomes part of the environment within which the ANS functions causing maladaptive responses.

Sympathetic

- Fight, flight, freeze
- Increases metabolism
- Uses body's resources regardless of cost
- Gastric and pelvic response since there are more sympathetic nerves in the abdomen and pelvis than anywhere else in the body
- Can inhibit the parasympathetic system

Parasympathetic

- Restorative
- Replenishes the body
- Increases the potential energy of the system
- Feelings of safety and peace and pleasure
- Rest and relaxation

The enteric (intestinal tract) system works independently of the central nervous system and is considered a specific aspect of the ANS. This may explain why the pain response can often come from the gut.

This approach provides temporary relief, reduces suffering, and increases quality of life but does not specifically target the cause of pain. In other words – it wears off just like pain medication and therefore needs to be provided in some sort of regular schedule.

2. **Massage targeting the cause of pain.** This is more of a mechanistic approach to massage. The methods attempt to change the anatomy or physiology that is causing the pain. Muscle tension can come from postural strain, scar tissue development, movement dysfunction, breathing dysfunction, trigger point activity, fascial tone issues, and circulation issues.

This approach provides stimulus for actual long term change in the body, removing or significantly altering the reason for the pain sensation.

The real world experience of massage combines these two approaches in a unique plan for each individual. The approach that is most effective is using the general full body massage as the foundation for care with judicious and target focused use of the more mechanical methods. The mechanical methods should be integrated into the general massage session with a dominance of time spent during the session with the full body massage application.

OUTCOMES FOR MASSAGE

The use of outcome statements is essential when evaluating the achievement of the quality and appropriateness of client care. A massage outcome can be identified by asking this question:

How do you want to feel or what do you want to be able to do?

Outcome statements are goals that require a target date for completion, which can vary greatly depending on the outcome desired. Once the date is established, we evaluate the client's progress toward achievement at regular intervals. Each evaluation of progress determines if the client is responding to the massage care plan or if the plan needs to be revised or extended. In some cases, a different plan needs to be developed.

Each outcome and massage application is individualized for the particular client, and progress (or lack of) is measured both qualitatively (behavior, e.g. able to climb stairs) and quantitatively (measurement, e.g. ROM increased to 70° of flexion).

The three basic outcomes for massage are:

- pleasure and palliation
- condition management
- therapeutic change.

While the massage strokes and other modes of application are similar for all three outcomes, the intent of the massage is quite different.

ASSESSMENT

Assessment is data collection. It is the process that identifies what is currently occurring, what are the effects, and what may be causing it. Assessment provides the data that are used to develop a plan of care that identifies the specific needs of the client and how those needs will be addressed. Assessment also identifies what interventions work, what methods do not work, and what progress the client is making.

Pain plan of care

A pain plan of care (i.e. treatment plan) should include a description of the pain treatment methods that will be utilized, their frequency, treatment goals, methods that will be used to measure progress towards the stated goals, and evidence that the person with pain was involved in the development of the pain treatment plan. The care plan needs to be reviewed and revised

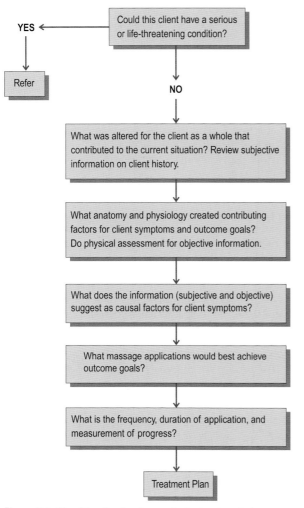

Figure 5.1 Algorithm for development of a treatment plan.

whenever significant changes in the person's condition are observed, or when the treatment methods selected have not been effective.

In order to determine the appropriate treatment for pain, several questions apply:

- What is the intensity?
- What is the location?
- What is the quality?
- Is it acute or chronic?
- What initiates or aggravates the pain?

Acute pain can generally be handled with rest, ice, elevation, compression, and anti-inflammatories and pain medications. However, chronic pain is more difficult to manage and might include any one of a combination of the treatments. Treatment is also governed by client preference and beliefs. It has been shown that people's treatment preference often is associated with a more favorable treatment outcome. Since massage therapy is highly desired by the public, it makes sense that this is a contributing factor to the success of our massages. Also, when planning treatment, you will use the above factors to assist in determining the treatment time, frequency, duration of care, and the appropriate time for a reassessment to determine the need for further care.

Outcomes measurement

Outcomes measurement involves collecting and analyzing information that is used to evaluate the efficacy of an intervention. Usually, in clinical settings, outcomes measures are collected before and after an intervention with the assumption that any changes observed in the measures can be attributed to the effects of the intervention.

Outcomes data can be used to direct treatment decisions to maximize success, and to generate pain treatment. Second, many government agencies, accreditation bodies, professional societies, and other organizations now require the collection and analysis of pain outcomes data.

Assessing pain

See Figure 5.2 for an example of a pain rating scale. The simplest measuring device, the verbal rating scale (VRS), records on paper, or a computer, what a patient reports whether there is 'no pain,' 'mild pain,' 'moderate pain,' 'severe pain,' or 'agonizing pain'.

Numerical rating scale (NRS)
This method uses a series of numbers (0–100 or 0–10).

- No pain would equal zero.
- Worst pain possible would equal the highest number on the scale.
- The patient is asked to apply a numerical value to the pain.
- This is recorded along with the date.

Using an NRS is a common and fairly accurate method for measuring the intensity of pain, but does not take account of the 'meaning' the patient gives to the pain.

Visual analogue scale (VAS)
This widely used method consists of a 10cm line drawn on paper, with marks at each end, and at each centimeter.

- The zero end of the line equals no pain at all.
- The 10cm end equals the worst pain possible.

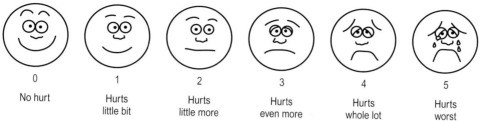

0	1	2	3	4	5
No hurt	Hurts little bit	Hurts little more	Hurts even more	Hurts whole lot	Hurts worst

Figure 5.2 Pain rating scale.

- The patient marks the line at the level of their pain.
- The VAS can be used to measure progress by comparing the pain scores over time. The VAS has been found to be accurate when used for anyone over the age of five.

Questionnaires
A variety of questionnaires exist, such as the McGill Pain Questionnaire and the Short McGill Questionnaire (and many others) (see Figs 5.3 & 5.4)

The shorter version lists a number of words that describe pain (such as throbbing, shooting, stabbing, heavy, sickening, and fearful).

Use of such questionnaires requires training so that accurate interpretation can be made of the patient's answers, therefore, apart from acknowledging that they can be very useful, the McGill (and other) questionnaires will not be discussed in this book.

There are a number of ways of getting further information, the simplest being to conduct a web search using 'McGill Questionnaire' as the key words.

Pain drawings
It can be useful for the patient to color the areas of their pain on a simple outline of the human body using a red pencil (see Fig. 5.3). The shaded or colored areas can be very useful when searching for trigger points during a massage.

The patient should write single word descriptions of the pain in different areas – throbbing, aching, etc., or a simple code can be used, for example:

xx = burning pain
!! = stabbing pain
00 = aching, and so on.

This records both the location and the nature of the person's pain, and can be compared with similar records at future visits.

A single sheet of paper can easily contain a VAS, a shortened McGill Questionnaire, as well as a series of simple questions such as those illustrated in Figure 5.4.

Pain threshold
- Applying pressure safely requires sensitivity.
- We need to be able to sense when tissue tension/ resistance is being 'met,' as we palpate, and when tension is being overcome.
- When applying pressure you may ask the patient 'Does it hurt?,' 'Does it refer?'
- To make sense of the answer it is important to have an idea of how much pressure you are using.
- The term 'pain threshold' is used to describe the least amount of pressure needed to produce a report of pain, and/or referred symptoms, when a trigger point is being compressed.
- It is important to know how much pressure is required to produce pain, and/or referred symptoms, and whether the amount of pressure being used has changed after treatment, or whether the pain threshold is different the next time the patient comes for treatment.
- It would not be very helpful to hear: 'Yes it still hurts' only because we are pressing much harder!

When testing for trigger point activity, we should be able to apply a moderate amount of force, just enough to cause no more than a sense of pressure (not pain) in normal tissues, and to be always able to apply the same amount of effort whenever we test in this way.

We should be able to apply enough pressure to produce the trigger point referral pain, and know that the same pressure, after treatment, no longer causes pain referral.

How can a person learn to apply a particular amount of pressure, and no more? It has been shown that using a simple technology (such as bathroom scales), physical therapy students can be taught to accurately produce specific degrees of pressure on request. Students are tested applying pressure to lumbar muscles. After training, using bathroom scales, the students can usually apply precise amounts of pressure on request (Keating et al 1993).

Algometer A basic algometer is a hand-held, spring-loaded, rubber-tipped, pressure measuring device

McGill Pain Questionnaire

Patient's name ______________________ Date ______________ Time __________ am/pm

PRI: S ________ (1–10) A ________ (11–15) E ________ (16) M ________ (17–20) PRI(T) ________ (1–20) PPI ________

1 FLICKERING __
QUIVERING __
PULSING __
THROBBING __
BEATING __
POUNDING __

2 JUMPING __
FLASHING __
SHOOTING __

3 PRICKING __
BORING __
DRILLING __
STABBING __
LANCINATING __

4 SHARP __
CUTTING __
LACERATING __

5 PINCHING __
PRESSING __
GNAWING __
CRAMPING __
CRUSHING __

6 TUGGING __
PULLING __
WRENCHING __

7 HOT __
BURNING __
SCALDING __
SEARING __

8 TINGLING __
ITCHY __
SMARTING __
STINGING __

9 DULL __
SORE __
HURTING __
ACHING __
HEAVY __

10 TENDER __
TAUT __
RASPING __
SPLITTING __

11 TIRING __
EXHAUSTING __

12 SICKENING __
SUFFOCATING __

13 FEARFUL __
FRIGHTFUL __
TERRIFYING __

14 PUNISHING __
GRUELLING __
CRUEL __
VICIOUS __
KILLING __

15 WRETCHED __
BLINDING __

16 ANNOYING __
TROUBLESOME __
MISERABLE __
INTENSE __
UNBEARABLE __

17 SPREADING __
RADIATING __
PENETRATING __
PIERCING __

18 TIGHT __
NUMB __
DRAWING __
SQUEEZING __
TEARING __

19 COOL __
COLD __
FREEZING __

20 NAGGING __
NAUSEATING __
AGONIZING __
DREADFUL __
TORTURING __

PPI

0 NO PAIN
1 MILD
2 DISCOMFORTING
3 DISTRESSING
4 HORRIBLE
5 EXCRUCIATING

BRIEF __ MOMENTARY __ TRANSIENT __	RHYTHMIC __ PERIODIC __ INTERMITTENT __	CONTINUOUS __ STEADY __ CONSTANT __

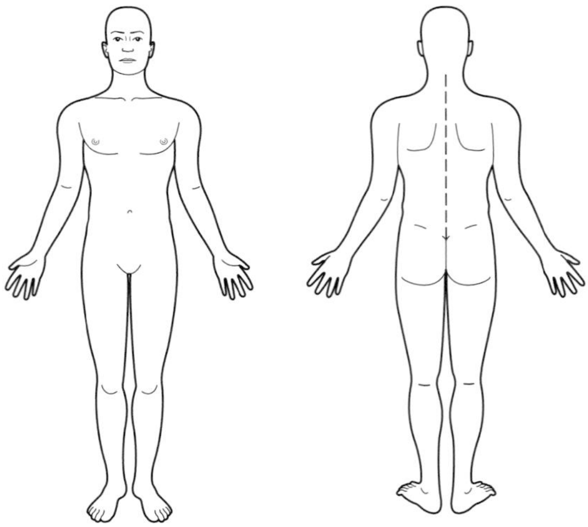

E = EXTERNAL

I = INTERNAL

COMMENTS:

(A)

Figure 5.3 A: McGill Pain Questionnaire.

that offers a means of achieving standardized pressure application.

Using an algometer, sufficient pressure to produce pain is to preselected points, at a precise 90° angle to the skin. The measurement is taken when pain is reported.

An electronic version of this type of algometer allows recording of pressures applied, however these

Short-form McGill Pain Questionnaire
Ronald Melzack

Patient's name _____   Date _____

	NONE	MILD	MODERATE	SEVERE
THROBBING	0)_____	1)_____	2)_____	3)_____
SHOOTING	0)_____	1)_____	2)_____	3)_____
STABBING	0)_____	1)_____	2)_____	3)_____
SHARP	0)_____	1)_____	2)_____	3)_____
CRAMPING	0)_____	1)_____	2)_____	3)_____
GNAWING	0)_____	1)_____	2)_____	3)_____
HOT-BURNING	0)_____	1)_____	2)_____	3)_____
ACHING	0)_____	1)_____	2)_____	3)_____
HEAVY	0)_____	1)_____	2)_____	3)_____
TENDER	0)_____	1)_____	2)_____	3)_____
SPLITTING	0)_____	1)_____	2)_____	3)_____
TIRING-EXHAUSTING	0)_____	1)_____	2)_____	3)_____
SICKENING	0)_____	1)_____	2)_____	3)_____
FEARFUL	0)_____	1)_____	2)_____	3)_____
PUNISHING-CRUEL	0)_____	1)_____	2)_____	3)_____

No pain |———————————————————————————————| Worst possible pain

PPI
0 NO PAIN   _____
1 MILD   _____
2 DISCOMFORTING   _____
3 DISTRESSING   _____
4 HORRIBLE   _____
5 EXCRUCIATING   _____

(B)

Figure 5.3 B: McGill Pain Questionnaire Continued.

forms of algometer are used independently of actual treatment, to obtain feedback from the patient, to register the pressure being used when pain levels reach tolerance, for example (see Fig. 5.5A & B).

A variety of other algometer designs exist, including a sophisticated version that is attached to the thumb or finger, with a lead running to an electronic sensor that is itself connected to a computer. This

NAME _____ DATE _____

Please tick any of the words that describes your pain under the column that describes its intensity.

	None	Mild	Moderate	Severe
Throbbing				
Shooting				
Stabbing				
Cramping				
Gnawing				
Hot-Burning				
Aching				
Heavy				
Tender				
Splitting				
Tiring-Exhausting				
Sickening				
Fearful				
Punishing-Cruel				

Your Pain is:

On Most Days ..... No Pain   Mild
                   Discomforting   Distressing
                   Horrible   Excruciating

At Its Worst .... No Pain   Mild
                   Discomforting   Distressing
                   Horrible   Excruciating

At Its Best .... No Pain   Mild
                   Discomforting   Distressing
                   Horrible   Excruciating

TODAY   No Pain   Mild
                   Discomforting   Distressing
                   Horrible   Excruciating

How many hours of the day are you in pain?   ....

How many days per week are you in pain?   ....

How many weeks per year are you in pain?   ....

What Drugs Have You Taken Today?   ....

....

Your Pain Today - Tick along scale below

No Pain [_____] **Worst Possible Pain**

PLEASE DRAW YOUR PAIN

xxx	Burning	= =	Numbness
!!	Stabbing	**	Cramping
oo	Aching	?	Other

Figure 5.4 McGill shortened Pain Questionnaire.

gives very precise readouts of the amount of pressure being applied by the finger or thumb during treatment (see Fig. 5.5C & D).

Baldry (2005) suggests that algometers should be used to measure the degree of pressure required to produce symptoms, 'before and after deactivation of a trigger point, because when treatment is successful, the pressure threshold over the trigger point increases.' If an algometer is not available, and in order to encourage only appropriate amounts of pressure being applied, it may be useful to practice simple palpation exercises.

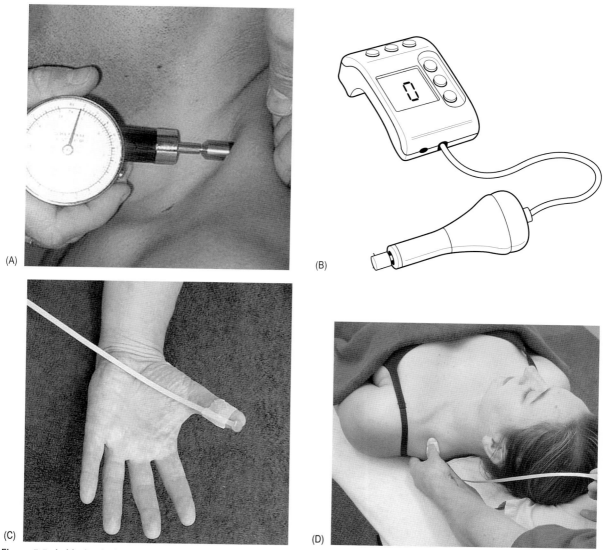

Figure 5.5 A: Mechanical pressure algometer being used to measure applied pressure. B: A version of an electronic algometer. C: Electronic algometer pressure pad attached to thumb (and to computer). D: Electronic algometer being used to evaluate pressure being applied to upper trapezius trigger point.

Performance measures Performance measures target areas of function, i.e. ability to perform. The function used for assessment can be related to daily activities such as ability to climb stairs, work functions such as ability to lift, push, or reach, or recreational activity such as gardening, golf, or knitting.

Performance measure can be more objective such as the time required to complete a task, the number of repetitions completed, or grip strength. Measurements during an assigned task are recorded before treatment and compared with performance during and after treatment.

Emotional distress

Significant pain often is accompanied or preceded by emotional distress and pain related fear. Emotional status and traits can have a significant impact on treatment outcome. Thus, comprehensive pain outcomes approaches should include methods to assess the varieties of emotional distress. There are numerous emotional distress instruments available for use and the psychologist is the most logical person to assess this area.

THE ASSESSMENT PROCESS

During assessment it is important to determine as many 'minor' signs and features of dysfunction as feasible rather than seeking one single 'cause.' The rationale for this process is that pain is usually multi-causal and massage is typically more beneficial for managing some factors more than others. By determining multiple factors involved in the condition, massage intervention can be focused to those areas best suited for massage application. Following are questions that will need to be answered:

- What's short?
- What's tight?
- What's contracted?
- What's restricted?
- What's weak?
- What's out of balance?
- What firing sequences are abnormal?
- What has happened, and/or what is the patient doing, to aggravate these changes?

- What relieves symptoms?
- And what can be done to help these changes to normalize?

Additional questions include:

- How did the injury occur?
- What activities increase or decrease the pain?
- How bad is the pain (pain scale)?
- When does the pain occur? Morning, afternoon, before, during, after activity, all the time?
- What are the characteristics of the pain?
  - Aching (impingement, swelling, inflammation),
  - Burning (nerve irritation, inflammation)
  - Sharp (acute injury).

First, massage application with stretching lengthens the short, tight areas. Coupled with therapeutic exercise, massage then stimulates the long, tight, and weak areas (Fritz 2008a).

The focus of massage intervention is to reduce the adaptive burden that is making demands on the structures related to pain symptoms and at the same time, to enhance the functional integrity of the body so that the structures and tissues involved can better handle the abuses and misuses to which they are routinely subjected.

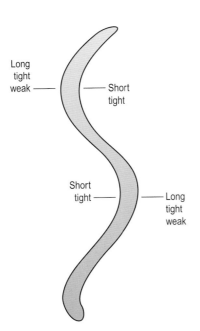

Figure 5.6 First, massage application with stretching lengthens the short, tight areas. Coupled with therapeutic exercise, massage then stimulates the long, tight, and weak areas. (From Fritz 2004.)

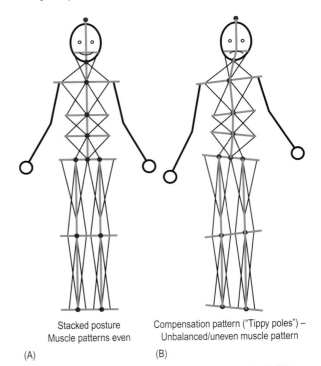

Stacked posture
Muscle patterns even

Compensation pattern ("Tippy poles") –
Unbalanced/uneven muscle pattern

(A)   (B)

Figure 5.7 Posture balance and imbalance. Stacked pole (A) versus tippy pole. B: postural influences on the body. (From Fritz 2004.)

Crossed syndrome patterns

As compensation occurs to overuse, misuse, and disuse of muscles of the head and neck, some muscles become overworked, shortened, and restricted, with others becoming inhibited and weak, and bodywide postural changes take place that have been characterized as 'crossed syndromes' (see Box 5.2.)

Among the commonest bodywide stress influences are postural patterns such as the upper and lower crossed syndromes (Janda 1982).

Trigger points are found in abundance in both postural and phasic muscles, but more abundantly in postural ones.These crossed patterns demonstrate the

imbalances that occur as antagonists become inhibited due to the overactivity of specific postural muscles. One of the main tasks in rehabilitation of pain and dysfunction is to normalize these imbalances, to release and stretch whatever is over-short and tight, and to encourage tone in those muscles that have become inhibited and weakened (Liebenson 1996).

In the upper crossed pattern we see how the deep neck flexors and the lower fixators of the shoulder (serratus anterior, lower and middle trapezius) have weakened (and possibly lengthened), while their antagonists the upper trapezius, levator scapulae, and the pectorals will have shortened and tightened.

Box 5.2 Crossed syndrome patterns

Among the commonest bodywide stress influences are postural patterns such as the upper and lower crossed syndromes (Janda 1996).

Upper crossed syndrome pattern

The upper crossed syndrome involves a round-shouldered, chin-poking, slumped posture that crowds the thorax and prevents normal breathing (Fig. 5.8).

The chest, neck, shoulder, and thoracic spine are all likely to be sites of pain and restrictions as a result.

The associated muscles, most particularly upper trapezius, levator scapulae, pectoralis major and minor, sternomastoid as well as most of the cervical and spinal muscles of the upper back, will either shorten, or weaken and lengthen (particularly deep neck flexor muscles), depending on their classification as a postural or phasic (see Box 5.3).

Lower crossed syndrome pattern

The lower crossed syndrome involves a typical 'sway-back' posture with slack abdominal and gluteal muscles, and over-tight erector spinae, quadrates lumborum, tensor fascia lata, piriformis and psoas (Fig. 5.9).

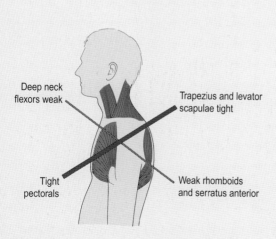

Figure 5.8 The upper crossed syndrome, as described by Janda. (From Chaitow 2001.)

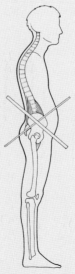

Figure 5.9 The lower crossed syndrome, as described by Janda. (From Chaitow 2001.)

Box 5.3 Different muscle types: postural (type 1) and phasic (type 2)

Janda (1986) and Lewit (1999) state that there are two basic muscle activities and types:

Type 1 – those muscles whose functions are mainly postural tend to shorten and become hypertonic when stressed, abused, or under - or overused.

Type 2 – those muscles whose functions are mainly phasic tend to hypotonia, weakening, and atrophy under conditions of under- or overuse, or abuse.

All muscles contain both type 1 and type 2 fibers. The muscles' type – postural or phasic – depends on which of the fiber types is greater.

There are other classification methods used to describe different muscle types and functions. In some the muscles are divided into 'stabilizers and mobilizers;' in others they are described as 'global' and 'local.' In this book the descriptors used by Janda and Lewit have been chosen (postural and phasic).

Postural muscles (Fig 5.10) include:

tibialis posterior
gastrocnemius-soleus
rectus femoris

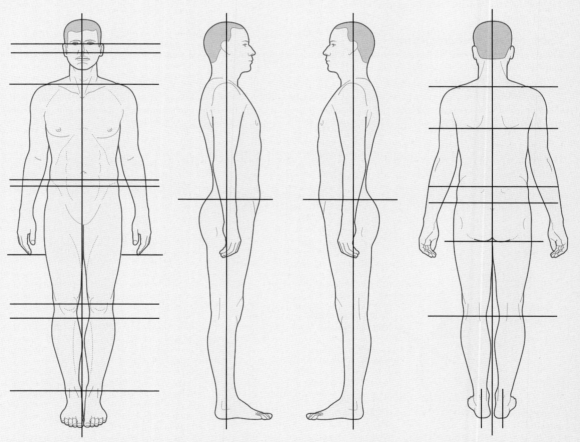

Figure 5.10 Postural evaluation recording form. This form may be photocopied for clinical or classroom use. (Adapted from NMT Center lower extremity course manual 1994.)

(Continued)

Box 5.3 (Continued)

- iliopsoas
- tensor fasciae latae
- hamstrings
- short thigh adductors
- quadratus lumborum
- piriformis
- some paravertebral muscles
- pectoralis major (and maybe minor)
- sternocleidomastoid
- upper trapezius
- levator scapulae
- flexors of the upper extremity.

A number of conditions exist in which specific patterns of dysfunction are associated with shortening of postural muscles (e.g. iliopsoas, piriformis, tensor fasciae latae, and iliotibial band). These muscles are particularly prone to development of trigger points, although trigger points are also found in phasic muscles.

Phasic muscles include:

- tibialis anterior
- the vasti
- the glutei
- abdominal muscles (mainly the recti)
- lower stabilizers of the scapulae
- some deep neck flexors
- extensors of the upper extremity.

Janda suggests that before any attempt is made to strengthen weakened muscles (using exercise), it is important for the shortened antagonists to be stretched and relaxed, removing inhibiting (weakening) influences. If a start is made exercising weakened phasic muscles this is likely to increase tone in the already tight antagonists.

Not shown in the illustration, but also short and tight, are the cervical extensor muscles, the suboccipitals, and the rotator cuff muscles of the shoulder.

In the lower crossed pattern, which is often found in conjunction with the upper crossed pattern, we find that the abdominal muscles have weakened, as have the gluteals, and at the same time psoas and erector spinae will have shortened and tightened. Not shown in the illustration, but also short and tight, are tensor fasciae latae, piriformis, quadratus lumborum, hamstrings, and latissimus dorsi.

Muscle function

Postural and phasic muscles

There are basically two types of muscles in the body – those that have as their main task stabilization, and those that have as their main task movement (Engel 1986, Woo et al 1987). These are known (in one of the many classification systems) as **postural** (also known as type 1 or 'slow twitch red') and

phasic (also known as type 2 or 'fast twitch white') (Janda 1982).

It is not within the scope of this book to provide detailed physiological descriptions of the differences between these muscle types, but it is important to know that:

- All muscles contain both types of fiber (type 1 and type 2) but the predominance of one type over the other determines the nature of that particular muscle.
- **Postural muscles** have very low stores of energy-supplying glycogen but carry high concentrations of myoglobulin and mitochondria. These fibers fatigue slowly and are mainly involved in postural and stabilizing tasks, and when stressed (overused, underused, traumatized) tend to shorten over time.
- **Phasic muscles** contract more rapidly than postural fibers, have variable but reduced resistance to fatigue, and when stressed (overused, underused, traumatized) tend to weaken, and sometimes to lengthen over time.

- Evidence exists of the potential for adaptability of muscle fibers. For example slow-twitch can convert to fast-twitch, and vice versa, depending upon the patterns of use to which they are put, and the stresses they endure (Lin 1994). An example of this involves the scalene muscles which Lewit (1999b) confirms can be classified as either a postural or a phasic muscle. If stressed (as in asthma) the scalenes will change from a phasic to become a postural muscle.
- Trigger points can form in either type of muscles in response to local situations of stress.

Postural muscles Those muscles that shorten in response to dysfunction include:

- trapezius (upper), sternocleidomastoid, levator scapulae and upper aspects of pectoralis major, in the upper trunk; and the flexors of the arms
- quadratus lumborum, erector spinae, oblique abdominals and iliopsoas, in the lower trunk
- tensor fascia lata, rectus femoris, biceps femoris, adductors (longus brevis and magnus) piriformis, hamstrings, semitendinosus, in the pelvic and lower extremity region.

Phasic muscles Those muscles that weaken in response to dysfunction (i.e. are inhibited) include:

- the paravertebral muscles (not erector spinae), scalenes, the extensors of the upper extremity, the abdominal aspects of pectoralis major
- middle and inferior aspects of trapezius; the rhomboids, serratus anterior, rectus abdominis; the internal and external obliques, gluteals, the peroneal muscles; and the extensors of the arms.

Box 5.4 is provided to chart changes (shortening) in the main postural muscles.

Palpation skills The ability of a therapist to regularly and accurately locate and identify somatic landmarks, and changes in function, lies at the heart of palpation skills.

Greenman (1996) has summarized the five objectives of palpation. You, the therapist, should be able to:

- detect abnormal tissue texture
- evaluate symmetry in the position of structures, both physically and visually
- detect and assess variations in range and quality of movement during the range, as well as the quality of the end of the range of any movement ('end feel')
- sense the position in space of yourself and the person being palpated
- detect and evaluate change, whether this is improving or worsening as time passes.

Box 5.4 NAME_____

Key:
E = Equal (circle both if both are short)
L & R are circled if left or right are short

Spinal abbreviations – indicating areas of flatness during flexion, and therefore reduced ability to flex – suggesting shortened erector spinae:

LL: low lumbar
LDJ: lumbodorsal junction
LT: low thoracic
MT: mid-thoracic
UT: upper thoracic

01. Gastrocnemius	E L R
02. Soleus	E L R
03. Medial hamstrings	E L R
04. Short adductors	E L R
05. Rectus femoris	E L R
06. Psoas	E L R
07. Hamstrings a/upper fires	E L R
b/lower fires	E L R
08. Tensor fasciae latae	E L R
09. Piriformis	E L R
10. Quadratus lumborum	E L R
11. Pectoralis major	E L R
12. Latissimus dorsi	E L R
13. Upper trapezius	E L R
14. Scalenes	E L R
15. Sternocleidomastoid	E L R
16. Levator scapulae	E L R
17. Infraspinatus	E L R
18. Subscapularis	E L R
19. Supraspinatus	E L R
20. Flexors of the arm	E L R
21. Spinal flattening	
a/seated legs straight	LL LDJ LT MT UT
b/seated legs flexed	LL LDJ LT MT UT
c/cervical spine extensors short?	Yes No

Perspectives
Stone (1999) describes palpation as the 'fifth dimension:'

Palpation allows us to interpret tissue function… a muscle feels completely different from a ligament, a bone and an organ, for example. There is a 'normal' feel to healthy tissues that is different for each tissue. This has to be learned through repeated exploration of 'normal' as the [therapist] builds his/her own vocabulary of what 'normal' is. Once someone is trained to use palpation efficiently, then finer and finer differences between tissues can be felt...one must be able to differentiate when something has changed from being 'normal' to being 'too normal'.

Maitland (2001) has commented:

In the vertebral column, it is palpation that is the most important and the most difficult skill to learn. To achieve this skill it is necessary to be able to feel, by palpation, the difference in the spinal segments – normal to abnormal; old or new; hypomobile or hypermobile – and then be able to relate the response, site, depth and relevance to a patient's symptoms (structure, source and causes). This requires an honest, self-critical attitude, and also applies to the testing of functional movements and combined physiological test movements.

Kappler (1997) explains:

The art of palpation requires discipline, time, patience and practice. To be most effective and productive, palpatory findings must be correlated with a knowledge of functional anatomy, physiology and pathophysiology. Palpation with fingers and hands provides sensory information that the brain interprets as: temperature, texture, surface humidity, elasticity, turgor, tissue tension, thickness, shape, irritability, motion. To accomplish this task, it is necessary to teach the fingers to feel, think, see, and know. One feels through the palpating fingers on the patient; one sees the structures under the palpating fingers through a visual image based on knowledge of anatomy; one thinks what is normal and abnormal, and one knows with confidence acquired with practice that what is felt is real and accurate.

ARTT

In osteopathic medicine the locality of a dysfunctional musculoskeletal area is noted as having a number of common characteristics, summarized by the acronym ARTT (sometimes rearranged as TART) (Gibbons & Tehan 2001).

This process is effectively adapted to the massage therapist. These characteristics describe the basis of osteopathic palpation, when assessing for somatic dysfunction:

- A relates to Asymmetry. This evaluates functional or structural differences when comparing one side of the body with the other.

- R relates to Range of motion. Alteration in range of motion can apply to a single joint, several joints, or a muscle. The abnormality may be either restricted or increased mobility, and includes assessment of range as well as quality of movement and 'end feel.'
- T relates to tissue Texture changes. The identification of tissue texture change is important in the diagnosis of somatic dysfunction. Palpable changes may be noted in superficial, intermediate, and deep tissues. It is important for a therapist to be able to distinguish 'normal' from 'abnormal', even if the nature of the change, or the cause(s), remain unclear.
- T relates to tissue Tenderness. Unusual levels of tissue tenderness may be evident. Pain provocation and reproduction of familiar symptoms are often used to localize somatic dysfunction such as trigger points.

Tissue 'levels' – palpation exercise

Pick (1999) has useful suggestions regarding the levels of tissue that you should be able to feel by application of pressure. He describes the different levels of tissues you should be aiming for as to be used in assessment and treatment:

- *Surface level:* This is the first contact, molding to the contours of the structure, no actual pressure. This is just touching, without any pressure at all and is used to start treatment via the skin.
- *Working level:* 'The working level...is the level at which most manipulative procedures begin. Within this level the practitioner can feel pliable counter-resistance to the applied force. The contact feels non-invasive...and is usually well within the comfort zone of the recipients.'
- *Rejection levels:* Pick suggests these levels are reached when tissue resistance is overcome, and discomfort/pain is reported. Rejection will occur at different degrees of pressure, in different areas, and in different circumstances.

So how much pressure should be used?

- When working with the skin – surface level.
- When palpating for trigger points – working level.
- When testing for pain responses, and when treating trigger points – rejection level.

When you are at this rejection level there is a feeling of the tissues pushing you away, you have to overcome the resistance to achieve a sustained compression.

Skin assessment and palpation

Changes in the skin, above areas of dysfunction ('hyperalgesic skin zones'), where the tissues may be inflamed, or where there is increased hypertonicity or spasm, or where there have been trigger point changes, are easily palpated (Bischof & Elmiger 1960, Reed & Held 1988).

- The skin adheres to the underlying fascia more efficiently, and is therefore more resistant to movements such as sliding (on underlying fascia), lifting, or rolling.
- The skin displays increased sympathetic activity, resulting in increased hydrosis (sweat). This sudomotor activity brings about a noticeable resistance during light stroking with (say) a finger. This resistance is known in clinical shorthand as 'skin drag.'
- The skin appears to be more 'compacted,' resisting effective separation, stretching, and lifting methods.
- The skin displays altered thermal qualities, allowing for some discrimination between such areas and normal surrounding tissue.

Tests

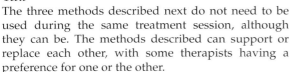

The three methods described next do not need to be used during the same treatment session, although they can be. The methods described can support or replace each other, with some therapists having a preference for one or the other.

Note: It is easier to displace skin against underlying tissue in slim individuals, with little fatty tissue. Obese individuals have a higher fat and water content subcutaneously, making displacement more difficult.

1. **Skin on fascia displacement**
   - The client/patient lies prone with the therapist standing to the side, at hip level, contacting the client/patient with both hands (or the pads of several fingers of each hand) flat against the skin bilaterally, at sacral level.
   - Only enough pressure should be used to produce adherence between the fingertips and the skin (no lubricant should be used at this stage).
   - The skin and subcutaneous tissues should be lightly moved ('slid') towards the head, simultaneously on each side, against the fascia by small pushing movements of the hands, assessing for the elastic barrier.
   - It is important that areas on both the left and right of the spine are examined at the same time.
   - The two sides should be compared for symmetry of range of movement of the skin and subcutaneous tissue, to the elastic barrier.

- The pattern of testing should be performed from inferior to superior.
- The degree of displacement possible should be symmetrical, if the deeper tissues are normal.
- It should be possible to identify local areas where the skin adherence to underlying connective tissue reveals restriction, compared with the opposite side.
- This is likely to be an area where the muscles beneath the skin being tested house active myofascial trigger points (TrPs), or tissue that is dysfunctional in some other way, or hypertonic.
- It is often possible to visualize these reflex areas as they may be characterized by being retracted or elevated, most commonly close to the lower thoracic border of the scapula and over the pelvic and gluteal areas.

2. **Skin stretching assessment** (Fig. 5.11) *Note:* At first, this method should be practiced slowly. Eventually, it should be possible to move fairly rapidly over an area that is being searched for evidence of reflex activity (or acupuncture points).
   - Choose an area to be assessed, where you identified abnormal degrees of skin on fascia adherence (see Test 1).
   - To examine the neck, shoulder, and midback region, place your two index fingers next to each other, on the skin, side by side or pointing toward each other, with no pressure at all onto the skin, just a contact touch.
   - Lightly and slowly separate your fingers, feeling the skin stretch to its 'easy' limit, to the barrier where resistance is first noted.
   - It should be possible – in normal tissue – to 'spring' the skin further apart, to its elastic limit, from that barrier.
   - Release this stretch and move both fingers 0.5 cm (between ¼ and ½ inches) to one side, or below, or above, the first test site, and repeat the assessment again, using the same direction of pull as you separate the fingers. Add a spring assessment once the barrier is reached.
   - Perform exactly the same sequence over and over again, until the entire area of tissue has been searched, ensuring that the rhythm you use is neither too slow nor too rapid. Ideally, one stretch per second should be performed.
   - When the segment of skin being stretched is not as elastic as it was on the previous stretch a potentially dysfunctional area will have been identified.
   - This should be marked with a skin pencil for future attention.

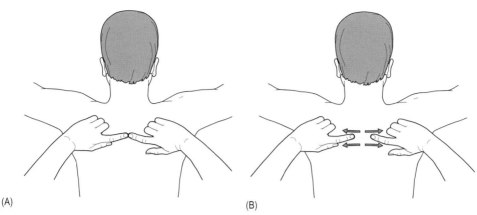

Figure 5.11 A: Fingers touch each other directly over skin to be tested – very light skin contact only. B: Pull apart to assess degree of skin elasticity – compare with neighboring skin area. (From Chaitow 1996.)

- Light digital pressure to the center of that small zone may identify a sensitive contracture which, on sustained pressure, may radiate or refer sensations to a distant site.
- If such sensations are familiar to the client/patient, the point being pressed is an active trigger point.

3. **Drag palpation assessment**
   - Sweat glands, controlled by the sympathetic nervous system, empty directly on the skin, creating increased hydrosis (sweat) presence, changing the behavior (e.g. elasticity) and 'feel' of the skin.
   - Lewit (1999b) suggests that reflex activity should be easily identified by assessing the degree of elasticity in the overlying skin, and comparing it with surrounding tissue.
   - The change in elasticity occurs at the same time as increased sweat activity. Before the days of electrical detection of acupuncture points, skilled acupuncturists could quickly identify 'active' points by palpation using this knowledge.
   - Measuring the electrical resistance of the skin can now find acupuncture points even more rapidly. Because the skin is moist, it conducts electricity more efficiently than when it is dry.

Method
- Using an extremely light touch ('skin on skin'), without any pressure, a finger or the thumb is stroked across the skin overlying areas suspected of housing dysfunctional changes (such as TrPS).

- The areas chosen are commonly those where skin-on-fascia movement (see Test 2) was reduced, compared with surrounding skin.
- When the stroking finger passes over areas where a sense of hesitation, or 'drag,' is noted, an area of increased hydrosis/sweat/sympathetic activity will have been identified.
- A degree of searching pressure, into such tissues, precisely under the area of drag, may locate a taut band of tissue, and when this is compressed a painful response is common.
- If pressure is maintained for 2–3 seconds a radiating or referred sensation (possibly pain) may be reported.
- If this sensation replicates symptoms previously noted by the client/patient, the point located is an active TrP.

Summary of skin palpation methods
- Movement of skin on fascia – resistance indicates general locality of reflexogenic activity, a 'hyperalgesic skin zone' such as a trigger point.
- Local loss of skin elasticity – refines definition of the location.
- Light stroke, seeking 'drag' sensation (increased hydrosis), offers pinpoint accuracy of location.

Therapeutic use of skin changes
1. **Releasing skin changes by stretching**
   - Return to a hyperalgesic skin zone identified by one of the tests described above. Gently stretch the skin to its elastic barrier and hold it at the elastic barrier for 10–15 seconds, without force.

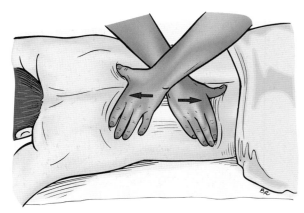

Figure 5.12 Light compressive force is applied, molding the hand to the skin. The hands are then separated without adding additional compressive force, providing a fascial stretch.

- You should feel the skin tightness gradually release so that, as you hold the elastic barrier, your fingers separate.
- If you now hold the skin in its new stretched position, at its new barrier of resistance, for a few seconds longer it should release a little more. This is, in effect, a mini-myofascial release process.
- The tissues beneath the 'released' skin will be more pliable and have improved circulation. You will have started the process of normalization.
- Larger areas, superficial to short tissues in the anterior thorax, for example, can be treated in much the same way as the small skin areas described above (Fig. 5.12).
- Using a firm contact, place the full length of the sides of both hands, from the little fingers to the wrists, onto an area of skin overlying tense muscles.
- Separate the hands slowly, stretching the skin with which they are in contact, until an elastic barrier is reached.
- After 15 seconds or so there should be a sense of lengthening as the superficial tissues release.
- If you then palpate the underlying muscles and areas of local tension you should be able to confirm that there has been a change for the better.

2. **Adding an isometric contraction**
   - If you had asked the client/patient to lightly contract the muscles under your hands for 5–7 seconds before starting the myofascial release, the tissues would probably have responded more rapidly and effectively.
   - The technique you would have been using is called muscle energy technique (MET), which is described in the next chapter.

3. **Positional release method** (Fig. 5.13).
   - Locate an area of skin that tested as 'tight' when you evaluated it, using one of the assessment tests described earlier.
   - Place two or three finger pads onto the skin and slide the skin superiorly and then inferiorly on the underlying fascia.
   - In which direction did the skin slide most easily and furthest?
   - Slide the skin in that direction and now, while holding it there, test the preference of the skin to slide medially and laterally.
   - Which of these is the 'easiest' direction?
   - Slide the tissue toward this second position of ease.
   - Now introduce a gentle clockwise and anticlockwise twist to these tissues.
   - Which way does the skin feel most comfortable as it rotates?
   - Take it in that direction, so that you are now holding the skin in three 'stacked' positions of ease.
   - Hold this for not less than 20 seconds.
   - Release the skin and retest; it should now display a far more symmetrical preference in all the directions which were previously 'tight.'
   - The underlying tissues should palpate as softer and less tense.

Findings
- You have now established that holding skin at its barrier (unforced) changes its function, as the skin releases.
- You will also have discovered that by adding a very light isometric contraction before the stretch it is even more effective.
- This last example will have shown you that moving tissues away from the barrier into ease (positional release technique) can also achieve a release. This last approach is more suitable for very painful, acute situations.

Neuromuscular technique assessment and treatment methods

The palpating hand(s) needs to uncover the locality, nature, degree, and if possible the age of dysfunctional soft tissue changes that may have taken place, and as we palpate we need to ask:

- Is this palpable change acute or chronic (or, as is often the case, an acute phase of a chronic condition)?
- If acute, is there any inflammation associated with the changes?

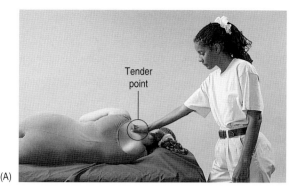

(A)

Tender
point

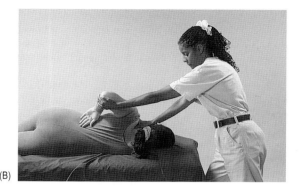

(B)

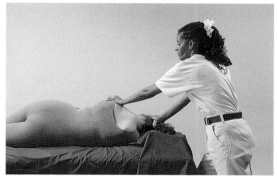

(C)

Figure 5.13 Procedure for generalized positional release. Repeat steps 1 through 5 until normal full resting length is obtained. A: Step 1. Locate the tender point. Step 2. Gently initiate the pain response with direct pressure. Remember, the sensation of pain is a guide. B: Step 3. Slowly position the body until the pain subsides. Ease off the pressure. Step 4. Wait at least 30 seconds or longer until the client feels the release. C: Step 5. Slowly reposition into the extended position.

- How do these palpable soft tissue changes relate to the client/patient's symptom pattern?
- Are these palpable changes part of a pattern of stress induced change that can be mapped and understood?
- Are these soft tissue changes painful and if so, what is the nature of that pain (constant, intermittent, sharp, dull, etc.)?
- Are these palpable changes active reflexively, and if so, are active or latent trigger points involved (that is, do they refer symptoms elsewhere, and if so, does the, client/patient recognize the pain as part of their symptom picture)?
- Are these changes present in a postural or phasic muscle group?
- Are these palpable changes the result of joint restriction ('blockage,' subluxation, lesion) or are they contributing to such dysfunction?
- In other words, we need to ask ourselves: 'What am I feeling, and what does it mean?'

Palpating for trigger points

In osteopathic medicine (works for massage as well) an acronym 'STAR' is used as a reminder of the characteristics of somatic dysfunction, such as myofascial trigger points.

STAR stands for:

- Sensitivity (or 'Tenderness') – this is the one feature that is almost always present when there is soft tissue dysfunction.
- Tissue texture change – the tissues usually 'feel' different (for example, they may be tense, fibrous, swollen, hot, cold, or have other 'differences' from normal).
- Asymmetry – there will commonly be an imbalance on one side, compared with the other, but this is not always the case.
- Range of motion reduced – muscles will probably not be able to reach their normal resting length, or joints may have a restricted range.

If two or three of these features are present this is enough to confirm that there is a problem, a dysfunction. It does not however explain why the problem exists, but is a start in the process toward understanding the patient's symptoms.

Research (Fryer 2004) has confirmed that this traditional osteopathic palpation method is valid. When tissues in the thoracic paraspinal muscles were found to be 'abnormal' (tense, dense, indurated) the same tissues (using a algometer) were also found to have a lowered pain threshold. Less pressure was needed to create pain (see Fig. 5.5) (Simons et al 1999).

While the 'tenderness,' altered texture, and range of motion characteristics, as listed in the STAR (or TART) acronym, are always true for trigger points, additional trigger point changes have been listed by Simons and colleagues (1999):

- The soft tissues housing the trigger point will demonstrate a painful limit to stretch range of motion – whether the stretching is active or passive (i.e. the patient is stretching the muscle, or you are stretching the muscle).
- In such muscles there is usually pain or discomfort when it is contracted against resistance, with no movement taking place (i.e. an isometric contraction).
- The amount of force the muscle can generate is reduced when it contains active (or latent) trigger points – it is weaker than a normal muscle.
- A palpable taut band with an exquisitely tender nodule exists, and this should be found by palpation, unless the trigger lies in very deep muscle and is not accessible.
- Pressure on the tender spot produces pain familiar to the patient, and often a pain response ('jump sign').

Treatment of trigger points is outlined and discussed in Chapter 7.

TESTS FOR MUSCLE WEAKNESS AND FIRING SEQUENCE

There are usually a number of causes and aggravating factors as well as different structures, involved in any case of head and neck pain, rather than just one cause.

The first objectives are to identify what these factors and tissues are, and to use treatment to enhance function and reduce the adaptive load.

- Functional tests (shoulder abduction, for example) demonstrate through observation and palpation which muscles are being overused, misused, or disused and are therefore likely to be shortened and/or weakened.
- These patterns of imbalance create crossed syndromes that can be recognized by observation (see Box 5.2).
- Tests for weakness indicate which muscles require toning – either through exercise, or through removal of inhibition from antagonists, or both.
- Tests for shortness indicate which muscles require releasing, relaxing, and stretching.
- Palpation methods using the STAR ingredients offer a useful way of identifying local dysfunction.
- Tests for the presence of trigger points help to locate and identify those in need of deactivation (active points).
- Breathing pattern disorders can disturb motor control of the spine and encourage postural problems with resulting pain. There are also chemical changes that occur with disordered breathing that can either cause or perpetuate pain.

By restoring balanced muscle activity, reducing tightness, increasing tone in weak structures, encouraging better breathing, and deactivating trigger points – normal function is encouraged.

Stages of care should include:

- relieving pain (massage, trigger point deactivation, ice, etc.)
- easing adaptive demands (better posture and use patterns)
- improving function (exercise, improved stability, etc.).

KEY POINTS

- It is useful to have a record of the level of a patient's pain from the first visit, so that comparisons can be made over time.
- There are a variety of ways of achieving a record, ranging from simple questions and answers, to use of various scales and questionnaires.
- The algometer (pressure gauge) is a tool that provides information as to how much pressure is needed to produce pain.
- It is possible to develop sensitive palpation skills that allow a uniform amount of pressure to be used when testing the sensitivity of a patient, or a local point.
- Various tests such as firing sequence strength/short or long assessment can be used to obtain data relevant to the condition.
- Information can and should be recorded so that progress (or no progress) can be measured accurately.

References

Baldry P: Accupuncture, trigger points and musculoskeletal pain, Edinburgh, 2005, Churchill Livingstone.

Bischof I, Elmiger G: Connective tissue massage. In Licht S, editor: Massage, manipulation and traction, New Haven, CT, 1960, Licht.

Chaitow L 1996: Palpation and assessment skills, ed2, Edinburgh, 1996, Churchill Livingstone.

Chaitow L 2001: Modern Neurological Techniques, ed 2, Edinburgh, 2001, Churchill Livingstone.

Chaitow L, DeLany J: Clinical application of neuromuscular techniques, vol 1 – the upper body, London, 2006, Churchill Livingstone.

Chaitow L, Fritz S: A massage therapist's guide to understanding, locating and treating myofascial trigger points, London, 2004, Churchill Livingstone.

Engel A, et al: Skeletal muscle types in mycology, New York, 1986, McGraw Hill.

Fritz S: Mosby's essential sciences for therapeutic massage: anatomy, physiology, biomechanics, and pathology, ed 2, St Louis, 2004, Mosby.

Fritz S: Mosby's fundamentals of therapeutic massage, ed 4, St Louis, 2008, Elsevier.

Fryer G, Hodgson L: The effect of manual pressure release on myofascial trigger points in the upper trapezius muscle, J Bodyw Mov Ther 9(4):248–255, 2005.

Fryer G, Morris T, Gibbons P: Relation between thoracic paraspinal tissues and pressure sensitivity measured by digital algometer, J Osteopath Med 7(2):64–69, 2004.

Gibbons P, Tehan P: Spinal manipulation, indications, risks and benefits, Edinburgh, 2001, Churchill Livingstone.

Greenman P: Principles of manual medicine, ed 2, Baltimore, 1996, Williams and Wilkins.

Janda V: Introduction to functional pathology of the motor system, Proceedings of VII Commonwealth and International Conference on Sport, Physiotherapy in Sport 3:39, 1982.

Kappler R: Palpatory skills. In Ward R, editor: Foundations for osteopathic medicine, Baltimore, 1997, Williams and Wilkins.

Keating J, et al: The effect of training on physical therapists ability to apply specific forces of palpation, Phys Ther 73(1):38–46, 1993.

Lewit K: Chain reactions in the locomotor system, J Ortho Med 21:52–58, 1999a.

Lewit K: Manipulation in rehabilitation of the locomotor system, ed 3, London, 1999, Butterworths.

Liebenson C: Rehabilitation of the spine, Baltimore, 1996, Williams and Wilkins.

Lin J-P: Physiological maturation of muscles in childhood, Lancet 4:1386–1389, 1994.

Maitland G: Maitland's vertebral manipulation, ed 6, Oxford, 2001, Butterworth-Heinemann.

Pick M: Cranial sutures: analysis, morphology and manipulative strategies, Seattle, 1999, Eastland Press.

Reed B, Held J: Effects of sequential connective tissue massage on autonomic nervous system of middle-aged and elderly adults, Phys Ther 68(8):1231–1234, 1988.

Simons D, Travell J, Simons L: Myofascial pain and dysfunction: the trigger point manual, vol 1: upper half of body, ed 2, Baltimore, 1999, Williams and Wilkins.

Stone C: Science in the art of osteopathy, Cheltenham, 1999, Stanley Thornes.

Woo SL-Y, et al: Injury and repair of musculoskeletal soft tissues. American Academy of Orthopedic Surgeons Symposium, Savannah, 1987.

Websites

The National Center for Complementary and Alternative Medicine: www.nccam.nih.gov

The National Pain Foundation: www.nationalpainfoundation.org

The Mayo Clinic: www.mayoclinic.com

Duke University's Center for Integrative Medicine: www.umassmed.edu/cfm/

The American Chronic Pain Association: www.theacpa.org

University of Maryland School of Medicine Center for Integrative Medicine: www.campain.umm.edu

The American Academy of Pain Management: www.aapainmanage.org

CHAPTER SIX
Outcome based massage

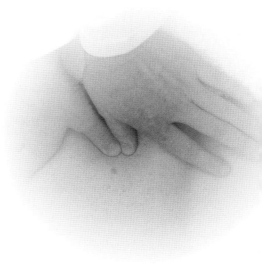

INTRODUCTION

When massage is used to address a specific problem or set of symptoms it is considered outcome based massage. Outcome based massage targets results instead of methods and modalities. Various methods can be combined to achieve outcomes. For example, if a massage therapist is working with a multidisciplinary health care team to treat pain, outcome based instructions to the massage therapist might include suggestions such as:

- increase pliability in connective tissue
- lengthen shortened muscles
- address trigger point referred pain
- reduce sympathetic arousal.

The instructions are unlikely to be 'apply Swedish massage with reflexology and energy based modalities.'

While the difference between massage modalities and massage based on outcome goals may seem simple, this is actually a major paradigm shift that the massage community continues to grapple with. Approaching therapeutic massage to address pain needs to be outcome based, since different massage modalities can be used alone, or in combination, and with other methods to achieve a positive change for those experiencing pain related problems.

To be proficient in outcome based massage it is necessary to be skilled in evaluation and clinical reasoning in order to develop appropriate treatment plans. The information in previous chapters provides the foundation upon which the massage therapist can make appropriate treatment plan decisions.

It is possible to include much of the assessment process in a general full body massage session. This is especially true of all the palpation based assessment. In fact it is desirable to consider the first few massage sessions as assessment. Then based on assessment information gathered during massage sessions, coupled with other information from a comprehensive history, tests performed outside the context of massage, together with information from other professionals involved with the patient, a specific treatment plan can be developed to achieve the outcome goals.

Because most people have preconceived ideas about what a massage should be (relaxing, passive, general) it becomes important to incorporate both assessment and treatment into the massage in such a way that the generalized full body experience of the massage is not compromised.

People enjoy massage because it feels good, and is a nurturing integrated experience. This major strength of massage needs to be preserved, not replaced. General nonspecific full body massage, based on the outcomes of decreased sympathetic arousal and maladaptive stress response, tactile pleasure sensation, and nurturing is effective in the treatment of pain symptoms even if nothing else is done (Yates 2004). It is prudent to preserve these qualities and benefits of massage when addressing specific pain conditions.

The massage therapist can increase the effectiveness of massage treatment by becoming more skilled in how to target a specific outcome, such as reducing pain and stiffness in the lumbar area. This is accomplished by incorporating assessment skills and targeted treatment methods based on that assessment information into the full body massage session. Targeted treatment such as for deactivation of trigger points can feel intense and/or uncomfortable. These methods are often better accepted and integrated by the patient when 'wrapped' in the pleasure and nurturing experience of a general massage session. Since chronic pain is so common and massage has been shown to be beneficial (see Chapter 2), the massage therapist needs to be skilled in this area.

Desired outcome

Based on many years of professional experience, client populations that often seek massage, typically experience pain symptoms.

Causal factors are typically a cumulative response to many different adaptive responses such as postural distortion, a combination of short soft tissue and long weak muscles or lax ligaments, various types of joint dysfunction especially instability, generalized stress and breathing dysfunction, repetitive strain, lack of movement – and the list goes on – as discussed in detail elsewhere in this book.

It is logical that individuals undergoing medical procedures such as surgery may develop pain secondary to the positioning required to perform the procedure, extended bed rest, reduced physical activity, anxiety, and other predisposing factors. Pain is a major treatment concern in health care in many populations including in children and adolescents, postural distortion during pregnancy, postural strain from obesity, and muscle pain as part of osteoporosis and other conditions related to aging (Yates 2004).

Management of pain and improvement in function requires lifestyle changes on the part of the client/patient and compliance with various treatment protocols. Chapter 8 also discusses lifestyle choices which could possibly be creating the symptom and be the cause of the dysfunction. Unfortunately, many people are not diligent when it comes to implementing these changes. For these individuals, pain, especially the types related to soft tissue dysfunction, can frequently be symptomatically managed with massage. This means that the massage outcome goal is pain management more so than targeting a change in the factors causing the condition. Just as pain medication will wear off, so will the effects of massage, so it may need to be more frequent in order to maintain symptom management.

Massage may actually be the treatment of choice for those people who will not be compliant with a multidisciplinary care plan for chronic pain conditions. Based on the assumption that they are not going to make behavioral changes, or do the necessary exercises, massage can replace – to some extent – the activities necessary to maintain pliability and flexibility in shortened soft tissue structures as well as reducing generalized stress. People can become discouraged, which increases the tendency to be noncompliant with self-treatment protocols. A massage twice a week can often manage the pain and dysfunction in these people by moving fluids, lengthening short structures, stimulating internal pain modulating mechanisms, and by reducing generalized motor tone by decreasing sympathetic autonomic nervous system actively, as well as by providing pleasurable relaxation experiences.

The goal is not to 'fix' the pain but to both mask it and superimpose short term beneficial changes in the tissue. If these patients are treated with medication they would take muscle relaxants, some sort of analgesic and anti-inflammatory, and possibly mood modulating drugs. All of these medications have potentially serious side effects with long-term use, making them undesirable in management of chronic pain. Massage may accomplish similar results to that achieved by medication, if applied frequently and consistently – and without the side effect problem.

Massage can replace or help reduce the dose of various medications, and it can be used indefinitely to treat the symptoms of chronic pain.

Massage has few if any side effects, is cost effective, produces at least short-term benefits and since people typically enjoy massage they tend to be compliant about attending sessions (Fritz 2008a,b). This situation is not ideal but it is not the worst-case situation either, and it is possible that eventually the patient/client will reach a point in their life when they are able and willing to be more responsible for the lifestyle and attitude changes necessary to manage pain syndromes.

DESCRIBING MASSAGE

There is an evolution taking place in massage. The shift from a modality focus (examples: Swedish massage, reflexology, deep tissue massage, Amma, Lomi Lomi) to an outcome focus requires a change in terminology and how massage application is described. One definition of massage is that it represents the manual manipulation of the soft tissues. Soft tissue manipulations create various mechanical forces which cause shifts in the form and function of the body. The physiological responses of the body to massage are not specific to the modality used, but to what is described as qualities of touch.

Qualities of touch

Massage application involves touching the body to manipulate the soft tissue, influence body fluid movement, and stimulate neuroendocrine responses.

How the physical contact is applied is considered the qualities of touch. Based on information from massage pioneer, Gertrude Beard, and current trends in therapeutic massage, the massage application can be described as follows (De Domenico & Wood 2007).

Depth of pressure

- Depth of pressure (compressive force), which is extremely important, can be light, moderate, deep, or variable.
- Most soft tissue areas of the body consist of three to five layers of tissue, including the skin; the superficial fascia; the superficial, middle, and deep layers of muscle; and the various fascial sheaths and connective tissue structures.
- Pressure should be delivered through each successive layer to reach the deeper layers without damage and discomfort to the more superficial tissues (see Fig. 6.1).
- The deeper the pressure, the broader the base of contact required on the surface of the body.
- It takes more pressure to address thick, dense tissue than delicate, thin tissue.
- Depth of pressure is important for both assessment and treatment of soft tissue dysfunctions. Soft tissue dysfunction can form in all layers of tissue.
- In order to treat various changes in soft tissue (such as a trigger point) it is necessary to be able to apply the correct level of pressure to both reach the location of the point, as well as compress the tissue to alter flow of circulation. Soft tissue dysfunctions located in surface tissue require less depth of pressure than those located in deeper muscle layers.

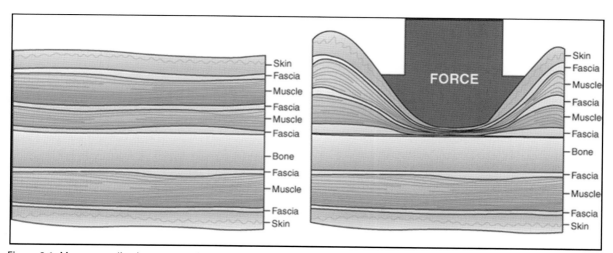

Figure 6.1 Massage applications systematically generate force through each tissue layer. This figure provides a graphic representation of force applied, which would begin with light superficial application, progressing with increased pressure to the deepest layer.

Drag

- Drag describes the amount of pull (stretch) on the tissue (tensile force).
- Drag is applicable for various types of palpation assessment for soft tissue dysfunctions, including skin drag assessment and functional technique used to identify areas of ease and bind.
- Ease is identified when tissue moves freely and easily while bind is where tissue palpates as stuck, leathery, or thick.
- Drag is also a component of connective tissue methods used to treat soft tissue dysfunctions and lymphatic drainage methods.

Direction

- Direction can move from the center of the body out (centrifugal) or in from the extremities toward the center of the body (centripetal).
- Direction can proceed from proximal to distal (or vice versa) of the muscle, following the muscle fibers, transverse to the tissue fibers, or in circular motions.
- Direction is a factor in stretching tissues containing soft tissue dysfunctions or in the methods that influence blood and lymphatic fluid movement.

Speed

- Speed is the rate that massage methods are applied.
- The speed can be fast, slow, or variable depending on the demands of the tissues being addressed and of the state of the client/patient. Faster and more energizing in situations where stimulation is called for, slower and more rhythmic where calming influences are needed.

Rhythm

- Rhythm refers to the regularity of application of the technique.
- If the method is applied at regular intervals, it is considered even, or rhythmic.
- If the method is disjointed or irregular, it is considered uneven, or arrhythmic.
- The on/off aspect of compression applied to a trigger point to encourage circulation to the area should be rhythmic, as should lymphatic drainage application.
- Jostling and shaking can be rhythmic or arrhythmic.

Frequency

- Frequency is the rate at which the method is repeated in a given time frame.

- This aspect of massage relates to how often the treatment, such as ischemic compression or gliding, is performed.
- In general, the massage practitioner repeats each method about three times before moving or switching to a different approach.
- The first application can be considered assessment, second treatment, and third post assessment.
- If the post assessment indicates remaining dysfunction, then the frequency is increased to repeat the treatment/post assessment application.

Duration

- Duration is the length of time that the method lasts, or that the manipulation stays focused on the same location.
- Typically, duration of a specific method is approximately 60 seconds although functional methods that position the tissue or joint in the ease (the way it wants to move) or bind (the way it does not want to move) can be an exception and may need to be applied for longer periods.
- Duration relates to how long compression is applied to soft tissue areas of dysfunction, or how long a stretch is held.

The following example describes how some of these qualities can be used to describe a massage modality. Myofascial/connective tissue methods may be indicated in the management and treatment of neck pain.

Massage used to influence superficial fascia can be explained as follows: Light pressure, with sustained drag, to create tension forces, stretching the tissues just past their end of range barriers (bind) in multiple directions, for a duration of 60 seconds and repeated 3 times (Fig. 6.2).

DELIVERY OF MASSAGE

- Through these varied qualities of touch, delivery of massage methods can be adapted to achieve the outcomes best suited to meet the needs of the client.
- The mode of application (e.g. gliding/effleurage, kneading/petrissage, compression) provides the most efficient way to apply the methods.
- Each method can be varied, depending on the desired outcome, by adjusting depth, drag, direction, speed, rhythm, frequency, and duration.
- In perfecting massage application, the quality of touch is as important as the method.

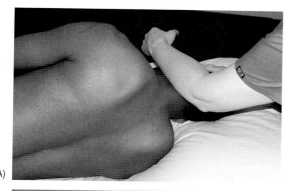

(A)

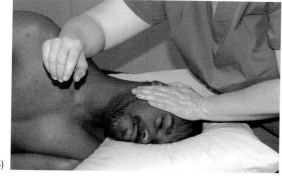

(B)

Figure 6.2 Example of using gliding method to affect fascia. (Reproduced with kind permission from Mosby's massage career development series, 2006).

- Quality of touch is altered when there is a contraindication or caution for massage.
- For example, when a person is fatigued, the duration of the application should be reduced; if a client has a fragile bone structure, the depth of pressure should be altered.

COMPONENTS OF MASSAGE METHODS

All massage methods introduce forces into the soft tissues. These forces stimulate various physiologic responses. Some massage applications are more mechanical than others; however, connective tissue and fluid dynamics are most affected by mechanical force.

Connective tissue is influenced by mechanical forces by changing its pliability, orientation, and length (Yahia et al 1993).

Fascia as a manifestation of connective tissue is a major target for massage application to achieve benefit. As a massage therapist, you will massage and therefore influence the fascia. It is impossible not to. There are adaptations to the application of massage that can target fascia. Simply, the tissue needs to be taken into the binding sensation and stretched away

from the bind/restriction and allowed to unravel – or both. In a real live body, muscles hardly ever transmit their full force directly via tendons into the skeleton as presented in textbook drawings. Instead, the force created by the muscle contraction (pulling) is distributed to the interconnected fascial network, which transmits these forces to synergistic as well as antagonistic muscles. The outcome affects the adjacent joint and regions several joints further away. For example, the muscles gluteus maximus and tensor fasciae latae both insert into the dense fascial sheet along the lateral thigh, called the iliotibial tract. This tissue is part of the fascial envelope of the thigh, called fascia lata, whose tension influences the lateral hamstrings and quadriceps, the knee joint, the whole lower leg, and the foot. Additionally, gluteus maximus has attachment to the lumbar dorsal fascia which influences the latissimus dorsi which in turn influences shoulder girdle function leading to specific muscle attachment points and isolated individual muscle function become almost obsolete. Muscles are not individual functional units, no matter how common this misconception may be.

It has been shown that fascia is densely innervated with many sensory nerve endings, including mechanoreceptors and nociceptors, which can become the source for acute myofascial pain syndromes. The fascial body is one large networking organ. Fascia is an active contractile tissue. Myofibroblasts are a unique group of smooth muscle-like fibroblasts (cells that forms connective tissue) that have a similar appearance and function regardless of the tissue type they are in. These cells are in fascia, and when they contract, they ball up, creating tautness, or a pulling force. It appears that the myofibroblasts contract very slowly in response to a superimposed force such as poor posture.

If the deep fascia contracts, it also needs to relax. By monitoring changes in muscular tension, joint position, rate of movement, pressure, and vibration, mechanoreceptors in the deep fascia are capable of initiating relaxation. Golgi tendon organs operate as a feedback mechanism by causing myofascial relaxation before the muscle force becomes so great that tendons might be torn. The implications of the research being carried on are huge for massage therapists (Liepsch 2006, Schleip et al 2006).

The movement of fluids in the body is a mechanical process – for example, the mechanical pumping of the heart.

- Forces applied to the body mimic various pumping mechanisms of the heart, arteries, veins, lymphatics, muscles, respiratory system, and digestive tract (Lederman 1997).

- Neuroendocrine stimulation occurs when forces are applied during massage that generate various shifts in physiology (Ernst & Fialka 1994).
- Massage causes the release of vasodilators, substances that then increase circulation in an area.
- Massage stimulates the relaxation response, reducing sympathetic autonomic nervous system dominance (Freeman & Lawlis 2001).
- Forces applied during massage stimulate proprioceptors, which alter motor tone in muscles (Lederman 1997).

Typically these two responses to massage (fluid dynamics and neuroendocrine) occur together, although the intent of the massage application can target one response more than the other.

Different forces

It is helpful to identify the different types of mechanical forces and to understand the ways in which mechanical forces applied during massage act therapeutically on the body. The forces created by massage are tension loading, compression loading, bending loading, shear loading, rotation or torsion loading, and combined loading.

How these forces are applied during massage becomes the mode of application. The historical/classic terms used to describe the application of these forces are effleurage, petrissage, tapotement, and so forth. These terms are gradually being replaced with the terms gliding, kneading, percussion, and oscillation. When force is applied to the tissue through the mode of application, this is called loading. The various forces listed above are outlined in more detail next.

Tension loading (Fig. 6.3)
- Tension forces (also called tensile forces) occur when two ends of a structure are pulled apart from one another.
- Tension force is created by methods such as traction, longitudinal stretching, and stroking with tissue drag.
- Tissues elongate under tension loading with the intent of lengthening shortened tissues.
- Tension loading is also effective in moving body fluids.
- Tension force is used during massage with applications that drag, glide, lengthen, and stretch tissue to elongate connective tissues and lengthen short muscles.
- Gliding and stretching make the most use of tension loading.
- The distinguishing characteristic of gliding strokes is that it is applied horizontally in relation to the tissues, generating a tensile force.

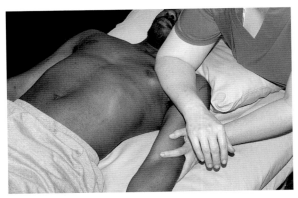

Figure 6.3 Gliding with compression.

- When applying gliding strokes, light pressure remains on the skin.
- Moderate pressure extends through the subcutaneous layer of the skin to reach muscle tissue but not so deep as to compress the tissue against the underlying bony structure.
- Moderate to heavy pressure that puts sufficient drag on the tissue mechanically affects the connective tissue and the proprioceptors (spindle cells and Golgi tendon organs) found in the muscle.
- Heavy pressure produces a distinctive compressive force of the soft tissue against the underlying or adjacent bone.
- Strokes that use moderate pressure from the fingers and toes toward the heart, following the muscle fiber direction, are excellent for mechanical and reflexive stimulation of blood flow, particularly venous return and lymphatics.
- Light to moderate pressure with short, repetitive gliding following the patterns for the lymph vessels is the basis for manual lymphatic drainage.

Note: The traditional term effleurage describes a gliding stroke.

Compression loading (Fig. 6.4)
- Compressive forces occur when two structures are pressed together.
- Compression moves down into the tissues, with varying depths of pressure adding bending and compressive forces.
- Compressive force is a component of massage application that is described as depth of pressure.
- The manipulations of compression usually penetrate the subcutaneous layer, whereas in the resting position they stay on the skin surface.
- Excess compressive force will rupture or tear muscle tissue, causing bruising and connective tissue damage. This is a concern when pressure is applied to deeper layers of tissue.

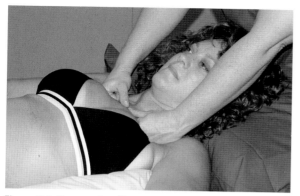

Figure 6.4 Compression. (Reproduced with kind permission from Mosby's massage career development series, 2006).

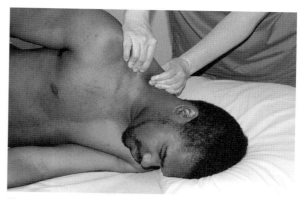

Figure 6.5 Using bend and torsion forces to stretch trigger point area. (Reproduced with kind permission from Mosby's massage career development series, 2006).

- To avoid tissue damage, the massage therapist must distribute the compressive force of massage over a broad contact area on the body. Therefore, the more compressive the force being used to either assess or treat the tissue, the broader the base of contact with the tissue should be, to prevent injury.
- Compressive force is used therapeutically to affect circulation, nerve stimulation, and connective tissue pliability.
- Compression is effective as a rhythmic pump-like method to facilitate fluid dynamics. Tissue will shorten and widen, increasing the pressure within the tissue and affecting fluid flow.
- Compression is an excellent method for enhancing circulation.
- The pressure against the capillary beds changes the pressure inside the vessels and encourages fluid exchange.
- Compression appropriately applied to arteries allows back pressure to build, and when the compression is released, it encourages increased arterial flow.
- Much of the effect of compression results from pressing tissue against the underlying bone, causing it to spread.
- Sustained compression will result in more pliable connective tissue structures and is effective in reducing tissue density and binding.
- Compression loading is a main method of trigger point treatment.

Bending loading (Fig. 6.5)
- Bending forces are a combination of compression and tension.
- One side of a structure is exposed to compressive forces while the other side is exposed to tensile forces.
- Bending occurs during many massage applications.

- Pressure is applied to the tissue, or force is applied across the fiber or across the direction of the muscles, tendons or ligaments, and fascial sheaths.
- Bending forces are excellent for direct stretching of tissue.
- Bending forces are very effective in increasing connective tissue pliability and affecting proprioceptors in the tendons and belly of the muscles.
- A variation of the application of bending force is skin rolling.
- Applying deep bending forces attempts to lift the muscular component away from the bone but skin rolling lifts only the skin from the underlying muscle layer.
- It has a warming and softening effect on the superficial fascia, causes reflexive stimulation of the spinal nerves, and is an excellent assessment method for trigger points.
- Areas of 'stuck' skin often suggest underlying problems (see Chapter 5).

Shear loading (Fig. 6.6)
- Shear forces move tissue back and forth creating a combined pattern of compression and elongation of tissue.
- Shearing is a sliding force.
- The massage method called friction uses shear force to generate physiological change by increasing connective tissue pliability and to ensure that tissue layers slide over one another instead of adhering to underlying layers, creating bind.
- Application of friction also provides pain reduction through the mechanisms of counterirritation and hyperstimulation analgesia (Yates 2004).
- Friction prevents and breaks up local adhesions in connective tissue, especially over tendons, ligaments, and scars (Gehlsen et al 1999).

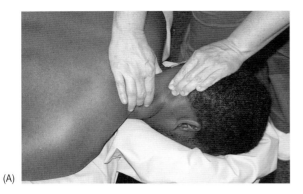

(A)

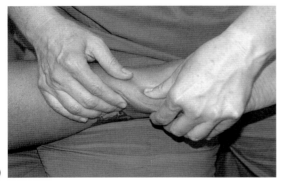

(B)

Figure 6.6 Shear. (Reproduced with kind permission from Mosby's massage career development series, 2006).

All of these outcomes of applying shear force during massage can address various factors influencing soft tissue pain. For example, the layers of soft tissue in the lumbar area can adhere to each other or develop local areas of fibrosis from microtrauma injury. The result is short inflexible tissues that can be a contributing factor in cervical, lumbar, and lower limb dysfunction. The fascia in the area can develop fibrotic changes that cause a decrease in pliability and shortening of the structure, which can also contribute to symptoms.

Trigger point referred pain patterns are aspects of pain symptoms and the tissues surrounding trigger points that have been in place a long time may be fibrotic.

Friction is beneficial in these situations as properly applied shear force loading of the tissues can create a controlled inflammatory response that stimulates a change in tissue structure.

- Friction consists of small, deep movements performed on a local area.
- The movement in friction is usually transverse to the fiber direction.
- It is generally performed for 30 sec – 10 min.
- The result of this type of friction is initiation of a small, controlled inflammatory response.

- The chemicals released during inflammation result in activation of tissue repair mechanisms together with reorganization of connective tissue.
- As the tissue responds to the friction, the therapist should gradually begin to stretch the area and increase the pressure and intensity of the method.
- The feeling for the client may be intense and typically described as burning, and if it is painful enough to produce flinching and guarding by the client, the application should be modified to a tolerable level so that the client reports the sensation as a 'good hurt.'

The recommended way to work within the client's comfort zone is to use pressure sufficient for him/her to feel the specific area, but not to feel the need to complain of pain.

The area being frictioned may be tender to the touch for 48 hours after use of the technique – the sensation should be similar to mild after-exercise soreness. Because the focus of friction is the controlled application of a small inflammatory response, heat and redness are caused by the release of histamine. Also, increased circulation results in a small amount of puffiness as more water binds with the connective tissue. The area should not bruise.

While using friction can be very beneficial there are cautions to applying excessive shear forces to tissues.

CAUTION: This method is not used during an acute illness, or soon after an injury, or close to a fresh scar, and should only be used if adaptive capacity of the client can respond to superimposed tissue trauma.

Excess friction (shearing force) may result in an inflammatory irritation that causes many soft tissue problems.

Friction will increase blood flow to an area but also cause edema from the resulting inflammation and tissue damage from the frictioning procedure. The method is best used in small localized areas of connective tissue changes and to separate layers of tissue that might have become adhered. The most common areas where more surface tissue becomes stuck to underlying structures are scars, pectoralis major muscle adhering to pectoralis minor, rectus femoris adhering to vastus intermedialis, gastrocnemius adhering to soleus, hamstring muscles adhering to each other, and overlapping areas of tendons and ligaments.

Rotation or torsion loading (Fig. 6.7)
This force type is a combined application of compression and wringing resulting in elongation of tissue along the axis of rotation. It is used where a combined effect to both fluid dynamics and connective tissue pliability is desired.

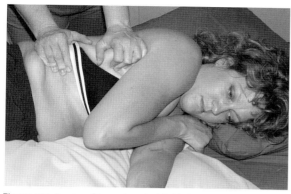

Figure 6.7 Torsion. (Reproduced with kind permission from Mosby's massage career development series, 2006).

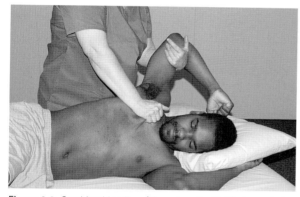

Figure 6.8 Combined loading. (Reproduced with kind permission from Mosby's massage career development series, 2006).

- Torsion forces are best thought of as twisting forces.
- Massage methods that use kneading introduce torsion forces.
- Soft tissue is lifted, rolled, and squeezed.
- Kneading soft tissue assesses changes in tissue texture and can be an aspect of treatment especially as an aspect of stretching tissue or encouraging circulation or fluid movement in soft tissue.
- Torsion force can be used therapeutically to affect connective tissue in the body.
- Changes in depth of pressure and drag determine whether the kneading manipulation is perceived by the client as superficial or deep.
- By the nature of the manipulation, the pressure and pull peak when the tissue is lifted to its maximum, and decrease at the beginning and end of the manipulation.

Note: Petrissage is another term for kneading.

Combined loading (Fig. 6.8)
- Tension – areas (stretched); bend – tissue lifted; torsion – tissue twisted.

- Combining two or more forces effectively loads tissue.
- The more forces applied to tissue, the more intense the response.
- Tension and compression underlie all the different modes of loading, therefore any form of manipulation is either tension, compression, or a combination.
- Tension is important in conditions where tissue needs to be elongated and compression where fluid flow needs to be affected.

JOINT MOVEMENT METHODS

- Joint movement is incorporated into massage for both assessment and treatment.
- Joint movement is used to position muscles in preparation for muscle energy methods and before stretching tissues.
- Joint movement also encourages fluid movement in the lymphatic, arterial, and venous circulation systems.
- Much of the pumping action that moves these fluids in the vessels results from rhythmic compression during joint movement and muscle contraction.
- The tendons, ligaments, and joint capsule are warmed from joint movement.
- This mechanical effect helps keep these tissues pliable.

Types of joint movement methods

- Joint movement involves moving the jointed areas within the physiologic limits of range of motion of the client.
- The two basic types of joint movement used during massage are active and passive. Active joint movement means that the client moves the joint by active contraction of muscle groups.
- The two variations of active joint movement are as follows:
  1. Active assisted movement, which occurs when both the client and the massage practitioner move the area.
  2. Active resistive movement, which occurs when the client actively moves the joint against a resistance provided by the massage practitioner.
- Passive joint movement occurs when the client's muscles stay relaxed and the massage practitioner moves the joint with no assistance from the client.
- Various forms of oscillation (rocking and shaking) involve passive joint movement.
- Since muscle energy techniques are focused on specific muscles or muscle groups, it is important to be able to position muscles so that the muscle attachments are either close together or in a lengthening phase with the attachments separated.

Box 6.1 Sequence of massage based on clinical reasoning to achieve specific outcomes

1. Massage application intent (outcome) determines mode of application and variation on quality of touch:
   Mode of application – influenced by type (gliding, kneading, oscillation, compression, percussion, movement, etc.)
   Quality of touch – location of application, depth of pressure (light to deep), tissue drag, rate (speed) of application, rhythm, direction, frequency (number of repetitions), and duration of application of the method.
2. Mode of application with variations in quality of touch generates mechanical forces.
3. Mechanical forces (tension, compression, bend, shear, torsion) affect tissue changes from physical loading, leading to influence on physiology.
4. Influence on physiology:
   Mechanical changes (tissue repair, connective tissue viscosity and pliability, fluid dynamics)
   Neurologic changes (stimulus response – motor system and neuromuscular, pain reflexes, mechanoreceptors)
   Psychophysiologic changes (changes in mood, pain perception, sympathetic and parasympathetic balance)
   Interplay with unknown pathways and physiology (energetic, meridians, chakras, etc.).
5. These factors contribute to development of treatment approach.
6. Treatment resulting in desired outcome.

- Joint movement is how this positioning is accomplished.
- Joint movement is effective for positioning tissues to be stretched.
- The more surface muscles are relatively easy to position during the massage using joint movement.
- The method can also be used for the smaller, deeper joints of the spine and surrounding muscles but the positioning needs to be precise and focused.
- Shortened tissue located in deep layers of muscle, or in a muscle that is difficult to lengthen by

moving the body, can be addressed with local bending, shearing, and torsion in order to lengthen and stretch the local area, and this is easy to accomplish during the course of the massage (see Box 6.1).

Regardless of the massage methods practiced, or the massage style, the previous explanations – qualities of touch, mode of application to apply mechanical forces to affect the body in various mechanical and reflexive ways, in order to achieve specific outcomes – should create a generic base for communicating and understanding massage application.

KEY POINTS

- Massage is outcome based, incorporating multiple methods to address pain.
- Outcome based massage relies on skilled evaluation and clinical reasoning in order to develop appropriate treatment plans.
- People enjoy massage because it feels good, and is a nurturing integrated experience. This major strength of massage needs to be preserved, not replaced.
- Massage application involves touching the body to manipulate the soft tissue, influence body

fluid movement, and stimulate neuroendocrine responses. How the physical contact is applied is considered the qualities of touch.
- Each method can be varied, depending on the desired outcome, by adjusting depth, drag, direction, speed, rhythm, frequency, and duration.
- Quality of touch is altered when there is a contraindication or caution for massage.
- All massage methods introduce forces into the soft tissues. These forces stimulate various physiologic responses.

References

De Domenico G, Wood E: Beard's massage, ed 4, Philadelphia, 1997, WB Saunders.

Ernst E, Fialka V: The clinical effectiveness of massage therapy – a critical review, *Forsch Komplementarmed* 1:226–232, 1994.

Freeman LW, Lawlis GF: Mosby's complementary and alternative medicine: a research-based approach, St Louis, 2001, Mosby.

Fritz S: Mosby's fundamentals of therapeutic massage, ed 4, St Louis, 2008a, Elsevier.

Fritz S: Mosby's essential sciences for therapeutic massage: anatomy, physiology, biomechanics, and pathology, ed 3, St Louis, 2008b, Elsevier.

Gehlsen G, Ganion L, Helfst R: Fibroblast responses to variation in soft tissue mobilization pressure, *Med Sci Sports Exerc* 31(4):531–535, 1999.

Lederman E: Fundamentals of manual therapy physiology, neurology, and psychology, New York, 1997, Churchill Livingstone.

Liepsch D: Fascia is able to contract in a smooth muscle-like manner and thereby influence musculoskeletal mechanics. In: Proceedings of the 5th World Congress of Biomechanics, Munich, 2006, pp 51–54.

Schleip R, Klingler W, Lehmann-Horn F: Fascia is able to contract in a smooth muscle-like manner and thereby influence musculoskeletal mechanics, *J Biomech* 39(S1):S488, 2006.

Yahia LH, Pigeon P, DesRosiers EA: Viscoelastic properties of the human lumbodorsal fascia, *J Biomed Eng* 15(5): 425–429, 1993.

Yates J: A physician's guide to therapeutic massage, ed 3, Toronto, 2004, Curties-Overzet.

CHAPTER SEVEN
Modalities working with massage

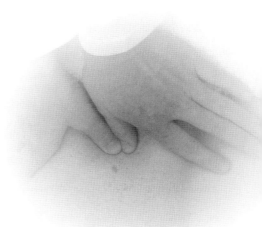

In this chapter a number of modalities that integrate well with massage therapy will be discussed. To support proficiency, practical examples and skill enhancement exercises are included. Let's begin by reviewing concepts from previous chapters.

MASSAGE AND PAIN MANAGEMENT

Let us summarize the application of massage to target pain.

The massage professional, as part of a health care team, can contribute valuable manual therapy in various pain conditions using direct tissue manipulation and reflex stimulation of the nervous system and the circulation. As a therapeutic intervention, massage may help reduce the need for pain medication, thus reducing the side effects of medication.

All medications, including over-the-counter medication available without a prescription, have some side effects. Obviously, with clients in extreme pain, the massage therapy must be monitored by a doctor or other appropriate health care professional. Most people experience pain in less severe forms occasionally throughout life. Massage may provide temporary symptomatic relief of moderate pain brought on by daily stress, replacing over-the-counter pain medications or reducing their use.

Acute pain and chronic pain are managed somewhat differently; therefore it is important to make the distinction between the two. Intervention for acute pain is less invasive and focuses on supporting a current healing process. Chronic pain is managed with either symptom relief or a more aggressive healing and rehabilitation approach that incorporates a therapeutic change process.

Various mechanisms influencing pain are affected during massage. The neurotransmitters that perpetuate and inhibit the pain response are affected by massage application. The neurochemical most recognized by clients is endorphin. Endorphins are part of a group of peptides that act as the body's internal pain modulator – like morphine. Endorphins have become recognized as part of the 'runner's high' phenomenon; actually, a combination of neurotransmitters and hormones work together to alter pain perception, both inhibiting it and/or enhancing it. Massage seems to alter the chemical interaction. The pain inhibiting chemicals influenced by massage are from the entire endorphin class, as well as serotonin, GABA, e-cannabinoids, and dopamine. The pain facilitating chemicals influenced by massage are adrenaline, noradrenaline, cortisol, and substance P. The research is still scant on just how this all works, but what we understand is sufficient for strategic development and justification of massage for pain modulation.

Massage also influences the nervous system, central and peripheral (somatic and autonomic). Application of massage that results in counterirritation and hyper-stimulation analgesia functions by activating the gate control for transmission of pain signals.

Reducing mechanical pressure on peripheral somatic nerves by increasing pliability in the tissues modulates pain sensation. Stimulation of nociceptors in tissues can be reduced by massage. Massage can inhibit the proprioceptors. When this occurs, joint function and the muscle tension–length relationship normalizes, decreasing pain. Supporting parasympathetic dominance increases pain tolerance.

Reducing hydrostatic pressure of edema using lymphatic drain application reduces interstitial fluid and decreases pressure on pain receptors. Similar results occur when tissue density is reduced, using connective tissue methods to increase ground substance pliability or to reduce adhesion from random connective tissue fiber distribution.

Pain can also occur if circulation is not appropriate. Ischemic tissues are sensitized to pain. Massage exerts a powerful influence on blood movement. Both arterial and venous circulation are involved and massage can target normalization. Massage also has a compassionate and comforting quality that can increase pain tolerance.

PAIN MANAGEMENT MASSAGE STRATEGIES

Massage application targeted to pain management incorporates the following principles:

1. General full-body application with a rhythmic and slow approach as often as feasible with 45–60 minute durations.
   Goal – Parasympathetic dominance with reduced cortisol.
2. Pressure depth is moderate to deep with compressive broad based application. No poking, frictioning, or application of pain-causing methods.
   Goal – Serotonin and GABA support and reduced substance P and adrenaline.
3. Drag is slight unless connective tissue is being targeted. Drag is targeted to lymphatic drain and skin stimulation.
   Goal – Reduce swelling and create counterirritation through skin stimulation.
4. Nodal points on the body that have a high neurovascular component are massaged with a sufficient depth of pressure to create a 'good hurt' sensation but not defensive guarding or withdrawal. These nodal points are the location of cutaneous nerves, trigger points, acupuncture points, reflexology points, etc. The foot, hands, and head, as well as along the spine, are excellent target locations.
   Goal – Gate control response, endorphin and other pain-inhibiting chemical release.
5. Direction of massage varies, but deliberately targets fluid movement.
   Goal – Improved circulation.
6. Mechanical force introduction of shear, bend, torsion, etc. are of an agitation quality to 'stir' the ground substance and not create inflammation.
   Goal – Increased tissue pliability and reduced tissue density.
7. Mechanical force application of shear, bend, and torsion is used to address adhesion or fibrosis but needs to be specifically targeted and limited in duration.
   Goal – Reduce localized nerve irritation or circulation reduction.
8. Muscle energy methods and lengthening are applied rhythmically, gently, and targeted to shortened muscles.
   Goal – Reduce nerve and proprioceptive irritation and circulation inhibition.
9. Stretching to introduce tension force is applied slowly, without pain and targeted to shortened connective tissue.
   Goal – Reduce nerve and proprioceptive irritation.
10. Massage therapists are focused, attentive, compassionate, but maintain appropriate boundaries.
    Goal – Support entrainment, bioenergy normalization, and palliative care.

Now that the massage application and mechanisms have been described, what else can be done?

Adjunctive treatment for pain: what else should you know, and what else might help?

Additional methods that modulate pain sensation and perception that can be incorporated into the massage are: simple applications of hot and cold hydrotherapy, analgesic essential oils, calming and distracting music, and so forth. Before highlighting a number of these important clinically associated topics, the fundamental process of adaptation needs to be revisited so that the role of therapeutic intervention is clearly established.

Remembering adaptation

1. *All* health problems can benefit from reducing the adaptive load(s) being coped with, i.e. all the stresses of living, whether these are:
   - biomechanical (poor posture, physically stressful activities, restricted or weakened soft tissues and joints, disturbed breathing function, etc.)
   - biochemical (allergy, toxicity, deficiency, infection, hormonal imbalance, etc.), or
   - psychosocial (anxiety, fear, depression, etc.) (see Fig. 7.1).
2. Additionally *all* health problems benefit from improved functionality – better circulation, mobility, strength, neural function, breathing, balance, posture, etc.
3. If the overall adaptive load is reduced, and/or if functions are improved, the self-regulating/self-repair systems and mechanisms of the body will be able to operate more effectively.

GENERAL ADAPTATION SEQUENCE (SEE FIG. 7.2)

Selye's (1978) General Adaptation Syndrome describes a process in which the individual, with his/her unique inherited and acquired characteristics, is responding to multiple variable or constant adaptive demands, resulting in:

- An initial *Alarm stage*. An example of this is the 'fight or flight' (sympathetic arousal) response that might be triggered by a single stress event, or by a number of minor stressors acting simultaneously (see Fig. 7.2). If the stressor(s) continue to operate the body's defense mechanisms move to what is known as:
- The *Adaptation phase* which continues until the ability of the body to compensate further is exhausted. This can be expressed as *homoeostatic exhaustion*, or a stage of *heterostasis*, where adaptation potential fails (think of a piece of elastic that has been stretched

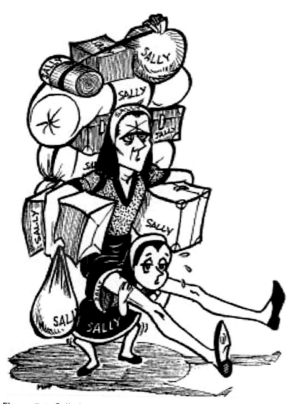

Figure 7.1 Sally has various health problems, including blinding headaches. She is carrying a number of adaptive burdens – some physical, some psychological/emotional, some biomechanical (malnourished etc.) – and she needs help to shed as many of these adaptive demands as possible, while also needing help to carry those that cannot be eliminated. This requires manual help (better tone, better posture, better breathing, fewer trigger points, etc.), as well as specific interventions to eliminate or reduce her chemical and psychological loads. (Reproduced with permission from *Journal of Bodywork and Movement Therapies* 192:107–116.)

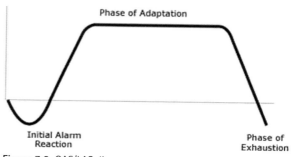

Figure 7.2 GAS/LAS diagram.

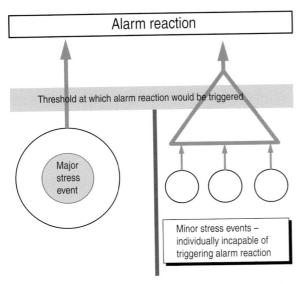

A combination of minor stresses, each incapable of triggering an alarm reaction in the general adaptation syndrome, can, when combined or sustained, produce sufficient adaptive demand to initiate that alarm. In fibromyalgia a combination of major and minor biochemical, biomechanical, and psychosocial stressors commonly seem to be simultaneously active.

Figure 7.3 Selye's alarm reaction.

until it starts to fray, and eventually snaps). When this occurs we have reached:

- The *Stage of exhaustion*. The individual's self-regulating/self-repair potentials will be exhausted (or severely strained) and chronic symptoms and frank disease follow. At this stage homoeostatic mechanisms may fail, decompensation features emerge, and treatment to slow, modify, or reverse the process is called for (Fig. 7.4).

Therapeutic choices available are limited to those that:

1. reduce the adaptive load
2. improve the ability of the body's systems to handle adaptive demands, or
3. treat symptoms.

What helps?

A wide range of methods, modalities, and techniques can be usefully employed by therapists to reduce the effects of adaptation influences, or to encourage better coping with these.

Those that will be considered, later in this chapter, in relation to pain include:

- acupuncture (what you should know about this)
- aromatherapy

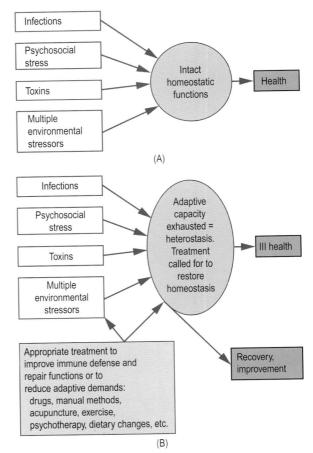

Figure 7.4 A: Homeostasis B: Heterostasis.

- emotion/stress management
- ergonomics
- high velocity manipulation (what you should know about this)
- hydrotherapy
- lifestyle changes, including nutrition, exercise posture
- respiration issues
- self-care
- soft tissue manipulation modalities.

Scope of practice limitations may not allow all massage therapists to utilize some of these methods, or to advise clients/patients specifically – for example, about nutritional influences on their symptoms; however, knowledge of these topics is important, so that at the very least, if they seem to apply in any given case, appropriate referral can be made. See Chapter 9 for more specific information on these methods.

General objectives based on an understanding of the adaptation process

There is a need:

1. To identify and help the individual to reduce the adaptive demands – the habits of life that are helping to create (or aggravate, or maintain) the dysfunctional state that allows minor trigger factors to activate the symptoms.
2. To enhance functionality by improving posture, breathing, mobility, etc.
3. To ease symptoms without adding to the person's adaptive burden, emphasizing the importance of remaining aware of just how sensitive and vulnerable this person is.
4. To support self-repair, self-regeneration, self-healing processes.
5. To take account of the whole person, the lifestyle, habits, attitudes, and behavior – and not just the symptoms.
6. To keep in mind that the more complex the condition, and/or the more sensitive and unwell the individual is, the less that should be done therapeutically at any given time.
7. To try to focus on causes – and, above all…
8. To do no harm.

INTERACTING CAUSES

Very few pain conditions arise from a single cause. Symptoms may emerge from a background involving very different stressors, interacting with the unique genetic, biomechanical, biochemical, and psychosocial characteristics of the individual.

Clearly any person whose system is coping with multiple types, levels, and degrees of compensation and adaptation, is likely to be susceptible to provocation by a variety of further stress factors – 'triggering' events or influences – including, as examples, additional physical and/or psychological strain, or a change in atmospheric pressure (such as occurs before a thunder storm), or a draft from air conditioning, or an infection, or an allergic response, or…a host of other possibilities.

- In such cases what's the real cause of pain?
- What's the real 'trigger'?
- Is the trigger really a 'cause,' or is it just a final straw?

Or, are the many interacting stresses the 'causes:' the biochemical, psychosocial, biomechanical factors to which the local area of pain (common locations are head, neck, low back, and lower limb joints) and the person as a whole, are adapting? What has led to the stage where a single additional stress (the trigger) can exacerbate the pain? Much depends on just how long adaptive stressor demands have been operating – weeks, months, years, or a lifetime? Two factors are commonly found regardless of the cause of pain. If massage can interact in these areas it is likely that pain intensity can be reduced and symptoms managed.

- Sensitization: as tissues respond to a variety of ongoing, or periodic, adaptive demands a degree of sensitization may occur, allowing minor stress factors (of any sort) to provoke pain. This feature of what is known as *central sensitization* is common to all forms of chronic pain and is discussed later in this chapter (Bendtsen et al 1996).
- Breathing pattern disorders: the common habit of upper chest breathing imposes physical stress (overuse) on the accessory breathing muscles, such as the scalenes, SCM, upper trapezius, as well as producing a wide range of biochemical and emotional changes (Fig. 7.5).

THE SENSITIZATION MODEL

Bendtsen (2000) has described a process of *central sensitization* (facilitation) that occurs after prolonged bombardment of pain messages from pain receptors (nociceptors) in myofascial tissues. At its simplest this means that nerves have become hyperirritable, so that even minor stimuli, that would previously not have caused any discomfort, can lead to a great deal of pain. This does not mean that the person is imagining the pain, but that the sensations reaching the brain are interpreted as being far stronger than would be the case under 'normal' conditions, before sensitization.

The research supporting this model demonstrates the need to understand how, over time, a reversible problem may become entrenched and chronic.

Once they exist, areas of facilitation/sensitization appear to be capable of being irritated by stressors of all types – physical, chemical, or psychological – even if there is no direct or obvious impact on the sensitized area (Bendtsen & Ashina 2000).

Example
Liem (2004) has explained a sequence that results from a degree of malocclusion, involving, as an example, the first molar on the left, where premature contact occurs on bringing the teeth together.

Figure 7.6 shows something of the chain reaction of adaptations resulting from this apparently minor structural imbalance, in which cranial modifications absorb the stresses of this dental misalignment, followed by bodywide muscular and fascial

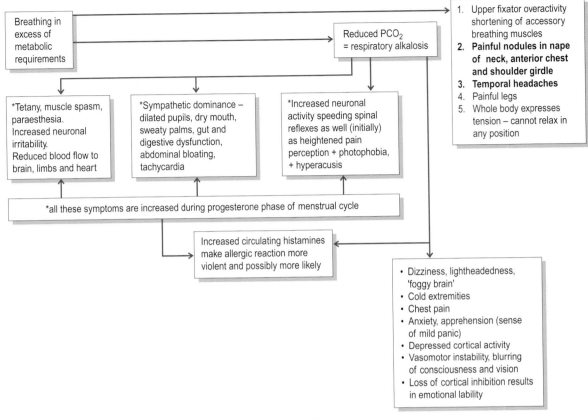

Figure 7.5 Bodywide adaptations in response to breathing pattern disorders.

adaptations that also include osseous changes involving the left clavicle, humerus, radius, ilium, patella, tibia, and foot.

This individual might therefore display a range of symptoms involving the foot, knee, pelvis, spine, neck, and/or head. Pain is likely to occur in multiple areas which can change over time as the adaptation continues. This is how a multitude of different pain symptoms can occur from one cause. If the initial adaptation was in the cranial area then the individual may experience headache. Over time the headaches may diminish but now the person has shoulder issues. Then months or years later the low back is stiff and painful and so on until there is little adaptive capacity left. Treatment of the areas of adaptation might offer short-term relief to such symptoms, however until the primary area of imbalance was addressed – the malocclusion – results would almost certainly be short-term.

Janda's example of adaptation and facial pain

Janda (1982) describes a typical postural pattern, in an individual with TMJ problems, involving changes in upper trapezius, levator scapulae, scalenii, sternocleidomastoid, suprahyoid, lateral and medial pterygoid, masseter, and temporalis muscles. In this pattern (described below) all these muscles will show a tendency to tighten and/or to develop tendencies to spasm, tenderness, and the evolution of trigger points.

The postural pattern associated with TMJ dysfunction might therefore involve:

1. hyperextension of the knees
2. increased anterior tilt of the pelvis
3. flexion of the hips
4. lumbar hyperlordosis
5. rounded shoulders and winged (rotated and abducted) scapulae
6. cervical hyperlordosis
7. compensatory overactivity of upper trapezius and levator scapulae
8. forward head position resulting in opening of the mouth and retraction of the mandible
9. intervertebral joint stress in the cervical spine
10. …and almost certainly pain.

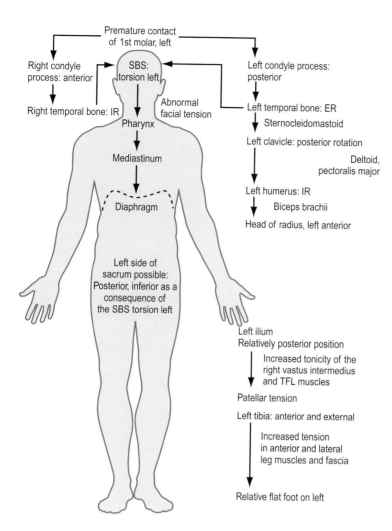

Figure 7.6 Bodywide adaptations in response to a left first molar malocclusion.

The message that can be drawn from these examples is that dysfunction patterns first need to be identified before they can be assessed for the role they might be playing in the person's pain and restriction conditions, and certainly before these can be successfully and appropriately treated.

Additionally, general full body massage that does not overtask the adaptive process is the intervention of choice when these adaptive patterns predominate. Initially (and maybe never) it is unlikely that we will know what is causing what. Where the current pain is located is likely not the causal factor of the pain but instead related to the adaptive response. We must realize that adaptation is important for function in the midst of the onslaught of life. The adaption that has occurred has been the best the body could do. Without this appreciation, the massage therapist may inadvertently unsettle a productive compensation pattern and the client

ends up in more pain. The lesson is to progress slowly and rely on the massage approach as presented in this text. As the massage continues for the individual it is imperative to gather information so that the general massage can be refined to best assist in pain management. Ongoing assessment needs to identify:

What's short? What's tight? What's weak? What's loose? What's affecting neighboring structures negatively? What's causing these changes, and what can be done about it without aggravating the situation?

What's to be done?

In any given case your role is to try to identify what can be done to help ease the current pain symptom (see previous chapters, and also Box 7.1), as well as what might be done, or what the person might do, to reduce the likelihood of further symptomatic episodes.

Box 7.1 Soft tissue modalities in a clinical management sequence

1. Identify local and general imbalances that may be contributing to the symptoms being presented (posture, patterns of use, local dysfunction).
2. Identify, relax, and stretch overactive, tight muscles, using massage and possibly muscle energy techniques (MET), positional release techniques (PRT), myofascial release techniques (MRT and others).
3. Mobilize restricted joints (possibly using MET, PRT).
4. Facilitate and strengthen weak muscles.
5. Reeducate (exercises, training, etc.) movement patterns, posture, and/or breathing function.

This sequence is based on sound biomechanical principles (Jull & Janda 1987, Lewit 1999) and serves as a useful basis for care and rehabilitation of the patient with musculoskeletal problems that may be contributing to pain. A variety of soft tissue normalization methods can be incorporated into this model (Greenman 1989, DiGiovanna 1991).

Box 7.2 Treatment as another form of stress

It is important that we remember that all forms of therapy, manual or otherwise, involving anything from the insertion of an acupuncture needle to modification of lifestyle or diet, to the taking of supplements or botanical substances, or application of manual techniques, demand a response from the systems or the tissues of the body. Treatments of all sorts – when appropriately applied – are therefore forms of what can accurately be termed 'therapeutic stress' (Selye 1978).

The objective should always be to use the least invasive, most appropriate form of *therapeutic stress* to achieve positive homoeostatic responses, ideally involving the least possible demand for additional adaptation – i.e. side effects.

In these examples, using a biomechanical model of care, incorporating massage and appropriate soft tissue modalities (see Box 7.1) and rehabilitation strategies (posture, breathing, etc.) should certainly help to alter/improve the soft tissue status, enhance circulation and lymphatic drainage, and, if appropriate, assist in the deactivating of trigger points that may be contributing to pain.

A broader model of care

The biomechanical model outlined in Box 7.1 is one way of managing such problems. Other proposed models for effective care of musculoskeletal dysfunction incorporate somatic, as well as behavioral features. For example, Langevin & Sherman (2006) have described a model in which a broader therapeutic approach to musculoskeletal dysfunction in general can be understood.

This is an 'integrative mechanistic' model that addresses both behavioral and structural aspects, as well as pain psychology, postural control, and neuroplasticity.

This model emphasizes the need, in many instances, for multidisciplinary treatment protocols, possibly including direct biomechanical/manual approaches including massage, movement reeducation, psychosocial interventions, and where necessary, pharmacological and/or nutritional treatment methods and modalities that meet the particular needs of the individual.

In this way long-term preventive approaches might also include:

- Enhanced standing, sitting and sleep postures.
- Greater care over work and leisure activity postures and positions (ergonomics); for example, consider the often prolonged periods of distorted or strained positioning involved in people working in dentistry, hairdressing, construction, massage, house-painting, automobile repair, plumbing, gardening, nursing, home-making, running, jumping, throwing, climbing, etc. Consider also that in such situations repetitive, and/or prolonged, stresses may be being loaded onto already compromised tissues, which may have become shortened and/or weakened, fibrotic, indurated, or in some other way dysfunctional, long before current stress patterns were imposed.
- Breathing rehabilitation strategies.
- Improved sleep patterns.
- Stress management (see Box 7.2), including learning relaxation techniques.
- Counseling or psychotherapy, if appropriate.
- Mobilization of restricted spinal structures and joints of the limbs – including self-help measures (see below).
- Stretching shortened associated musculature – including self-help measures (see below).
- Improved nutrition and/or detoxification.

THE MODALITIES

A number of modalities that integrate well with massage therapy will be discussed, together with some practical examples and skill enhancement exercises.

The methods that will be outlined in this way include:

1. Neuromuscular technique
2. Muscle energy technique
3. Positional release technique
4. Integrated neuromuscular inhibition (for trigger point deactivation)
5. Spray-and-stretch chilling methods
6. Rehabilitation exercise methods.

NEUROMUSCULAR TECHNIQUE ASSESSMENT AND TREATMENT METHODS

The palpating hand(s) needs to uncover the locality, nature, degree, and, if possible, the age of dysfunctional soft tissue changes that may have taken place, and as we palpate we need to ask:

- Is this palpable change acute or chronic (or, as is often the case, an acute phase of a chronic condition)?
- If acute, is there any inflammation associated with the changes?
- How do these palpable soft tissue changes relate to the client/patient's symptom pattern?
- Are these palpable changes part of a pattern of stress induced change that can be mapped and understood?
- Are these soft tissue changes painful and if so, what is the nature of that pain (constant, intermittent, sharp, dull, etc.)?
- Are these palpable changes active reflexively, and if so, are active or latent trigger points involved (that is, do they refer symptoms elsewhere, and if so, does the client/patient recognize the pain as part of their symptom picture)?
- Are these changes present in a postural or phasic muscle group?
- Are these palpable changes the result of joint restriction ('blockage,' subluxation, lesion) or are they contributing to such dysfunction?
- In other words, we need to ask ourselves 'What am I feeling, and what does it mean?'

Neuromuscular technique (NMT) evolved in Europe in the 1930s as a blend of traditional Ayurvedic (Indian) massage techniques and soft tissue methods derived from other sources. Stanley Lief DC and his cousin, Boris Chaitow ND DO, developed the techniques now known as NMT into an excellent and economical diagnostic (and therapeutic) tool (Youngs 1962, Chaitow 2003a). There is also an American version of NMT that emerged from the work of chiropractor Raymond Nimmo (Cohen & Gibbons 1998).

Trigger points

The major sites of trigger points are often close to the origins and insertions of muscles and this is where NMT probes for information more effectively than most other systems.

Lief (Chaitow 2003a) advocated that the same sequence of contacts be followed at each treatment session, whether assessing or treating, the difference between these modes (assessment and treatment) being merely one of repetition of the strokes, with a degree of added pressure when treating.

Lief's recommendation did not, however, mean that the same treatment was given each time, for the essence of NMT is that the pressure applied, both in diagnosis and in therapy, is variable, and that this variability is determined by the changes located in the tissues themselves.

Basics of NMT

- A light lubricant is always used in NMT, to avoid skin drag.
- The main contact is made with the tip of the thumb(s), more precisely the medial aspect of the tip.
- In some regions the tip of the index or middle finger is used instead as this allows easier insertion between the ribs for assessment (or treatment) of, for example, intercostal musculature.

Neuromuscular thumb technique
The therapist uses the medial tip (ideally) of the thumb to sequentially 'meet and match' tissue density/tension and to insinuate the digit through the tissues seeking local dysfunction (Fig. 7.7).

Neuromuscular finger technique
The therapist utilizes the index or middle finger, supported by a neighboring digit (or two), to palpate and assess the tissues between the ribs for local dysfunction. This contact is used instead of the thumb if it is unable to maintain the required pressure (Fig. 7.8).

Posture and positioning

- The therapist's posture and positioning are particularly important when applying NMT, as the correct application of forces dramatically reduces the energy expended and the time taken to perform the assessment/treatment.
- The examination table should be at a height which allows the therapist to stand erect, legs separated

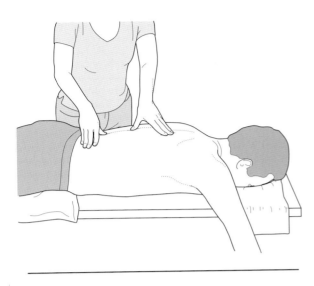

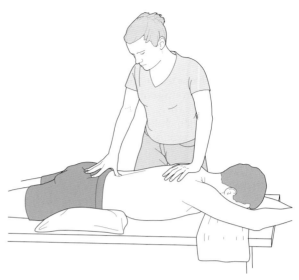

Figure 7.9 Neuromuscular technique (NMT) practioners posture should ensure a straight treating arm for ease of transmission of body weight, as well as leg positions that allow for easy transfer of weight and center of gravity. These postures assist in reducing energy expenditure and ease spinal stress. (From Chaitow 2003a.)

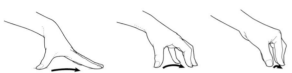

Figure 7.7 Neuromuscular (NMT) thumb technique. (From Chaitow 2003a.)

The NMT thumb stroke

- It is important that the fingers of the assessing/treating hand act as a fulcrum and that they lie at the front of the contact, allowing the stroke made by the thumb to run across the palm of the hand, toward the ring or small finger as the stroke progresses (Fig. 7.7).
- The finger/fulcrum remains stationary as the thumb draws intelligently toward it, across the palm. This is quite different from a usual massage stroke, in which the whole hand moves. Here the hand is stationary and only the thumb moves.
- Each stroke, whether it be diagnostic or therapeutic, extends for approximately 4–5 cm before the thumb ceases its motion, at which time the fulcrum/fingers can be moved further ahead in the direction the thumb needs to travel.
- The thumb stroke then continues, feeling and searching through the tissues.
- Another vital ingredient, indeed the very essence of the thumb contact, is its application of variable pressure (diagnostic pressure is in ounces or grams initially) which allows it to 'insinuate' and tease its way through whatever fibrous, indurated, or contracted structures it meets.
- A degree of vibrational contact, as well as the variable pressure, allows the stroke and the contact to

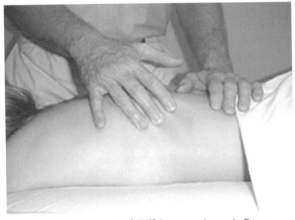

Figure 7.8 Neuromuscular (NMT) intercostal muscle finger technique. (From Chaitow 2003a.)

for ease of weight transference, with the assessing arm straight at the elbow. This allows the therapist's body weight to be transferred down the extended arm through the thumb, imparting any degree of force required, from extremely light to quite substantial, simply by leaning on the arm (Fig. 7.9).

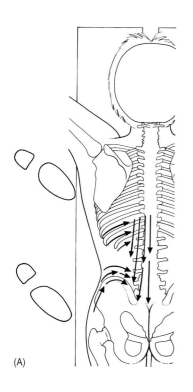
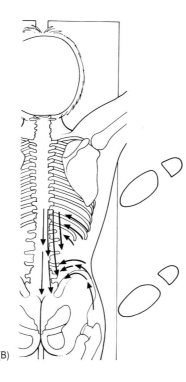

(A)   (B)

Figure 7.10 Sixth positions of suggested sequence of applications of neuromuscular technique (NMT). (From Chaitow 2003a.)

have an 'intelligent' feel and seldom risk traumatizing or bruising tissues, even when heavy pressure is used.

Patterns: NMT maps

The pattern of strokes which Lief and Chaitow evolved allows maximum access to potential dysfunction in the shortest time and with least demand for altered position and wasted effort.

These strokes are applied to the low back area with the suggested therapist foot positions shown in Figures 7.10 and 7.11.

Application of NMT

- Diagnostic assessment involves one superficial and one moderately deep contact only.
- If treatment is decided on at that time then several more strokes, applied from varying angles, would be used to relax the structures, to stretch them, to inhibit contraction, or to deal with trigger points discovered during the examination phase.
- When assessing (or treating) joint dysfunction, it is suggested that all the muscles associated with a joint receive NMT attention to origins and insertions, and that the bellies of the muscles be searched for evidence of trigger points and other dysfunctions (fibrosis, contractions, etc.).
- A full spinal NMT assessment can be accomplished in approximately 15 min with ease, once the method is mastered.
- However, a diagnostic evaluation of a localized region, e.g. covering the area above and below the crest of the pelvis, accompanied by other diagnostic and assessment modalities and methods, may be all that is necessary.
- With effective use of NMT, not only would localized, discrete 'points' be discovered, but also patterns of stress bands, altered soft tissue mechanics, contractions, and shortenings.

NMT exercises: finger and thumb strokes

- Apply a light lubricant, position yourself (Figs 7.9 & 7.10), and place your treating hand with your fingers acting as a fulcrum, and the thumb (medial tip) feeling through the tissues, slowly and with variable pressure.
- Practice this, in no particular sequence of strokes, until the mechanics of the body-arm-hand-thumb positions are comfortable and require no thought.

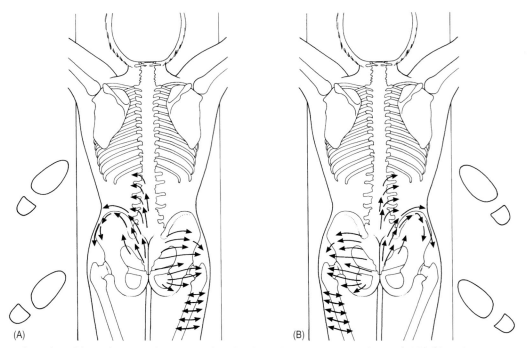

Figure 7.11 Seventh positions of suggested sequence of applications of neuromuscular technique (NMT). (From Chaitow 2003a.)

- Pay attention to varying the pressure, to *meeting and matching tension in the tissues*, and to using body weight, transferred through a straight arm, to increase pressure when needed.
- Also practice the use of the finger stroke, especially on curved areas, by drawing the slightly hooked and supported (by one of its neighboring digits) finger toward yourself, in a slow, deliberate, searching manner.
- Follow the strokes precisely as illustrated in Figures 7.10 and 7.11, although the direction of strokes need not follow arrow directions.
- The objective is to obtain information, without causing excessive discomfort to the client/patient, and without stressing your palpating hands.
- In its treatment mode NMT involves using greater pressure in order to modify dysfunctional tissues, but in these sequences you can, if you wish, focus on 'information gathering' only, not treating.
- In time, with practice, treatment and assessment meld seamlessly together, with one feeding the other.
- Chart any findings you make: tender areas, stress bands, contracted fibers, edematous areas, nodular structures, hypertonic regions, trigger points, and so on.

- If trigger points are located, note their target area as well.

MUSCLE ENERGY TECHNIQUE

Are the tissues you are assessing tense or relaxed? Can your palpating hands identify 'ease' and 'bind'?

The tissues provide the palpating hands or fingers with a sense of these states, and there can never be enough focus on these two characteristics, which allow the tissues to speak as to their current degree of activity, comfort, or distress. Ward (1997) states that 'Tightness suggests tethering, while looseness suggests joint and/or soft tissue laxity, with or without neural inhibition.'

Most problems of the musculoskeletal system involve, as part of their etiology, dysfunction related to muscle shortening (Janda 1978, Liebenson 1996).

Where weakness (lack of tone) is apparently a major element, it will often be found that antagonists are shortened, reciprocally inhibiting their tone, and that prior to any effort to strengthen weak muscles, hypertonic antagonists should be dealt with by appropriate means (such as MET, see below), after which spontaneous toning occurs in the previously hypotonic or relatively weak muscles.

If tone remains reduced, then, and only then, should there be specific focus on toning weak muscles (Lewit 1999).

Which method should you choose, PIR or RI?

The presence of pain is frequently the deciding factor in choosing one or other of the methods described (post isometric relaxation, PIR, or reciprocal inhibition, RI) – contracting the agonist or the antagonist.

When using PIR, the very muscles which have shortened are being contracted.

If the condition of the area is one in which there is a good deal of pain, where any contraction could well trigger more pain, it might be best to avoid using these muscles, and choose the antagonists instead. Use of the antagonists (inducing RI) might therefore be your first choice for MET when the shortened muscles are very sensitive.

Later, when pain has been reduced by means of MET (or other) methods, PIR techniques (which use isometric contraction of the already shortened muscles rather than the antagonists used in RI methods) could be tried.

To a large extent, just how acute or chronic a condition is helps to decide the method best suited to treating it.

Both methods (PIR and RI) will produce a degree of increased tolerance to stretch.

The essential variables of MET

- The amount of effort used in the contraction effort.
- Other major variables that are controllable are, how long the contraction is allowed to continue, and how often it is repeated.
- The degree of effort in isometric contractions should always be much less than the full force available from the muscles involved.
- The initial contraction should involve the use of a quarter or less of the strength available.
- This is never an exact measurement, but indicates that we do not ever want a wrestling match to develop between the contracting area controlled by the client/patient, and the counterforce offered by you.
- After the initial slowly commenced contraction, subsequent contractions may involve an increase in effort, but should never reach more than half of the full strength of that muscle.
- We want above all to achieve a controlled degree of effort at all times, and this calls for the use of only

part of the available strength in a muscle or muscle group.

- The timing of isometric contractions is usually such as to allow around 7 seconds for the contraction, from beginning to end.
- It is important to remember that the start and the end of contraction should always be slow. There should never be a rapid beginning or end to the contraction.
- Always attempt a smooth build-up of power in the muscle(s) and a slow switch-off of the contraction at the end. This will prevent injury or strain, and allows for the best possible results.
- Contractions should always commence with the shortened muscle held close to its end of range, but, for comfort, never while it is already at stretch.
- After the isometric contraction, assisted by the client/patient, you should move the muscle past its previous barrier, into a slight stretch, and this should be held for not less than 30 seconds to achieve slow lengthening.
- No pain should be caused.
- If there is pain you may have taken the muscle into an excessive degree of stretch.
- Each stretch should be repeated twice.

MET exercises

Before starting this exercise (Greenman 1996, Goodridge & Kuchera 1997), ensure that the client/patient lies supine, so that the nontested leg is abducted slightly, with the heel over the end of the table (Fig. 7.12).

Post isometric relaxation (PIR)
- The leg to be tested should be close to the edge of the table.
- Ensure that the tested leg is in the anatomically correct position, knee in full extension and with no external rotation of the leg, which would negate the test.
- Holding the client/patient's foot/ankle, you slowly ease the straight leg into abduction.
- Stop the abduction when you sense that a barrier of resistance has been reached.
- This 'first barrier' is sensed by an increase in the amount of effort as you move the leg into abduction (Fig. 7.12A).
- Your other (palpating) hand rests passively on the inner thigh, palpating the muscles which are being tested (adductors and medial hamstrings).
- This palpating hand must be in touch with the skin, molded to the contours of the tissues being assessed, but should exert no pressure, and should be completely relaxed.

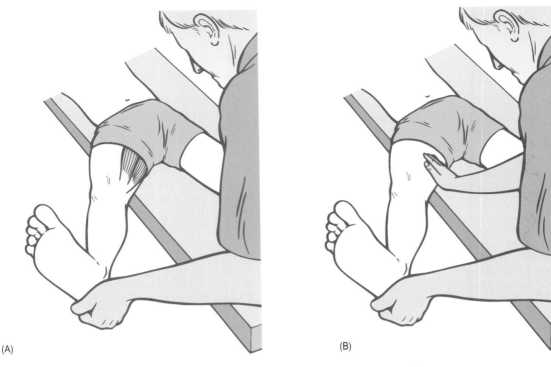

(A)   (B)

Figure 7.12 Position for treatment of shortness in adductors of the thigh. (From Chaitow 2001a.)

- That palpating hand should also sense the barrier, by virtue of a feeling of increased tension/bind (Fig. 7.12B).
- Normal excursion of the straight leg into abduction is around 45°.
- By testing both legs it is possible to evaluate whether the inner thigh muscles are tight and short on both sides, or whether one is and the other is not.
- Even if both are tight and short, one may be more restricted than the other. This is the one to treat first using MET.
- The point at which the very first sign of bind was noted is the resistance barrier.
- Identification and appropriate use of the first sign of resistance (i.e. where bind is first noted) is a fundamental part of the successful use of MET.

Treatment of shortness using MET
- The client/patient is asked to use no more than 20% of available strength to attempt to take the leg gently back toward the table (i.e. to adduct the leg) against firm, unyielding resistance offered by you.
- In this example, the client/patient is trying to take the limb away from the barrier, while you hold the

limb firmly (or place yourself between the leg and the table, as in Fig. 7.13).
- The client/patient will be contracting the agonists, the muscles which require release (and which, once released, should allow greater and less restricted abduction).
- The isometric contraction should be introduced slowly, and resisted without any jerking, wobbling, or bouncing.
- Maintaining the resistance to the contraction should produce no strain in the therapist.
- The contraction should be held for between 7 and 10 seconds. (This is thought to place 'load' on the Golgi tendon organs, neurologically influencing intrafusal muscle spindle fibers, inhibiting muscle tone, and providing the opportunity for the muscle to be taken to a new resting length/resistance barrier without effort; Scariati 1991.)
- An instruction is given to the client/patient, 'Release your effort, slowly and completely,' while the therapist maintains the limb at the same resistance barrier.
- The client/patient is asked to breathe in and out, and to completely relax, and as he/she exhales, stretch is introduced which takes the tissues

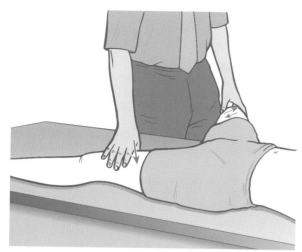

Figure 7.13 Position for treatment of shortness in adductors of the thigh. (From Chaitow 2001a.)

to a point just beyond the previous barrier of resistance.

- It is useful to have the client/patient gently assist in taking the (now) relaxed area toward and through the barrier.
- The stretch is held for 30 seconds.
- The procedure of contraction, relaxation, followed by client/patient assisted stretch is repeated (ideally with a rest period between contractions) at least once more.

Reciprocal inhibition (RI)
This example involves abduction of the limb (i.e. shortened adductors), against resistance.

- The barrier, first sense of restriction/bind, is evaluated as the limb is abducted, at which point the limb is returned a fraction toward a midrange position (by a few degrees only).
- From this position, the client/patient is asked to attempt to abduct the leg, using no more than 20% of strength, taking it toward the restriction barrier, while the therapist resists this effort.
- After 7 seconds, following the end of the contraction, the client/patient is asked to 'release and relax,' followed by inhalation and exhalation and further relaxation, at which time the limb is guided through the new barrier, with the client/patient's assistance.
- This stretch is held for at least 30 seconds.

MET: some common errors and contraindications

Greenman (1996) summarizes several of the important elements of MET as follows.

There is a client/patient-active muscle contraction:

- from a controlled position
- in a specific direction
- met by therapist-applied distinct counterforce
- involving a controlled intensity of contraction.

Client/patient errors during MET usage
Commonly based on inadequate instruction from the therapist:

1. Contraction is too strong (*remedy:* give specific guidelines, e.g. 'use only 20% of strength,' or whatever is more appropriate).
2. Contraction is in the wrong direction (*remedy:* give simple but accurate instructions).
3. Contraction is not sustained for long enough (*remedy:* instruct the client/patient to hold the contraction until told to ease off, and give an idea ahead of time as to how long this will be).
4. The client/patient does not relax completely after the contraction (*remedy:* have them release and relax, and then inhale and exhale once or twice, with the suggestion 'now relax completely').

Therapist errors in application of MET
1. Inaccurate control of position of joint or muscle in relation to the resistance barrier (*remedy:* have a clear image of what is required and apply it).
2. Inadequate counterforce to the contraction (*remedy:* meet and match the force).
3. Counterforce is applied in an inappropriate direction (*remedy:* ensure precise direction needed for best results).
4. Moving to a new position too hastily after the contraction (*remedy:* take your time to have the client/patient relax completely before moving to a new position).
5. Inadequate client/patient instruction is given (*remedy:* get the instructions right so that the client/patient can cooperate).
6. The therapist fails to maintain the stretch position for a period of time that allows soft tissues to begin to lengthen (ideally 30 seconds, but certainly not just a few seconds).

Contraindications and side effects of MET

- If pathology is suspected, no MET should be used until an accurate diagnosis has been established.
- Pathology (osteoporosis, arthritis, etc.) does not rule out the use of MET, but its presence needs to be established so that dosage of application can be modified accordingly (amount of effort used, number of repetitions, stretching introduced or not, etc.).

- There are no other contraindications except for the injunction to cause no pain.

Pulsed MET

There is another MET variation, which is powerful and useful: pulsed MET (Ruddy 1962). This simple method has been found to be very useful since it effectively accomplishes a number of changes at the same time, involving the local nerve supply, improved circulation and oxygenation of tissues, reduction of contraction, etc.

This method depends for its effectiveness on the 'pulsed' efforts of the person producing them being very light indeed, with no 'wobble' or 'bounce,' just the barest activation of the muscles involved. The following is an example of self-applied pulsed MET:

- Sit at a table, rest your elbows on it, and tilt your head forwards as far as it will go comfortably and rest your hands against your forehead.
- Use a pulsing rhythm of pressure of your head pushing against your *firm* hand contact, involving about 2 pulsations per second (against your hands) for 10 seconds.
- After 20 pulsations, retest the range of forward bending of your neck. It should go much further, more easily than before.
- This method will have relaxed the muscles of the region, especially those involved in flexion, and will have produced 20 small reciprocal inhibition 'messages' to the muscles on the back of your neck which were preventing easy flexion.
- Pulsed MET may be used for restricted muscles or joints in any part of the body.
- The simple rule is to have the client/patient engage the restriction barrier, while you provide a point of resistance (with your hands) as the client/patient pulses toward the barrier rhythmically.
- No pain should be felt.
- After 20 contractions in 10 seconds, the barrier should have retreated and the process can be repeated from the new barrier.
- The pulsing method should always be against a fixed resistance, just as in other MET methods.

POSITIONAL RELEASE TECHNIQUE

Positional release technique (PRT) is itself made up of a number of quite different methods, but the one that is probably most suitable for use in a massage therapy context is called strain–counterstrain (SCS). In order to understand this method, a brief explanation is needed (D'Ambrogio & Roth 1997, Deig 2001, Chaitow 2003b). Jones (1981) described the evolution

of strain–counterstrain as depending upon identification of 'tender' points found in the soft tissues associated with joints that have been stretched, strained, or traumatized.

- These tender points are usually located in soft tissues shortened at the time of the strain or trauma (i.e. in the antagonists to those that were stretched during the process of injury).
- For example, in spinal problems following on from a forward bending strain, in which back pain is complained of, the appropriate 'tender' point will be found on the anterior surface of the body (Fig. 7.14).
- The same process of tender point development in shortened structures takes place in response to chronic adaptation.
- Tender points are exquisitely sensitive on palpation but usually painless otherwise.
- Once identified, such points are used as monitors (explained below) as the area, or the whole body, is repositioned ('fine tuned') until the palpated pain disappears or reduces substantially.
- Tissue tension almost always eases at the same time as the easing of pain in the palpated point,

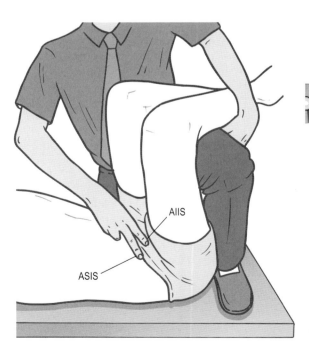

Figure 7.14 Position of ease for flexion strain of T9 to lower lumbar regions involves flexion, side bending, and rotation until ease is achieved in monitored tender point on the lower abdominal wall or the ASIS area.

making it possible to palpate the person, or part, into an ease position.

- If the 'position of ease' is held for some 90 seconds, there is often a resolution of the dysfunction which resulted from the trauma.

Positional release exercise

- Using one of the skin assessment methods discussed earlier in this chapter, or NMT, or whatever palpation method you are used to, palpate the musculotendinous tissues that are antagonists to those that were being stretched during a joint or spinal trauma or strain, or which are chronically shortened as part of a longstanding problem.
- The area being assessed should be one that is not being complained of as being painful.
- Any localized, unusually tender area in such tissue can be used as a 'tender point.'
- You should apply sufficient pressure to that point to cause mild discomfort and then slowly position the joint or area in such a way as to remove the tenderness from the point (Figs 7.15 & 7.16).
- Creating 'ease' in the tissues housing the point usually involves producing some degree of increased slack in the palpated tissues.
- Hold this position for 90 seconds and then slowly return to a neutral position and repalpate.
- The tenderness should have reduced or vanished, and functionality should be improved.

Main features of PRT

- All movements should be passive (therapist controls the movement, client/patient does nothing), and movements are painless, slow, and deliberate.

- Existing pain reduces, and no additional or new pain is created.
- Movement is *away* from restriction barriers.
- Muscle origins and insertions are brought together, rather than being stretched.
- Movement is away from any direction, or position, that causes pain or discomfort.
- Tissues being palpated relax.
- Painful tissues being palpated (possibly a trigger point) reduce in pain.
- It is often the case that the position of ease is a replica of a position of strain that started whatever problem the client/patient now has.

Guidelines for PRT use

1. For treatment of tender points on the anterior surface of the body, flexion, sidebending, and rotation should be *toward* the palpated point, followed by fine tuning to reduce sensitivity by at least 70%.
2. For treatment of tender points on the posterior surface of the body, extension, sidebending, and

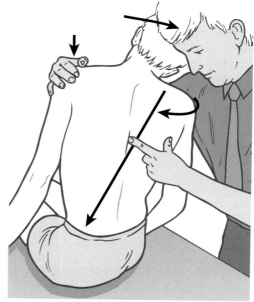

Figure 7.16 Treatment of thoracic region dysfunction (in this example tissue tension to the right of the 6th thoracic vertebra). One hand monitors tissue status as the patient is asked to 'sit straight' and to then slightly extend the spine. The operator then introduces compression from the right shoulder toward the left hip which automatically produces sidebending and rotation to the right. If ease is noted in the palpated tissues, the position is held for 30–90 seconds.

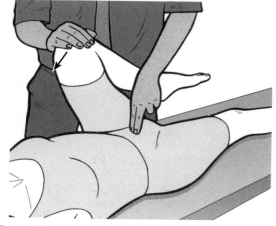

Figure 7.15 Treatment of pubococcygeus dysfunction.

rotation should be *away* from the palpated point, followed by fine tuning to reduce sensitivity by 70%.

3. The closer the tender point is to the midline, the less sidebending and rotation should be required, and the further from the midline, the more sidebending and rotation should be required, in order to effect ease and comfort in the tender point (without any additional pain or discomfort being produced anywhere else).

4. The direction toward which sidebending is introduced when trying to find a position of ease often needs to be away from the side of the palpated pain point, especially in relation to tender points found on the posterior aspect of the body.

The SCS process described step-by-step

- To use the strain–counterstrain (SCS) approach a painful point is located.
- This can be a 'tender' point or an actual trigger point.
- Sufficient pressure is applied to the point to cause some pain.
- If it is a trigger point, ensure that just enough pressure is being applied to cause the referred symptoms.
- The client/patient is told to give the pain being felt a value of 10.

Note: This is not a situation in which the client/patient is asked to ascribe a pain level out of 10, instead it is one in which the question asked is 'Does the pressure hurt?' If the answer is 'Yes,' then the client/patient is told: 'Give the level of pain you are now feeling a value of 10, and as I move the area around and ask for feedback, give me the new pain level – whatever it is.'

- It is important to ask the client/patient to avoid comments such as 'The pain is increasing' or 'It's getting less,' or any other verbal comment, other than *a number out of 10*. This helps to avoid undue delay in the process.
- In this example, we can imagine that the tender, or trigger, point is in the gluteus medius (Fig. 7.17).
- The client/patient would be prone, and the therapist would be applying sufficient pressure to the point in the gluteus medius to register pain which he/she would be told has a value of 10.
- The supported leg on the side of pain would be moved in one direction (say extension at the hip) as the client/patient is asked to give a value out of 10 for the pain.
- If the pain reduces, another direction might be introduced (say adduction) – and the question is repeated.
- If the pain increases, a different movement direction would be chosen.

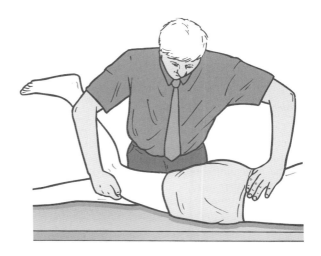

Figure 7.17 Position of ease for a tender point associated with an extension strain of the lumbar strain involves use of the legs of the prone patient as means of achieving extension and fine tuning.

- By gradually working through all the movement possibilities, in various directions, and possibly adding compression and distraction, a position would be found where pain drops by at least 70% (i.e. the score reaches 3 or less).
- Once this 'position of ease' has been found, after all the careful slow motion fine tuning, it is maintained for not less than 90 seconds – and sometimes more – after which a slow return is made to the starting position.
- Range of motion and degree of previous pain should have changed for the better.
- In different tissues, the possible directions of movement might include flexion, extension, rotation one way or the other, side flexion one way or the other, translation (shunting, or evaluating joint-play), as well as compression or distraction – to find the position of maximum ease.

When tissues are at ease
What happens when tissues are at ease (whether for 90 seconds or much longer)?

1. Pain receptors (nociceptors) reduce in sensitivity, something that is of importance where pain is a feature, whether this involves trigger points or not (Van Buskirk 1990, Bailey & Dick 1992).

2. In the comfort/ease position there is a marked improvement in blood flow and oxygenation through the tissues.

3. Facilitated areas (spinal or trigger points) will be less active, less sensitized, calmer, and less painful.

Box 7.3 Summary of skin palpation methods

- Movement of skin on fascia: resistance indicates general locality of reflexogenic activity, a 'hyperalgesic skin zone' such as a trigger point
- Local loss of skin elasticity: refines definition of the location
- Light stroke, seeking 'drag' sensation (increased hydrosis), offers pinpoint accuracy of location

Summary of muscle energy technique

- By lightly contracting a short, tight muscle isometrically (the agonist) for approximately 7 seconds, an effect known as post isometric relaxation (PIR) is produced. This offers an opportunity to stretch the previously shortened muscle(s) more effectively
- By lightly contracting the antagonists to tight/short muscles, an effect known as reciprocal inhibition (RI) is produced in the affected muscle(s), and this also offers an opportunity to stretch the previously shortened muscle(s) more effectively
- A process known as 'increased tolerance to stretch' (ITS) is produced by isometric contractions (i.e. MET) of the agonist(s), the muscle(s) needing lengthening, or their antagonists. This ITS effect means that you can more easily (because the muscle will be more relaxed) introduce greater force into a stretch than you could have done without the isometric contraction, because a neurological change will have taken place, reducing the sensitivity of the client/patient (Ballantyne et al 2003, Rowlands et al 2003)

The aim is to contract the shortened muscles, or their antagonists, in order to achieve the release of tone and to then be able, with greater ease, to stretch the muscle(s).

Positional release is used as part of the integrated neuromuscular inhibition (INIT) sequence described below, for trigger point deactivation.

INTEGRATED NEUROMUSCULAR INHIBITION (FOR TRIGGER POINT DEACTIVATION)

An integrated treatment sequence has been developed for the deactivation of myofascial trigger points. The method is as follows:

1. The trigger point is identified by palpation.
2. Ischemic compression is applied in either a sustained or intermittent manner.
3. When referred or local pain starts to reduce in intensity, the compression treatment stops.
4. The client/patient should be told, e.g:
   I am going to press that same point again, and I want you to give the pain that you feel a 'value' of 10. I will then gently reposition the area and you will feel differences in the levels of pain. In some positions the pain may increase, in others it will decrease. When I ask you for feedback as to what's happening to the pain, please give me a number out of 10. If the pain has increased it may go up – to say 11 or 12. Just give me the number you are feeling. We are aiming to find a position in which the pain drops to 3 or less, and the more accurately you give me the 'pain score' the faster

I will be able to fine tune the process, so that we can get to the 'comfort position.'

5. Using these methods (as described in the section above, on PRT) the tissues housing the trigger point are then carefully placed in a position of ease.
6. This ease position is held for approximately 20–30 seconds, to allow neurological resetting, reduction in pain receptor activity, and enhanced local circulation/oxygenation.
7. An isometric contraction is then focused into the musculature around the trigger point to create post isometric relaxation (PIR), as discussed in the MET section earlier in this chapter.
8. The way this is done varies with the particular part of the body being treated. Sometimes all that is necessary is to say to the client/patient, 'Tighten the muscles around the place where my thumb is pressing.'
9. At other times, if the client/patient is being supported in a position of ease, it may be helpful to say something like: 'I am going to let go of your leg (or neck, or arm, or whatever else you are supporting) and I want you to hold the position on your own for a few seconds.' In one way or another you need to induce a contraction of the muscle tissues surrounding the trigger point, so that they can be more easily stretched afterwards.
10. After the contraction (5–7 seconds, with the client/patient using only a small amount of

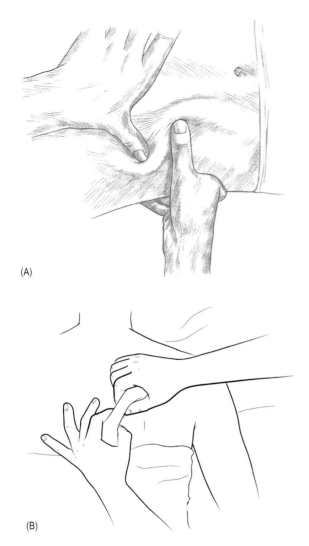

(A)

(B)

Figure 7.18 A: 'S' bend pressure applied to tense or fibrotic musculature. B: The lower trapezius fibers are treated in the same way.

effort), the soft tissues housing the trigger point are stretched locally (Fig. 7.18).

11. The local stretch is important because it is often the case in a large muscle that stretching the whole muscle will effectively lengthen it, but the tight bundle where the trigger point is situated will be relatively unstretched, like a knot in a piece of elastic which remains knotted even though the elastic is held at stretch.

12. After holding the local stretch for approximately 30 seconds, the entire muscle should then be contracted and stretched – again holding that stretch for at least 30 seconds.

13. The client/patient should assist in stretching movements (whenever possible) by activating the antagonists and so facilitating the stretch.

14. A towel that has been wrung out in warm/hot water placed over the treated tissues for 5 min helps to ease the soreness that may follow this treatment.

15. Within 24 hours, the trigger should have reduced in activity considerably, or no longer be active.

16. Retesting immediately after the INIT sequence may not offer evidence of this, as tissues will be tender.

SPRAY-AND-STRETCH METHODS

An effective method for deactivation of trigger points, and also for easing pain and releasing chronic muscle spasm, is use of spray-and-stretch methods (Mennell 1975).

- A container of vapocoolant spray with a calibrated nozzle that delivers a fine jet stream, or a source of ice, is needed.
- The jet stream should have sufficient force to carry in the air for at least 3 ft. A mist-like spray is less desirable (Fig. 7.19).
- Ice can consist of a cylinder of ice formed by freezing water in a paper cup and then peeling this off the ice. A wooden handle should be frozen into the ice to allow for its ease of application, as it is rolled from the trigger toward the referred area in a series of sweeps.
- A piece of ice may also be used, directly against the skin, for the same purpose, although this tends to be messy as the ice melts.
- Whichever method is chosen, the client/patient should be comfortably supported to promote muscular relaxation.
- If a spray is used, the container is held about 2 ft (60 cm) away, in such a manner that the jet stream meets the body surface at an acute angle or at a tangent, not perpendicularly. This lessens the shock of the impact.
- The stream/ice massage is applied in one direction, not back and forth.
- Each sweep is started at the trigger point and is moved slowly and evenly outward over the reference zone. The direction of chilling should be in line with the muscle fibers toward their insertion.
- The optimum speed of movement of the sweep/roll over the skin seems to be about 4 in (10 cm) per second.
- Each sweep is started slightly proximal to the trigger point and is moved slowly and evenly through the reference zone to cover it and extend slightly beyond it.

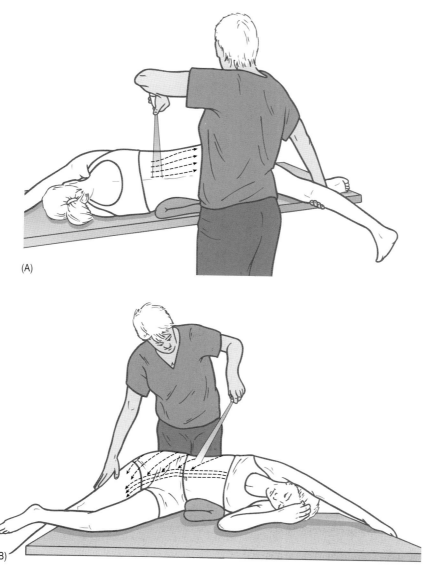

Figure 7.19 Anterior and posterior views of application of vapocoolant spray to trigger point (quadratus lumborum in this illustration). Muscles housing trigger points are placed at stretch while a coolant spray is utilized to chill the point and the area between it and the target reference area.

- These sweeps are repeated in a rhythm of a few seconds on and a few seconds off, until all the skin over the trigger and reference areas has been covered once or twice.
- If aching or 'cold pain' develops, or if the application of the spray/ice sets off a reference of pain, the interval between applications is lengthened.
- Care must be taken not to frost or blanch the skin.
- During the application of cold or directly after it, the taut fibers should be stretched passively.

- The fibers should not be stretched in advance of the cold.
- Steady, gentle stretching is usually essential if a satisfactory result is to be achieved.
- As relaxation of the muscle occurs, continued stretch should be maintained for 20–30 seconds, and after each series of cold applications active motion is tested.
- An attempt should be made to restore the full range of motion, but always within the limits of

pain, as sudden overstretching can increase existing muscle spasm.

- The entire procedure may occupy 15–20 minutes and should not be rushed. The importance of re-establishing normal motion in conjunction with the use of the chilling is well founded.

REHABILITATION EXERCISE METHODS

Norris (1999) advises the following guidelines for reestablishing back stability, using stabilization exercises for the different triage groups:

- *Simple backache:* begin stability exercises and continue until fully functional.
- *Nerve root compression:* begin exercise as pain allows, but refer to specialist if there has been no improvement within 4 weeks.
- *Serious pathology:* use back stabilization exercises only after surgical or medical intervention.

There are many interlocking rehabilitation features (Liebenson 1996) that may be involved in any particular case:

- normalization of soft tissue dysfunction
- deactivation of myofascial trigger points
- strengthening weakened structures
- proprioceptive reeducation using physical therapy methods
- postural and breathing reeducation
- ergonomic, nutritional, and stress management strategies
- psychotherapy, counseling, or pain management techniques
- occupational therapy which specializes in activating healthy coping mechanisms
- appropriate exercise strategies to overcome deconditioning.

A team approach to rehabilitation is called for where referral and cooperation between health care professionals allow the best outcome to be achieved. You are encouraged to develop an understanding of the multiple disciplines with which you can interface so that the best outcome for the client/patient can be achieved.

Core stability and breathing rehabilitation exercises are described in Chapter 9.

KEY POINTS

- Good palpation skills allow a therapist to rapidly and accurately localize and identify dysfunctional tissues.
- Neuromuscular technique (NMT) offers a unique way of searching tissues for local changes (such as trigger points) in a sequential way, and then treating whatever is located.
- Muscle energy techniques (MET) offer useful ways of encouraging length into previously tight, short, soft tissues.
- Positional release technique (PRT) offers painless ways for encouraging release of hypertonicity and spasm.

- Spray-and-stretch chilling methods are of proven value in trigger point deactivation and easing spasm.
- Integrated neuromuscular inhibition (INIT) is a sequence involving pressure methods, together with MET and PRT for trigger point deactivation.
- Rehabilitation exercise methods are vital for ultimate recovery and prevention.
- Massage combines with any of these approaches and has unique attributes of its own in pain care.

References

Adams T, Steinmetz M, Heisey S, et al: Physiologic basis for skin properties in palpatory physical diagnosis, *JAOA* 81(6):366–377, 1982.

Bailey M, Dick L: Nociceptive considerations in treating with counterstrain, *JAOA* 92:334–341, 1992.

Ballantyne F, Fryer G, McLaughlin P: The effect of muscle energy technique on hamstring extensibility: the mechanism of altered flexibility, *J Osteopath Med* 6(2):59–63, 2003.

Bendtsen L: Central sensitization in tension-type headache. Possible pathophysiological mechanisms, *Cephalalgia* 20:486–508, 2000.

Bendtsen L, Ashina M: Sensitization of myofascial pain pathways in tension-type headache. In Olesen J, Tfelt-Hansen P, Welch KMA, editors: The headaches, ed 2, Philadelphia, 2000, Lippincott Williams & Wilkins, pp 573–577.

Bendtsen L, Jensen R, Olesen J: Qualitatively altered nociception in chronic myofascial pain, *Pain* 65:259–264, 1996.

Bischof I, Elmiger G: Connective tissue massage. In Licht S, editor: Massage, manipulation and traction, New Haven, 1960, Licht.

Chaitow L: Muscle energy techniques, ed 2, Edinburgh, 2001, Churchill Livingstone.

Chaitow L: Modern neuromuscular techniques, ed 2, Edinburgh, 2003a, Churchill Livingstone, pp 120–131.

Chaitow L: Positional release techniques, ed 2, Edinburgh, 2003b, Churchill Livingstone.

Chaitow L, DeLany J: Clinical applications of neuromuscular techniques, vol 1 – the upper body, Edinburgh, 2001, Churchill Livingstone.

Cohen J, Gibbons R: Raymond Nimmo and the evolution of trigger point therapy, *J Manipulative Physiol Ther* 21(3):167–172, 1998.

D'Ambrogio K, Roth G: Positional release therapy, St Louis, 1997, Mosby.

Deig D: Positional release technique, Boston, 2001, Butterworth-Heinemann.

DiGiovanna E: Osteopathic diagnosis and treatment, Philadelphia, 1991, Lippincott.

Gibbons P, Tehan P: Spinal manipulation: indications, risks and benefit, Edinburgh, 2001, Churchill Livingstone.

Goodridge J, Kuchera W: Muscle energy treatment techniques. In Ward R, editor: Foundations of osteopathic medicine, Baltimore, 1997, Williams and Wilkins.

Greenman P: Principles of manual medicine, Baltimore, 1989, Williams and Wilkins.

Greenman P: Principles of manual medicine, ed 2, Philadelphia, 1996, Lippincott Williams & Wilkins.

Janda V: Muscles, central nervous motor regulation, and back problems. In Korr IM, editor: Neurobiologic mechanisms in manipulative therapy, New York, 1978, Plenum.

Janda V: Introduction to functional pathology of the motor system. In: Proceedings of the VII Commonwealth and International Conference on Sport, *Physiotherapy in Sport* 3:39, 1982.

Jones L: Strain and counterstrain, Colorado Springs, 1981, Academy of Applied Osteopathy.

Jull G, Janda V: Muscles and motor control in low back pain. In Twomey L, Taylor J, editors: Physical therapy for the low back. Clinics in physical therapy, New York, 1987, Churchill Livingstone.

Kappler R: Palpatory skills. In Ward R, editor: Foundations for osteopathic medicine, Baltimore, 1997, Williams and Wilkins.

Langevin H, Sherman K: Pathophysiological model for chronic low back pain integrating connective tissue and nervous system mechanisms, St Louis, 2006, Elsevier.

Lewit K: Manipulative therapy in rehabilitation of the locomotor system, ed 3, London, 1999, Butterworth-Heinemann.

Liebenson C, editor: Rehabilitation of the spine, Baltimore, 1996, Williams and Wilkins.

Liem T: Cranial osteopathy: principles and practice, Edinburgh, 2004, Churchill Livingstone, p 340.

Maitland G: Maitland's vertebral manipulation, ed 6, Oxford, 2001, Butterworth-Heinemann.

Mennell J: Therapeutic use of cold, *JOAO* 74(12):1146–1158, 1975.

Norris CM: Functional load abdominal training, *J Bodyw Mov Ther* 3(3):150–158, 1999.

Reed B, Held J: Effects of sequential connective tissue massage on autonomic nervous system of middle-aged and elderly adults, *Phys Ther* 68(8):1231–1234, 1988.

Rowlands AV, Marginson VF, Lee J: Chronic flexibility gains: effect of isometric contraction duration during proprioceptive neuromuscular facilitation stretching techniques, *Res Q Exerc Sport* 74(1):47–51, 2003.

Ruddy TJ: Osteopathic rapid rhythmic resistive technique, Carmel, 1962, Academy of Applied Osteopathy Yearbook, pp 23–31.

Scariati P: Myofascial release concepts. In DiGiovanna E, editor: An osteopathic approach to diagnosis and treatment, London, 1991, Lippincott.

Selye H: The stress of life, revised ed, New York, 1978 & 1999, McGraw Hill.

Stone C: Science in the art of osteopathy, Cheltenham, 1999, Stanley Thornes.

Van Buskirk R: Nociceptive reflexes and the somatic dysfunction, *J Am Osteopath Assoc* 90:792–809, 1990.

Ward R: Foundations of osteopathic medicine, Baltimore, 1997, Williams and Wilkins.

Youngs B: Physiological basis of neuro-muscular technique, *British Naturopathic Journal* 5(6):176–190, 1962.

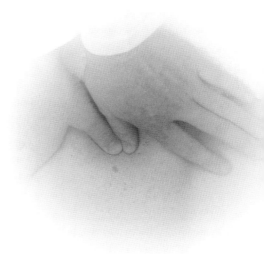

CHAPTER EIGHT
Full body massage

CHAPTER CONTENTS

INTRODUCTION

The protocol described in this chapter is used as a foundation for using massage to address pain. Any of the various positions and method applications found throughout the textbook can be incorporated into the massage. Do not be limited by the illustrations in the sequence.

Massage should have pleasurable aspects to the application. It should feel good and effectively produce results. The assessment and massage application should not produce a guarding response. During active treatment, the sensations can be intense and reproduce symptoms such as trigger point referral pain patterns, or burning sensation for some forms of connective tissue application. However, depending on the client outcomes there are times when uncomfortable methods are necessary to achieve results, and while the actual massage application may be intense, the result will indicate improvement.

As long as the client is able to respond to a full body massage, all of the following areas need to be assessed and intervention provided. It is not necessary to be done in this order but all need to be addressed during a comprehensive full body massage. Due to interconnected fascial networks and neuromuscular reflex patterns, massage in one area influences the entire body just as dysfunction or compensation in a body area has an influence on the whole body. Observation for whole body influence needs to be maintained. There will be many instances when this protocol is too intensive and the modified palliative protocol is more appropriate.

The following protocol is a comprehensive sequential approach that is suggested as a basis of massage. It does not need to be performed in this exact manner and once learned will almost always need to be altered for each individual client.

This protocol should not be used 48 hours prior to any medical procedure requiring any form of anesthesia including locals. Do not use this protocol post surgery or if the client is fragile, fatigued, etc. Use the modified palliative care protocol as a base instead and modify as needed.

GENERAL PROTOCOL

A general pattern approach is used during the massage session. The general approach consists of assessing each area, then addressing the outcome goals with appropriate massage methods.

The sequence is as follows:

- Skin, superficial fascia, and edema
- Deeper fascial structures, muscle layers, circulation, and edema
- Tissue density, ground substance, and fluid
- Joint end feel and intrinsic joint play
- Motor tone
- Reflex mechanisms
- Firing patterns (muscle activation sequences)
- Flexibility.

This massage assessment/treatment protocol will require 60 minutes. This time frame is okay if the client is healthy but remember most of the patients in health care (or should it be called sick care?) are not healthy. Sometimes 30 minutes is a better length for the massage. Instead of doing one long massage break it up into shorter sessions.

Rehabilitative methods found in the previous chapter should be incorporated into this general approach to ensure full body normalization. While it is appropriate to use some isolated spot work on specific target areas the response is improved when incorporated into full body application.

FACE AND HEAD

Thorough massage of the face and head is very important and very comforting. It is not uncommon to spend 10 minutes on the head and face.

Many connective tissue structures are anchored and originate in the area. Since there is a fascial connection from the feet to the top of the head, connective tissue bind patterns can either originate in the head area or be the location of the symptom of the various tension patterns from other parts of the body.

The muscles of the head and face are highly innervated and some of them, such as the masseter, are very strong. Many pressure sensitive structures (nerves, blood, and lymph vessels) are in close proximity to the head and face muscles and connective tissue structures. This sensitivity to pressure, combined with high sensation awareness, often results in pain in the head and face area.

The facial features should look symmetrical with little creasing of the skin from underlying increases in bind, tension, or tone in the myofascial structures.

The scalp should move easily on the skull in all directions. There are connective tissue bands that circle the head. The larger muscles (temporalis, occipital frontalis, and masseter) should be resilient to palpation with no observable or palpable trigger point activity. If there is evidence of sinus congestion, careful work on the small muscles of the face may allow better drainage.

The hair should not pull out during general massage of the scalp. If it does, this could indicate systemic illness fatigue or nutritional deficiencies and should be referred for evaluation by the appropriate professional.

The skin should be resilient, soft, supple, and mostly free from blemishes. Changes in skin texture are indications of increased systemic strain. Increased blemishes may indicate an increased cortisol and androgen level which is also associated with the stress response. If the skin is oily, be cautious about the type of lubricant that is used or work without it.

It is appropriate to massage the head and face muscles in all directions. It is interesting that when the muscles of the face that create a smile are activated, the neurochemical response can shift. Therefore, when massaging the face it may be beneficial to stroke in the direction that helps to create the shape of a smile.

Procedures for the face

The direction of the lymphatic stroking should be toward the neck and have sufficient drag to gently pull the skin. Address this area with the client in the supine or sidelying position (Fig. 8.1).

- Lightly and systematically, stroke the face to assess for temperature changes, tissue texture, and areas of dampness. If there are identified areas, note them for further investigation.
- Use light compression to assess for bogginess or swelling. If an increase in interstitial fluid is suspected, use lymphatic drain techniques to assist in fluid flow. If in doubt, assume that there is fluid stagnation and perform the methods. (Remember when moving fluid, you cannot push a river. Moving fluid is deliberate work.)
- As mentioned previously, the direction of the lymphatic stroking should be toward the neck and have sufficient drag to gently pull the skin.

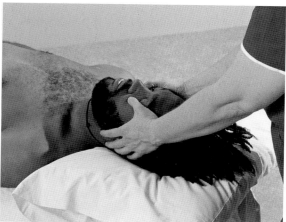

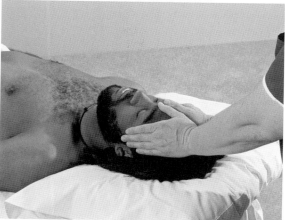

Figure 8.1 Massage of the sinuses.

Figure 8.2 Focused intention.

- When the area is drained, remassage in the direction of the smile.
- Continuing with the face, carefully move the skin to identify any areas of bind in the superficial connective tissue. Be aware of any bind areas that correspond to the areas identified by the light stroking. Pay particular attention to any areas containing scars, as connective tissue bind is common in areas of scar tissue. Be aware that the soft tissues of the neck weave directly and indirectly into the soft tissues of the head and face. When palpating the soft tissue of the face, observe for tissue movement or bind in adjacent areas.
- Areas of bind can be addressed by slowly moving the tissue into ease, which is the way it most wants to go. Multiple load directions can be used. For example, if the skin and superficial fascia want to move up and to the right between the eyebrows, then that would be the direction of the forces introduced. Hold the tissue at ease for up to 30 seconds and reassess. Subtle changes in the lines of force serve to load and unload the tissue, resulting in hysteresis. Usually the area will improve in pliability.
- Next, address the muscle structures. The facial muscles are only one or two layers deep; therefore, light to moderate compressive force is adequate.
- If muscle tone has increased from sustained isometric contraction, use direct pressure to inhibit the spindle cells and the Golgi tendons. This pressure is applied in a broad based compression with sufficient intensity to elicit tenderness or reproduce the symptoms, but not so intense that a muscle tenses or breathing changes occur (Fig. 8.2).

- Muscle energy methods can be used in combination with the compression by having the client contract the muscle against the pressure applied by the hand. It may take a few experimental contractions before the right muscle pattern is discovered. When the correct muscle contracts, the area will tense or seem as if it is pushing against the massage therapist's pressure. Pulsed muscle energy, where a repeated contract–relax, contract–relax pattern is used, is especially effective for the facial muscles.
- Positional release is possible by using eye positions until the pain is reduced in the compressed area.
- Apply pressure to the painful area until the client can feel the tenderness or the reproduced symptoms. Maintain the pressure while the client slowly moves the eyes in different positions until pain, tenderness, or symptom sensation is reduced. When the tone begins to reduce, a bending or tension force can then be applied to the muscle fibers.
- To finish the face, return to the initial light stroking to reassess for temperature changes etc. There should be a normalization of areas that were hot, cold, damp, rough, or binding.

Working with the face is relaxing. Therefore, if the face is done first, it can set the stage for a calming whole-body massage; if the face is done at the end of the session, it will gently finish the massage.

Procedures for the head

It is important that the scalp moves freely in all directions on the skull to reduce pressure on muscle, nerves, and vessels. Address this area with the client in the prone, supine, and sidelying positions (Fig. 8.3).

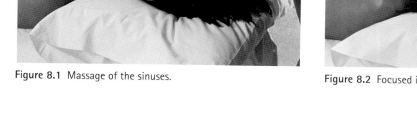

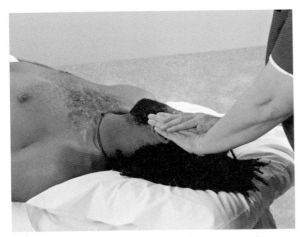

Figure 8.3 Head turned to the side to allow access to the muscles of mastication.

- Place the hands on either side of the head by the ears. Turning the head to the side facilitates pressure application. Move the scalp in various directions to assess for bind.
- If an area binds, it can be addressed by slowly moving the tissue into ease, dragging it the way it most wants to go. Multiple load directions can be used.
- Next, move tissues into bind and repeat back and forth to increase pliability.

The muscle structure of the head is very strong. The temporalis is part of the chewing mechanism and is often increased in tone due to gum chewing and gritting and clenching of the teeth. The suboccipital muscles weave into the posterior neck extensors via connective tissue attachments. The occipital muscles often become locked in isometric contraction patterns and then eventually become fibrotic.

The frontalis and occipitalis are actually one muscle, connected by connective tissue called the galea aponeurotica, which attaches at the base of the skull and neck tissues, and runs to the forehead. The two portions of this muscle have to be balanced, or an uneven pull force and/or pain can occur. If the occipitalis shortens, then pain can be felt in the forehead, and sometimes there is the sensation that the eyebrows are being pulled back. Squinting, scowling, and grimacing can increase tension in the frontalis and exert pull in the back of the head.

- If muscle tone has increased in any muscles of the head from sustained isometric contraction use broad based direct pressure to inhibit the spindle cells and the Golgi tendons.

- Apply pressure using broad based compression with sufficient intensity to elicit tenderness or reproduce the symptoms, but not so intense that any muscle tensing or breathing changes occur.
- Muscle energy methods can be used in combination with the compression by having the client contract against the pressure applied by the hand or forearm. It may take a few experimental contractions before the right muscle pattern is discovered.
- Some clients enjoy having their hair gently pulled. The hair can be used as a handle to pull the scalp away from the skull. Make sure that a large bunch of hair is grasped, a gentle pull introduced to bind is held, and is then released. Systematically done, this application addresses the entire scalp.
- Compression to the sides of the head and to the front and back of the head, coupled with a scratching motion to the scalp, can be very pleasant.

NECK

The joints in this area are the atlas and the axis and remaining cervical vertebrae. Local muscles are involved in the stability of this area and consist primarily of the suboccipital group. These muscles also act as proprioceptive feedback stations on the position of the head in relationship to the rest of the body, and are involved with the ocular, tonic neck, and pelvis reflexes for maintaining posture and balance. In some instances, the suprahyoid may also work to balance the head, exerting a small counterforce to the suboccipitals. The global muscles that can influence the occipital base are the sternocleidomastoid, platysma, semispinalis, splenius capitis, and trapezius. Besides the muscles that attach to the cervical area, we will also discuss the muscles that do not attach to the head, such as the scalenes, levator scapulae, longissimus cervicis, semispinalis cervicis, iliocostalis cervicis, spinalis, longus colli, and infrahyoids, as well as the multifidi, rotatores, interspinales, and intertransversarii at each individual vertebra.

There are many vessels and nerves in this area, including the brachial plexus. Impingement is common, with referral patterns in the neck, down to the chest, and to the arms. This is the area where thoracic outlet syndrome occurs. Preventative care is needed for this condition.

If a client had impact trauma in the head, then the neck will have absorbed the force and restrained the motion.

The neck is involved in many reflex patterns, including the tonic neck reflex. The muscles that insert on the ribs often become short with upper chest breathing patterns. The outcome of this may be

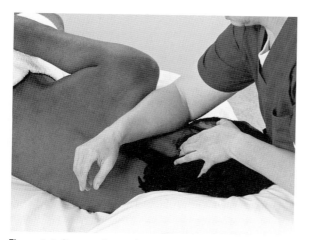

Figure 8.4 Compression to the lower cervical area and upper shoulder; the patient moves the shoulder to achieve combined loading.

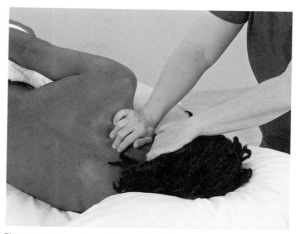

Figure 8.5 Kneading of the neck and upper shoulder (patient sidelying).

chronic overbreathing and breathing pattern syndrome symptoms.

It is difficult to list individual muscles that can influence any particular area because the body is such an interconnected structure; however, these are the main muscles that affect the local joint stability and proprioceptive information and global movement of this area. The local muscles are deep, and the global muscles, being more superficial, comprise the first and second layer of tissue.

The cervical and brachial plexus and vessels supplying the head and upper limb are located in this area. Impingement is common. It is essential that this area functions normally to ensure proper positional reflexes necessary for agility and precise movement. Sympathetic dominance will increase muscle tone in the area. The area most often shows decreased connective tissue pliability.

Address this area with the client prone and in a sidelying position (Fig. 8.4).

- Systematically, lightly stroke the area to assess for temperature changes, skin texture, and damp areas. Observe for skin reddening (histamine response) and gooseflesh (pilomotor). These signs indicate possible changes in skin pliability and accumulation of interstitial fluid, as indicated by boggy or edematous tissue and/or increased skin pressure (like a water balloon).
- If increased fluid pressure is evident, drain the area using a combination of light pressure to drag the skin and deeper, rhythmic, broad based compression and kneading to stimulate the deeper vessels.

- Begin with lighter pressure directed toward the collar bone, covering the entire area. Then introduce pumping broad based compression combined with active and passive movement by having the client slowly rotate the head in circles first one way and then the other.
- Next, address the superficial fascia by assessing for tissue bind, always observing for involvement in adjacent areas such as the upper back, chest, head, and face.
- Address areas of bind, slowly moving the tissue into ease, dragging it the way it most wants to go. Multiple load directions can be used.
- Bending force can also be introduced.
- By lifting the tissue much in the way that a mother cat would carry or lift a kitten by the neck, maintain the drag on the tissue until the thixotropic nature of the ground substance is affected and becomes more pliable. Subtle changes in the lines of force serve to load and unload the tissue resulting in hysteresis.
- Work slowly and deliberately, interspersing lymphatic drain type stroking every minute or so. The posterior tissue is very thick, and work in this area can be relatively aggressive, whereas the anterior tissue between the chin and hyoid is more delicate, and gentler methods need to be used in this area.

The musculature in the posterior region needs to be addressed in layers, systematically moving from superficial to deep. Depending on the size of the neck, the depth to the suboccipitals can be more than 2 in (Fig. 8.5).

- The upper trapezius area can be grasped, lifted, kneaded, and shaken, all of which will influence the fluid, connective tissue, and neuromuscular elements. Work the upper trapezius tissue all the way to the proximal attachments at the head.
- Use a wave-like motion over the area to assess for the sliding. If the tissues are adhered, reintroduce connective tissue methods by grasping the surface layer, lifting it off the underlying tissue and systematically shearing the tissue until it is freed from the underlying area. If the area is very adhered, it may take many sessions before the layers separate sufficiently to allow proper muscle action. Work for up to 3 min on an area or until it gets warm.
- Maintaining a broad based contact, increase the compressive force and contact the next layer of tissue. Again, glide and drag the tissue from proximal attachment to distal attachment and then reverse. Repeat three or four times.
- Because this area is extremely active in proprioceptive functions, muscle energy methods are effective, especially using motion and position of the eyes. Depending on the situation, use varying degrees of intensity. The gentlest method is positional release using the eye position to locate the position of release as follows: Locate the tender point and then, while maintaining pressure on the area, have the client slowly move his/her eyes in circles until the tenderness dissipates.
- Hold for up to 30 seconds.
- Next, if the area is not acutely painful, while maintaining the same pressure contact with the tender area, have the client look hard, moving only the eyes toward the pain. This will initiate a tensing of the muscles. Have the client hold this position for a few seconds and then look in the opposite direction; this will activate opposing antagonist patterns and initiate reciprocal inhibition.
- Have the client hold this position for a few seconds and then slowly turn the head in the direction of the eyes, as far as possible from the pain. When the end of range is reached, apply a small overpressure to lengthen the muscles. After a few seconds, apply a bit more tension to the bind and stretch the connective tissue.
- The most aggressive muscle energy pattern used in this area involves appropriate facilitation and inhibition of muscle contraction.
- The client's head should be in a natural position. The client can be in the supine, prone, sidelying, or seated position.
- Place hands on either side of the client's head just above the ears and stabilize the head. Instruct the client to push against one of your hands and look hard in that direction. Apply sufficient resistance so that the contraction remains isometric.
- Next, have the client continue to push but to turn only the eyes in the opposite direction to inhibit the contracting muscles. Apply a slightly increased pressure to determine if the area is inhibited. The client should not be able to hold against the increased pressure unless using other muscles or holding the breath.
- If the area does not inhibit, apply sufficient overpressure to move the head 1 in. Slowly let go and repeat until the area inhibits easily.
- If a change is not noted in two or three attempts, it is likely that the problem is more global and connected to some other reflex or proprioceptive pattern. Leave it alone.
- Repeat on the other side. This series of moves can substantially reduce the sensation of tightness in the neck, especially the need to 'crack' the neck.
- Gentle rocking rhythmic ranges of motion of the area (oscillation) may be used to continue to relax the area. The more global muscles can be remassaged gently or lymphatic drain massage can complete the procedure.

ANTERIOR TORSO

The anterior torso is best addressed before the posterior torso because it is the location of the structures causing most of the aching and dysfunction in the posterior torso.

This area consists of the ribcage, which protects the vital organs, and the abdominal contents. The muscles in the anterior torso area are primarily responsible for breathing. The pectoralis major and pectoralis minor provide the arm and scapula with both movement and stability. The abdominal muscles are layered and quite intricate in design, as well as being extensively encased and supported by fascia structures. This is an important area of core stability, and an understanding of how the abdominal group functions in posture is necessary.

Attachments of the muscles from the neck (platysma, sternocleidomastoid, scalenes) and the connective tissue connections that unify the body are situated in the upper chest. The muscles of the anterior torso are in functional units with the head and neck flexors. The muscles of this area are involved in flexion and adduction movements in the frontal and sagittal planes. The fiber orientation of the muscles and fascia is multidirectional with a strong diagonal and perpendicular focus.

Three major cross sections of tissue in the transverse plane define this area. First, the muscles of the neck overlap with the muscles of the upper thorax and the back of the neck and torso, to form the thoracic diaphragm. Second, the diaphragm muscle itself separates the upper and lower torso, and third, the pelvic floor is closed by the crisscross design of the pelvic floor muscles. These transverse layers of tissue are involved in stability and respiration.

Procedures for the anterior torso

Massage begins with superficial work, progresses to deeper tissue layers, and then finishes off with superficial work. Initial applications are palpation assessment to identify temperature and superficial tissue changes. This area can be massaged while the client is sidelying or supine. A combination of both is most desirable (Figs 8.6 & 8.7).

- Systematically lightly stroke the area to assess for temperature changes, skin texture, and damp areas. Observe for skin reddening (histamine response) and gooseflesh (pilomotor). These signs indicate possible changes in connective tissue, muscle tone, or circulation patterns.
- Increase the pressure slightly and assess for superficial fascial bind, changes in skin pliability, and accumulation of interstitial fluid, as indicated by boggy or edematous tissue and/or increased skin pressure (like a water balloon.)
- If increased fluid pressure is evident, drain the area using a combination of light pressure to drag the skin and deeper, rhythmic, broad based compression and kneading to stimulate the deeper vessels.
- Begin with lighter pressure in the direction of the axilla while working above the waist, or toward the groin while working below the waist, covering the entire area. Then introduce pumping broad based compression, which can be combined with active and passive movement of the area.
- Next, address the superficial fascia by assessing for tissue bind, observing for adjacent areas involved, such as the tissue leading into the shoulder and pelvic girdles.
- Move the skin to identify any areas of bind in the superficial connective tissue. Notice whether any bind areas correspond to the areas of skin reddening or gooseflesh identified by the light stroking. Pay particular attention to any scars, because connective tissue bind is common at these sites.
- Treat areas of superficial fascial bind with myofascial release methods. Address these areas by slowly moving the tissue into ease, dragging it the way it most wants to go.
- Multiple load directions can be used. For example, if the skin and superficial fascia want to move up and to the right at the sternum, then that would be

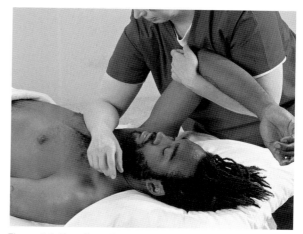

Figure 8.6 Kneading of the pectoralis major.

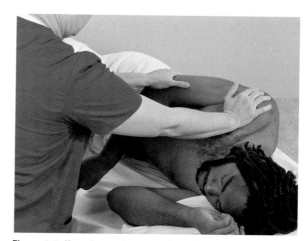

Figure 8.7 Kneading and compression using counterpressure.

the direction of the forces introduced. Hold the tissue in ease position until release is felt, or for up to 30 seconds.

Next work into the bind:

- Use a slow, sustained drag on the binding tissues, with the lines of tension being introduced at each end of the binding tissue.
- Place your forearm or flat hand (finger pads if the hand is too large) at one end of the bind and the other forearm and hand at the other end of the bind.
- Contact the tissue gently but firmly, pressing only as deep as the superficial fascial layer, and separate the forearms or hands, creating a tension force into the binding tissue.

- The musculature in the anterior thorax is addressed in layers, systematically, moving from superficial to deep. It is important to make sure that muscle layers are not adhered to each other. The most common occurrence is pectoralis major stuck to pectoralis minor. One muscle layer should be sheared off the next deeper layer. It is helpful to place the client so that the surface layer is in a slack position by positioning the attachments of the muscle close together and bolstering the clients so that he/she can remain relaxed.
- Because the fascia in the chest covers the pectoralis major, which extends into the arm, the arm can be used to increase or release the tension force on the tissue.
- Use gliding with a compressive element, beginning at the shoulder, and work from the distal attachment of the pectoralis major at the arm toward the sternum, following the fiber direction. This can be done in a supine or sidelying position with the client rolled. Repeat three or four times, each time increasing the drag and moving slower.
- Any areas that redden may be housing trigger point activity. Because latent trigger points can cause muscles to fire out of sequence, it is important to restore as much normalcy to the tissue as possible.
- To increase circulation to the area and shift neuroresponses of latent trigger points, move the skin over the point into multiple directions of ease, and hold the ease position for up to 30 seconds.
- If this does not relieve the tenderness, positional release is the next option, followed by muscle energy methods, if necessary. Local lengthening of the tissue containing the trigger points is effective, and authorities have found that it is needed to complete the release of trigger points. Local lengthening is accomplished by using tension, bending, or torsion force on the tissue with the trigger point and taut band.

Avoid direct pressure or transverse friction because these methods have the potential for creating tissue damage. If the trigger point does not release with the methods described, then it is part of a compensation pattern that must be dealt with, and the trigger point is likely serving a useful function. Leave it alone.

Once the surface tissue is addressed, then the second layer of muscle is massaged. It is important to make sure that the surface tissue and the fascial separation between muscle layers is not adhered together in any way. Assess by lifting the surface tissue and moving it back and forth in a wave-like movement.

The main muscles being addressed are the pectoralis minor, anterior serratus, and external and internal abdominal obliques.

- Use compression with gliding deep enough to address this layer of tissue.
- Broaden the base of contact so that the surface tissue does not tighten to guard against poking.
- Glide in various directions, both with and against the grain of the muscle fibers.
- Repeat three or four times, with each application slower and at a slightly different angle to access the multiple fiber directions of these muscles.
- Next, knead slowly across the fiber direction, using enough pressure and lift to ensure that you are affecting muscle fiber in this layer. The methods address both connective tissue and neuromuscular elements of the muscle.
- Repeat three or four times, increasing the depth and drag each time and being aware of the muscle moving with the application. Work the entire length of the area, and repeat.
- Narrow the focus to address the third tissue layer to include the intercostals. Make sure the surface muscles slide over these muscles. This is commonly a ticklish area, so do not use a hesitant touch.
- Glide and drag the tissue using the fingers. These are not long moves since the span of these muscles is between ribs.
- Repeat three or four times.
- Tender points are treated with positional release. Many times the position of release can be reached by different compressive forces on the ribs to change the shape of the rib cage.

If bones are brittle in this area, be cautious. If direct movement of the ribcage is not possible, moving the hips or shoulders also changes the position of the ribs. It is very important to address these tender points since they can interfere with effective movement of the ribs during breathing.

When addressing deeper tissue layers always remember to protect the more superficial muscles by applying pressure gradually and with as broad a base of contact as the area will allow. Muscle energy methods are introduced by having the client inhale and exhale.

The abdominal organs can be rolled to encourage peristalsis. Specific massage to the large intestine can support normal bowel elimination. To complete the area, rhythmic compression of the entire anterior torso area can be used. This stimulates lymphatic flow and supports breathing function (Fig. 8.8).

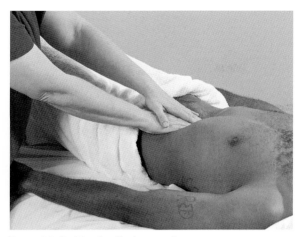

Figure 8.8 Position for diaphragm release.

POSTERIOR TORSO

The posterior torso consists of the thoracic vertebrae, ribs, lumbar vertebrae, sacrum, and coccyx, and the structures that attach to these bones. The most superficial layer of muscle serves to connect, stabilize in force couples, and move the limbs. These soft tissue structures are relatively global. The second, third, and fourth layers of muscle attach intrinsically on the vertebral column and ribs. These muscles and soft tissue structures become progressively more local the deeper they are oriented.

The middle layer of muscles has multiple attachments on the vertebrae and ribs orienting in a direction parallel to the spine. These muscles, collectively called the sacrospinal or erector spinae, function to extend and stabilize the back. Because the degree of movement for these muscles is limited, the stabilization of posture becomes their primary function. Stabilization involves smaller concentric and eccentric muscle function with sustaining isometric contraction, therefore these muscles will often feel tense to the client.

Major connective tissue structures begin at the head and cover the entire posterior trunk. These structures spread into the shoulder and pelvis as part of the supporting structures of limbs.

The deeper layer of muscles – multifidi, rotatores, intertransversarii, and interspinales – are primarily stabilizers with important proprioceptive function for the position of the spine. The deep muscles, which attach from one vertebra to the next, shorten and become hypersensitive to movement. They are difficult to stretch and tense, and often the client feels as if he/she wants to 'crack' the back.

Many nerves exit the spine and the potential for entrapment exists. The most common locations where this may occur in the lumbar area are at the lumbar and sacral plexuses.

The quadratus lumborum is a deep muscle that often has trigger point activity, with referred pain to the low back causing difficulty during the firing pattern of leg abduction.

The functions of the soft tissue in the posterior torso include extension, rotation, and lateral flexion, but the main function is maintaining an upright posture.

The posterior torso is often the location of many complaints. The reason for the tension, binding, trigger points, and so forth is usually compensatory and adaptive to some sort of postural strain. Direct massage work in the area without also addressing the causal factors is purely palliative, and its effects only last a short period of time. Anterior flexion, internal rotation, and adduction patterns are usually more likely to be involved in the actual cause of backaches because they are pulling forward in the sagittal and transverse planes toward the midline.

When these movement patterns are shortened, posterior thorax structures become inhibited, long, and tight. There are exceptions, usually in the lumbar area where muscles and connective tissue can shorten.

Be cautious in addressing trigger points and connective tissue bind in inhibited and long muscles of the posterior torso because these conditions may be part of a resourceful compensation pattern. Instead, focus treatment on the anterior thorax and then reassess posterior structures. Use general massage methods in the inhibited and long areas to reduce symptoms.

Procedures for the posterior torso

As described previously, massage begins with superficial work, progresses to the deeper tissue layers, and then finishes off with superficial work. Initial applications are palpation assessments to identify temperature and surface tissue changes.

- Systematically lightly stroke the area to assess for temperature changes, skin texture, and damp areas (Fig. 8.9). Observe for skin reddening (histamine response) and gooseflesh (pilomotor). These signs indicate possible changes in connective tissue, muscle tone, or circulation patterns.
- Increase the pressure slightly and assess for superficial fascial bind, changes in skin pliability, and accumulation of interstitial fluid, as indicated by boggy or edematous tissue and increased skin pressure (like a water balloon).

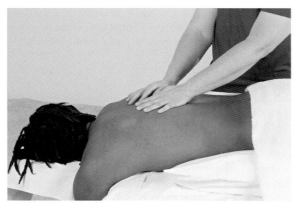

Figure 8.9 Palpation and assessment of the skin.

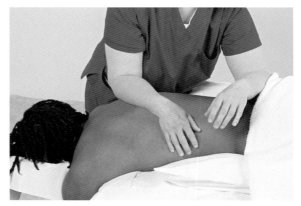

Figure 8.10 Tension force applied to the skin and superficial fascia. Primary focus: connective tissue pliability.

- If increased fluid pressure is evident, then lymph-drain the area using a combination of light pressure to drag the skin and deeper, rhythmic, broad based compression and kneading to stimulate the deeper vessels.
- Begin with lighter pressure in the direction of the axilla while working above the waist, and toward the groin while working below the waist, covering the entire area. Then introduce pumping broad based compression. If in doubt about the presence of fluid retention, then assume it is there and drain the area.

Next, address the superficial fascia by assessing the tissue bind, always observing for involvement in adjacent areas, such as the tissue leading into the shoulder and pelvic girdles.

- Move the skin to identify any areas of bind in the superficial connective tissue. Notice whether any bind areas correspond to the areas of skin reddening or gooseflesh identified by the light stroking. Pay particular attention to any scars, because connective tissue bind is common at these sites.
- Areas of superficial fascial bind are treated with myofascial release methods. Address these areas by slowly moving the tissue into ease, dragging it the way it most wants to go.
- Multiple load directions can be used. For example, if the skin and superficial fascia want to move up and to the right between the scapulae then that would be the direction of the forces introduced. Hold tissue in ease position for 30–60 seconds.
- Then work into the bind with a slow, sustained drag on the binding tissues and the lines of tension being introduced at each end of the binding tissue.
- Place your forearms or flat hands at one end of the bind and the other hand at the other end of the bind (Fig. 8.10).

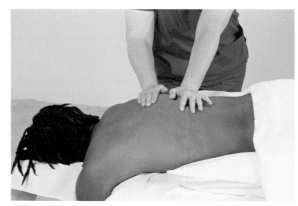

Figure 8.11 Palm gliding – light, medium, or deep pressure. Light to moderate drag, slow speed. Primary focus: assessment of tissue texture and movement of tissue layers.

- Contact the tissue gently but firmly, pressing only as deep as the superficial fascial layer, and separate the forearms or hands, creating a tension force into the binding tissue. Bending force can also be introduced (Fig. 8.11).
- Maintain the drag on the tissue until the thixotropic nature of the ground substance is affected and it becomes more pliable. Subtle changes in the lines of force serve to load and unload the tissue.
- Next, grasp as much of the binding tissue as possible and lift it until the resistance is identified (Fig. 8.12). Slowly load and unload with torsion and shear force until the tissue becomes warm and more pliable. This method is intense and the client should feel a pulling or slight burning sensation. The client should not feel the need to tense or change breathing in order to endure the application. Work slowly, interspersing lymphatic

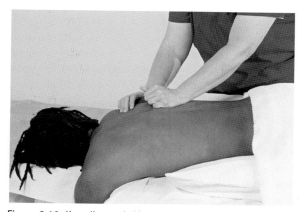

Figure 8.12 Kneading and skin rolling. Primary focus: assessment of skin and superficial fascia.

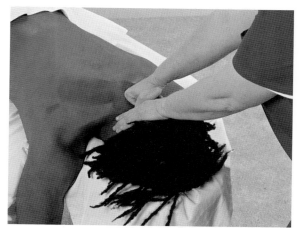

Figure 8.13 Fist gliding or compression of the upper shoulder and neck region. Primary focus: assessment and treatment.

drain-type stroking every minute or so. The posterior fascia tissue is very thick, especially at the thoracolumbar aponeurosis, and work in this area can be more intense than in other areas of the body.

The musculature in the posterior thorax region needs to be addressed in layers, systematically, moving from superficial to deep. It is important to make sure that muscle layers are not adhered to each other. One layer of muscle should be sheared off the next deeper layer.

- Use gliding with a compressive element, beginning at the iliac crest, and work diagonally along the fibers of the latissimus dorsi, ending at the axilla. Repeat three or four times, each time increasing the drag and moving slower.
- Move up to the thoracolumbar junction and repeat the same sequence on the lower trapezius.
- Then, beginning near the tip of the shoulder, glide toward the middle thoracic area to address the middle trapezius. Repeat three or four times, increasing drag and decreasing speed.
- Begin again near the acromion and address the upper trapezius with one or two gliding stokes to complete the surface area.
- If any area binds against the drag, working across the grain of the muscle and in the opposite direction may be beneficial (Fig. 8.13).

Any areas that redden may be housing trigger point activity. Because latent trigger points can cause muscles to fire out of sequence, it is important to restore as much normalcy to the tissue as possible.

To increase circulation to the area and shift neuroresponses of latent trigger points, move the skin over the latent trigger point into multiple directions of ease, and hold the ease position for up to 30 seconds. If this does not relieve the tenderness, positional release is

the next option, followed by muscle energy methods, if necessary.

Local lengthening of the tissue containing the trigger points is effective, and leading authorities have found it is necessary to complete the release of trigger points. Local lengthening is accomplished by using either tension, bending, or torsion force on the tissue with the trigger point and taut band.

Avoid direct pressure or transverse friction, because these methods have the potential for creating tissue damage. If the trigger point does not release using these methods described, then it is part of a compensation pattern. In this situation, the trigger point is likely serving a useful function, especially in the posterior muscles that are often in a long and taut state. The trigger point areas would serve to shorten the tissue and add some counterforce to the areas that are short and pulling (Fig. 8.14).

- Finish off the area with kneading, making sure that the muscle tissue easily lifts off the layer underneath it.
- Once the surface tissue is addressed, target the second layer of muscle. It is important to assess to make sure that the surface tissue and the fascial separation between muscle layers is not adhered together in any way.

The main muscles being addressed at this time are spinae, serratus posterior inferior and superior (especially if the client is coughing, sniffing, or has any other breathing dysfunction), and rhomboids.

- Begin at the iliac crest and use gliding deep enough to address this layer of tissue, following the tissue fiber direction. Maintain a broad base of

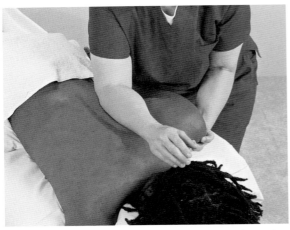

Figure 8.14 Position for combined loading: compression and movement of the scapular region.

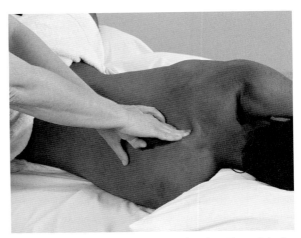

Figure 8.15 Massage of the deep muscles along the vertebral column.

contact so that the surface tissue does not tighten to guard against poking. Glide toward the scapula, ending just past the rhomboids.

- Repeat three or four times, each stroke slower at a slightly different angle to access the multiple fiber direction of these muscles. Then reverse the direction and work from superior to inferior.
- Next, knead slowly across the fiber direction using enough pressure and lift to ensure that you are affecting muscle fiber in this layer. These methods will address both the connective tissue and the neuromuscular elements of the muscle.
- Repeat three or four times increasing the depth and drag each time and being aware of the muscle moving with the application. Work the entire length of the area and repeat.

Narrow the focus to address the next layer, which includes the multifidus, rotators, intertransversarii, and interspinales, etc.

- Make sure that the more superficial surface muscles slide over these muscles. Glide and drag the tissue, using the forearm and fingers, from the proximal attachment to the distal attachment, and then reverse. These are not long moves as the span of these muscles is between one and three vertebrae.
- Repeat three or four times. A prone or sidelying position can be used successfully.

By changing the angle of the contact, the compression can identify any area where short muscle structures are impinging the nerves. When the area is located, the symptoms that are bothering the client will be reproduced. Compression is then combined with muscle energy methods, starting from the least invasive of

positional release, using the eyes, and then progressing to the more invasive contract, relax, and antagonist contract methods. Rotary movements of the torso while the client is in the sidelying position work well in this area to isolate muscles for muscle energy methods. The goal is to temporarily inhibit the motor tone of the problematic muscle bundle so that it can be lengthened to the appropriate resting length and reduce pressure on the nerves or vessels.

These small muscles respond to compression in the muscle belly. This serves to bend the belly as well as exert tension force at the insertion, to affect the proprioceptors in these locations (Fig. 8.15).

When addressing deeper tissue layers, always remember to protect the more superficial tissue by applying pressure gradually and with as broad a base of contact as the area will allow.

SHOULDER

The shoulder is a complex musculoskeletal unit. The joint structure is so mobile that it relies more than other major joints on muscles and fascia to provide stability. The movement of the scapula, acromioclavicular (AC), sternoclavicular (SC), and glenohumeral joints in a coordinated fashion is necessary for both maximal mobility and stability of the area. The inner (local) muscle unit, rotator cuff muscles, and coracobrachialis hold and guide the humerus in the glenoid fossa, using the scapula as a broad based attachment. The deltoid muscle is expansive and actually functions as three separate units. It also acts as a protective cover for the shoulder. Other muscles of the torso and arm such as the rhomboids, anterior serratus, pectoralis minor, trapezius, and triceps both stabilize and move the scapula, performing a series of muscle actions and working together in force couples. The pectoralis major and latissimus dorsi form global units that extend the range of motion of the arm.

Muscle/fascial components from the torso and neck affect the stability and mobility of the shoulder. Involvement of gate reflexes necessitates that the shoulders and hip function in coordinated movement patterns.

Nerve impingement of the brachial plexus refers pain to the shoulder and arm.

Procedures for the shoulder (Fig. 8.16)

The shoulder is massaged with the client in supine, prone, sidelying, and seated positions. Massage of the torso and neck naturally progresses to the shoulder.

Assessment of all range of motion patterns and muscle strength will indicate which structures are short and which are long.

- Move the shoulder actively and passively through flexion, extension, internal and external adduction and abduction, and full circumduction (Fig. 8.17). Compare active and passive movements.
- Gently compress the joint to make sure that there is no intercapsular involvement. If pain occurs, refer the client to an appropriate specialist. Massage can still be performed, but be aware that muscle tension patterns may be a guarding response creating appropriate compensation.

It is necessary to make sure that the scapula is mobile on the scapulothoracic junction and that appropriate movement is occurring at the AC and SC joints.

- Systematically lightly stroke the area to assess for temperature changes, skin texture, and damp areas. Observe for skin reddening (histamine response) and gooseflesh (pilomotor). These signs indicate possible changes in connective tissue, muscle tone, or circulation patterns.
- Increase the pressure slightly and assess for superficial fascial bind, changes in skin pliability and accumulation of interstitial fluid, as indicated by boggy or edematous tissue and/or increased skin pressure/turgor (like a water balloon).
- If increased fluid pressure is evident then drain the area using the lymphatic drain procedure.
- Begin with lighter pressure directed toward the axilla, covering the entire area.
- Then introduce pumping broad based compression, which is more efficient when followed by or combined with active and passive movements.
- If in doubt about the presence of fluid retention, assume it is there and drain the area.

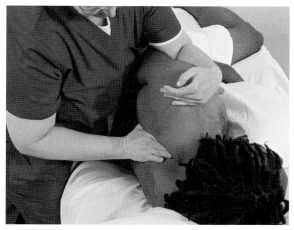

Figure 8.16 Position for addressing the scapular border and for providing movement to the scapula with the patient in the sidelying position.

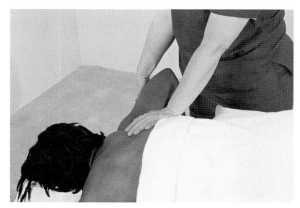

Figure 8.17 Shoulder area: position for active and passive range of motion, muscle testing, and muscle energy methods for lengthening and stretching.

Next, address the superficial fascia by assessing for tissue bind. Always observe for superficial fascia involvement in adjacent areas, such as the tissue leading into the torso and neck.

- Move the skin to identify any areas of bind in the superficial connective tissue. Notice whether any bind areas correspond to the areas of skin reddening or gooseflesh identified by the light stroking. Pay particular attention to any scars, because connective tissue bind is common at these sites.
- Treat any superficial fascial bind with myofascial release methods. Address these areas by slowly moving the tissue into ease, applying drag to move it the direction it most easily wants to go.

- Multiple load directions can be used. For example, if the skin and superficial fascia want to move up and to the left on the deltoid, that would be the direction of the forces introduced. Hold ease position for up to 30 seconds. Reassess.

The musculature needs to be addressed in layers systematically, moving superficial to deep.

- Begin on the posterior aspect to address the midthorax region that connects with the shoulder. This area is covered by the trapezius (first layer of the muscle). This area was addressed while massaging the torso, but now is massaged again in relationship to the shoulder. Carry the strokes into the posterior deltoid.
- Use gliding with a compressive element from the upper, middle, and lower aspects of the trapezius, slowly dragging tissue toward its distal attachment at the shoulder. Repeat with the latissimus dorsi again in relationship to shoulder function and carry the stroke into the posterior deltoid. If any area binds against the drag, working across the grain of the muscle and in the opposite direction may be beneficial.
- Any areas that redden may be housing trigger point activity. Trigger points can cause muscles to fire out of sequence, so it is important to restore as much normalcy to the tissue as possible. Address using the least invasive methods first.
- Finish the area with kneading, making sure that the muscle tissue easily lifts off the layer underneath it.
- If adhesions are identified, introduce a bend, shear, or torsion force until the tissue becomes more pliable.
- Repeat this sequence bilaterally. Once the surface tissue is addressed, then the second layer of muscle is massaged.

The main muscles being addressed in this sequence are the rhomboids, infraspinatus, teres major and minor, subscapularis, and the deeper layers of the deltoid muscle.

- Begin at the vertebral attachments of the rhomboids and use a compressive gliding parallel to the muscle fibers, deep enough to address this layer of tissue. Maintain a broad base of contact so that the surface tissue does not tighten to guard against poking.
- Glide toward the scapula. Repeat three or four times, each time slower and at a slightly different angle.
- Knead slowly across the fiber direction using enough pressure and lift to ensure that you are

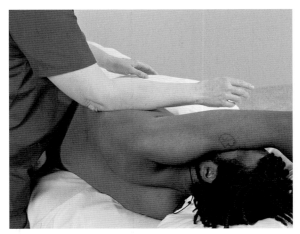

Figure 8.18 Position for addressing rib movement (especially effective for the anterior serratus).

affecting muscle fiber in this layer. These methods address both the connective tissue and neuromuscular elements of the muscle. Repeat three or four times, increasing the depth and drag each time and being aware of the muscle moving with the application.

- Next, address the supraspinatus. Glide from the medial border of the scapula toward the acromion. Work above the spine of the scapula to access the supraspinatus. The soft heel of the palm of the hand may fit better in these areas than the forearm. Reverse the direction and then slowly and deeply knead the area. Make sure the upper trapezius is not binding on the supraspinatus.
- Repeat sequence from the medial and lower medial border to address the infraspinatus and the teres major and minor.
- Using gliding and kneading, massage the triceps toward the attachment on the lateral border of the scapula.
- Next, slowly and deeply knead the posterior and medial deltoid.

This sidelying position is effective for addressing the latissimus and teres major and minor attachment on the arm (Fig. 8.18).

- Repeat the sequences described and add placement of the arm over the head. Perform active and passive movements while the area is being massaged.
- Finish by gliding and kneading the entire area. Add oscillation (shaking and rocking) in various positions. As a finishing stroke, drain the area.

ARMS

The arm functions as an open chain most of the time. This means that the wrist, elbow, and shoulder joints can function independently of each other. However, even in open chain function, the joints and tissues influence each other. When the hands are fixed, as when doing a pushup or some sort of handspring, the chain is closed, meaning that the wrist, elbow, and shoulder function in a coordinated movement.

The muscles of the arm primarily work at the elbow. The triceps and biceps cross two joints and function at the shoulder, as well. Some of the muscles of the forearm also cross the elbow.

The gait reflexes coordinate interaction between the arms and legs with flexor, adductor, and internal rotation pattern on the left arm and right leg during forward motion (concentric contraction) working together. Antagonists are functioning eccentrically, decelerating the movement with some inhibition to allow stability and agility during movement. Movement then reverses to the right arm and left leg and the opposite pattern is activated. At the same time, the extensor, abductor, and external rotation pattern is facilitating in concentric contraction in the opposite pattern while the antagonist pattern is functioning eccentrically. This back and forth gait movement is necessary for agility and postural balance. It can become disrupted during illness and injury or repetitive training activities especially if the movement patterns are altered.

It is often necessary to work with the arms and legs in some sort of coordinated pattern to increase the effectiveness of the massage. For example, the client can actively swing the knee back and forth in an open chain position while massage is being applied to the opposite arm. The flow of the massage application can proceed from the left arm to the right leg and then from the right arm to the left leg. Another example is to work with the right biceps and the left hamstring, then work with the right triceps and the left quadriceps, and vice versa. The sidelying position gives the best access for optimal body mechanics but the supine or prone position can be used as well.

The muscles of the arm are in two layers. The two heads of the biceps and the three heads of the triceps are thick muscles, each with attachments on the shaft of the humerus that can bind. The brachialis and anconeus constitute the second layer of muscles.

The arm can be massaged in all basic positions and is often addressed more than once during the massage. The back of the arm is accessible when the client is in the prone position. The lateral and medial aspects can be reached when the client is in the sidelying position. With the client in the supine position, the anterior arm

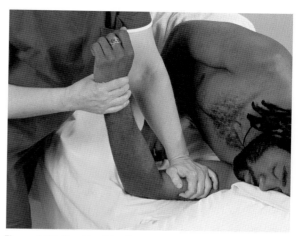

Figure 8.19 Combined loading: compression and movement. Internal and external rotation, effective alternative for kneading methods.

is easily reached, and the lateral, medial, and posterior regions can be massaged as well.

These muscles need to glide over the bone, so it is important to make sure that the tissues roll over the humerus (Fig. 8.19).

Procedures for the arms

- Massage of the arm naturally progresses from the shoulder to the forearm and then to the hand. Assessing all range of motion patterns and muscle strength will indicate which structures are short and which are long.
- The arm can be massaged in the supine (Fig. 8.20), sidelying, or prone position. Massage begins with superficial work and progresses to deeper layers and then finishes off with superficial work. Initial applications are palpation, range of motion, strength, and neurologic assessment. This sequence focuses on massage of the arm in the prone and sidelying position.
- Move the arm actively and passively through all joint motion patterns. Compare active and passive movements of the arms for balanced function.
- Gently compress the elbow joint to make sure there is no intracapsular involvement. If pain exists, refer. Massage can be performed but be aware that muscle tension patterns may be guarding the response, creating appropriate compensation.

Any areas that are not functioning optimally should be noted and reassessed after they are massaged.

- Systematically, lightly stroke the area to assess for temperature changes, skin texture, and damp

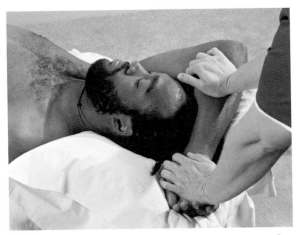

Figure 8.20 Position for massage of the arm (patient supine).

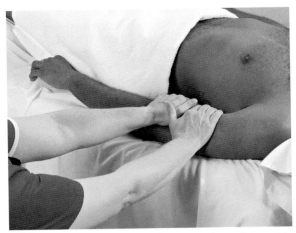

Figure 8.21 Kneading of the arm (patient supine and therapist kneeling).

areas. Observe for skin reddening (histamine response) and gooseflesh (pilomotor).

- Increase the pressure slightly and assess for superficial fascial bind, changes in skin pliability, and accumulation of interstitial fluid. If increased fluid pressure is evident, use lymphatic drain.
- Next address the superficial fascia by assessing for tissue bind, always observing for involvement in adjacent areas such as the tissue leading into the shoulder.
- Move the skin to identify any areas of bind in the superficial connective tissue. Notice whether any bind areas correspond to the areas of skin reddening or gooseflesh identified by the light stroking. Pay particular attention to any potential connective tissue bind in areas of scar tissue.
- Treat areas of superficial fascial bind with myofascial release methods. Address these areas of bind by slowly moving the tissue into ease, dragging it the way it most wants to go.
- Multiple load directions can be used.
- Bending and torsion forces using compression and kneading can also be introduced (Fig. 8.21).
- Begin at the elbow, with the client prone. Carry the strokes into the posterior deltoid and into the scapular attachment.
- Reverse the direction, using compression ending at the elbow and then glide again toward the shoulder. Repeat three or four times, each time slower and deeper while maintaining a broad based contact to protect the more superficial tissue and reduce the potential for guarding.
- If any area binds against the drag, working across the grain of the muscle and in the opposite direction may be beneficial.

Any areas that redden may be housing trigger point activity. Because trigger points can cause muscles to fire out of sequence, it is important to restore as much normalcy to the tissue as possible.

Once the surface tissue is addressed, the deep surface of the triceps muscle is massaged. It is important to make sure that the surface tissue and the fascial separation between muscle segments are not adhered together in any way.

- Use compressive gliding parallel to the fibers and deep enough to address this layer of tissue. Broaden the base of contact so that the surface tissue does not tighten, to guard against poking. Adding passive movement to the compression serves to move the bone a bit against the deep tissue, creating combined loading. Repeat three or four times, each time slower and with a slightly different angle.
- Next, glide and knead slowly across the fiber direction, using enough pressure and lift to ensure that you are affecting muscle fiber and that the tissue can slide around the bone. These methods address both the connective tissue and neuromuscular elements of the muscle. Repeat three or four times, increasing the depth and drag each time and being aware of the muscle moving with the application.
- With the client in the sidelying position, place the client's arm on the torso. This makes it easier for the massage therapist to use the forearm to massage the client's arm.
- Systematically lightly stroke the area to assess for temperature changes, skin texture, and damp areas. Observe for skin reddening (histamine response) and gooseflesh (pilomotor).

- Increase the pressure slightly and assess for superficial fascial bind, changes in skin pliability, and accumulation of interstitial fluid.
- Begin with lighter pressure directed toward the shoulder, covering the entire area.
- Then introduce pumping broad based compression, combined with active and passive movement, by having the client flex and extend the elbow and shoulder, and then performing passive movement.
- If in doubt about the presence of fluid retention, assume it is there and drain the area. Drainage direction would be toward the axilla.
- Next, address the superficial fascia by assessing for tissue bind, always observing for involvement in adjacent areas such as the tissue leading into the shoulder, neck, and forearm.
- Tension force can be added. Have the client actively or passively move the arm into slight flexion and extension and then back into the original position while the massage is applied. Repeat the movement back and forth until a change is noted. Work slowly and deliberately, interspersing lymphatic drain type stroking every minute or so.
- When an area that is bothering the client is located, familiar symptoms will be reproduced. Compression combined with muscle energy methods, from the least invasive of positional release to the more aggressive integrated methods, can be used to create a shift in function. The goal is to temporally inhibit the motor tone of the muscle bundle that is problematic so that it can be lengthened to the appropriate resting length and the client feels reduced pressure on the nerves or vessels.
- Finish by gliding and kneading the entire area in the supine position. Add oscillation (rocking and shaking) in various positions. As a finishing stroke, drain the area.

FOREARM, WRIST, AND HAND

The forearm muscles function to work the wrist and fingers. They also weakly assist elbow movements. This can be an issue when the elbow, wrist, and fingers are functioning as a unit, as while throwing a ball, when the fingers have to grasp (isometric) but the wrist and elbow have to move (concentric and eccentric), thus creating the potential for rubbing at the attachments. The end result from repetitive movements like these can be tendonitis and bursitis. Muscles near the elbow and wrist allow supination and pronation of the hand. Repetitive movement is common for these tissues, as is repetitive strain illness and injury. The goal of the massage is to maintain normal tissue

function so that repetitive movement does not become repetitive strain.

The muscles of the forearm are categorized as superficial, intermediate, and deep, and are best addressed as three layers that include the supinator, pronator teres, and pronator quadratus. The muscles can also adhere to each other, both one on top of the other and in the side-by-side positions. Because the movements of the fingers have a slightly different range than the wrist, it is essential that these muscles glide easily over one another. The superficial muscle layer primarily functions at the wrist, with some activity at the elbow, whereas the deep layers work the fingers, with some activity at the wrist.

The bellies of these muscles are closer to the elbow, and they taper to the tendons in the wrist and fingers. It is important to gauge pressure of the massage, which is more intense along the proximal half of the forearm where the muscle bulk is located. Connective tissue binding often shows up in the distal half of the forearm and into the hand.

Typically, the forearm or flat, soft palm of the hand is used to massage the client's forearm, but the foot also works very well to apply compression. The arch of the foot fits nicely over the muscle bulk and the client can provide active movement of the wrist and finger while the compression is being applied. This is effective in reducing tone and connective tissue bind in the muscles resulting from repetitive movements.

Procedures for the forearm, wrist, and hand

The massage pattern is very similar to that presented for all body areas. Massage of the wrist and hand initially involves working with the muscles of the forearm in relationship to the action of the wrist, fingers, and thumb (Fig. 8.22).

- Systematically compress the muscles of the forearm, beginning at the elbow and working toward the wrist while the client moves the wrist and fingers, back and forth in circles, or makes and releases a fist.
- To isolate a particular muscle function related to a wrist or finger action, have the client move the wrist or finger in the way that creates the symptom and then palpate the forearm muscles to see which ones are activated. Then use compression or gliding while the client moves the wrist or fingers to affect the identified area. Occasionally, trigger point type application is necessary.

Once this is complete, address range of motion of the wrist. The wrist is often jammed, with a reduction in joint play. A general method to restore joint play is to

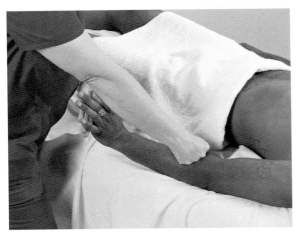

Figure 8.22 Loose fist compression of the wrist extensors with active movement.

use the 'mobilization with movement' sequence. This sequence involves the traction of a joint and moving the joint into the ease and pain free position by the therapist. The client is passive while the position is found. The position is then maintained by the therapist, and the client actively moves the joint through a range of motions. For the wrist, having the client move the wrist in a circle will be effective.

Next, address the intrinsic muscles of the hand.

- Systematically work the area, using compression and gliding of the soft tissues between the fingers and the web of the thumb and on the palm.
- To assist lymphatic movement, use rhythmic compression to stimulate the network of lymphatic vessels in the palm.
- Trigger points are commonly found in the opponens pollicis and other muscles of the palm near the wrist. Positional release works well: apply compression on the point while the client moves the associated finger or thumb.
- Direct pressure or tapping can stimulate the acupuncture points at the side of each nail. An easy way to do this is to squeeze, release, and repeat three or four times, on the lateral and medial side of each finger- and thumbnail.
- There is also a major acupuncture point in the web of the thumb used for pain control, nausea, and other dysfunction. Use rhythmic on/off compression to this point to aid general homoeostasis.
- The finger and thumb joints often become jammed, and the 'mobilization with movement' sequence described previously can be used on each joint of the fingers and thumb. The fingers are hinge joints, as is the distal joint of the thumb. Once traction is applied

and the ease position found, the client moves the area back and forth. The thumb is a saddle joint; therefore circular movement is more effective.

- Finally, address the metacarpal joints. Moving the carpal bones back and forth is effective.
- To finish off, use oscillation (rocking and shaking) and lymphatic drain.

HIP

The hip is a complex musculoskeletal unit. The joint structure is mobile, relying on a deep joint capsule, ligaments, muscles, and fascia to provide stability. It is less mobile than the shoulder. The movement of the sacroiliac (SI) and femoral joints in a coordinated fashion is necessary for both maximal mobility and stability of the area.

The inner (local muscle) unit (deep lateral rotator muscles), coupled with an extensive ligament structure, holds and guides the femur in the acetabulum, using the bones of the pelvis as a broad based attachment point. The gluteus maximus is an expansive outer unit (global muscles) interacting with the contralateral latissimus dorsi and ipsilateral tensor fasciae latae and IT band to provide stability and force closure from the lumbar back and SI joint area down into the knee. Combined with the gluteus medius and minimus, the gluteus maximus can be compared to the deltoid muscle of the shoulder.

The gluteal muscles interact with the adductors to provide a force couple arrangement during gait.

The psoas and gluteus maximus can become dysfunctional if core stability is inadequate. The gluteus maximus is often inhibited, caused by a short and tight psoas. Muscle activation sequences of the global muscles of the hip are affected if the lower abdominal group does not fire normally. In this type of dysfunction, the psoas and rectus abdominus will fire too soon (synergistic dominance) and inhibit the gluteus maximus. The hip extension firing pattern will in turn become dysfunctional, causing lumbar and hamstring shortening. The knee can be affected. Calf muscles, especially the gastrocnemius, then begin to dominate, leading to both knee and ankle dysfunction.

Muscle fascial components in the torso affect the stability and mobility of the hip. Involvement of gait reflexes necessitates that the shoulders and hips function in coordinated movement.

Nerve impingement by the lumbar and sacral plexus refers pain to the hip and leg.

Procedures for the hip

The hip is usually massaged with the client in the prone positions. Massage of the torso naturally

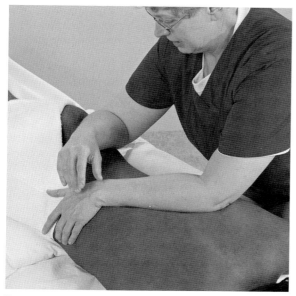

Figure 8.23 Forearm gliding using various pressure depths, directions, and speeds to assess the gluteal area.

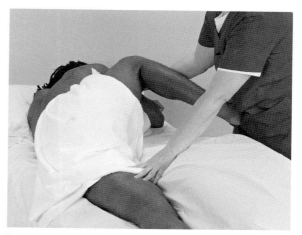

Figure 8.24 Position for movement methods for hip (patient sidelying): flexion and external rotation.

progresses to the hip. Assessment of all range of motion patterns and muscle strength will indicate which structures are short and which are long.

Massage begins with superficial work, and progresses to deeper layers, and then finishes off with superficial work. Initial applications are palpation, range of motion, strength, and neurologic assessment (Fig. 8.23). The hip should be first actively and then passively moved though flexion, extension, internal and external rotation, adduction, and abduction as well as full circumduction (Fig. 8.24). This part of assessment can most easily be done, with least restriction and greatest range of motion, with the client in the sidelying position. Active and passive movement of left and right hip should be compared.

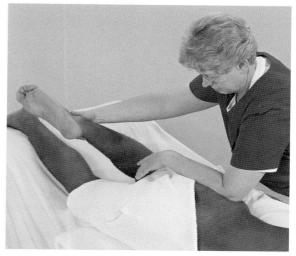

Figure 8.25 An example of inhibitory pressure combined with joint movement to create a combined loading effect. Movement can be passive to introduce mechanical force or active to introduce muscle energy methods.

- Compress the joint gently to make sure that there is no intracapsular involvement. If there is, refer the client to the appropriate specialist. Massage can be performed, but be aware that muscle tension patterns may be guarding, creating appropriate compensation.
- Bend the client's knee and internally and externally rotate the leg (Fig. 8.25). Initial movement occurs in the hip joint, and secondary movement occurs at the SI joint. In general, 45° of internal and external rotation in this position indicates normal function. Any alteration in this pattern indicates potential for both SI joint and hip joint dysfunction.

Any areas that are not functioning optimally should be noted and reassessed after the massage of the area. If the pattern does not normalize, referral to appropriate medical personnel is necessary.

Systematically, lightly stroke the area to assess for temperature changes, skin texture, and damp areas. Observe for skin reddening (histamine response) and gooseflesh (pilomotor). Increase the pressure slightly and assess for superficial fascial bind, changes in skin pliability, and accumulation of interstitial fluid, as indicated by boggy or edematous tissue and/or increased skin pressure (like a water balloon).

- If in doubt about the presence of fluid retention, assume it is there and drain the area.
- Next, address the superficial fascia by assessing for tissue bind, always observing for involvement in adjacent areas such as the tissue leading into the torso and leg.
- Move the skin to identify any areas of bind in the superficial connective tissue. Notice whether any bind areas correspond to the areas of skin reddening or gooseflesh identified by the light stroking. Pay particular attention to any scars because connective tissue bind is common at these sites.
- Treat areas of superficial fascial bind with myofascial release methods. Address these areas by slowly moving the tissue into ease, dragging it the way it wants to go. Multiple load directions can be used. For example, if the skin and superficial fascia want to move up and to the right near the sacrum, then that would be the direction of the forces introduced. Hold the ease position for up to 30 seconds
- Then work into the bind with a slow, sustained drag on the binding tissues, with the lines of tension being introduced at each end of the binding tissue. Place your flat forearm or hand at one end of the bind and the other forearm or hand at the other end of the bind.
- Contact the tissue gently but firmly, pressing only as deep as the superficial fascial layer, and separate the forearms or hands, creating a tension force into the binding tissue.
- Maintain the drag on the tissue until the thixotropic nature of the ground substance is affected and becomes more pliable. Subtle changes in the lines of force serve to load and unload the tissue, resulting in hysteresis. Active and passive range of motion can serve to load and unload tissues.
- The musculature needs to be addressed in layers, moving from superficial to deep. It is important to make sure that muscle layers are not adhered to each other. If adhesions exist, one muscle layer should be sheared off the next, deeper layer. Layers tend to stick where the gluteus maximus weaves into the IT band at a lengthy musculotendinous junction. Use a wave-like motion to assess the tissue. It is helpful to place the client so that the surface layer is in a slack position with the attachments of the muscle close together, and bolstering the client so that he/she stays relaxed. In some situations, the sidelying position may be better for this.

Begin on the posterior side to address the lumbar region that connects with the hip. This area was addressed while massaging the torso but now is massaged in relationship to the hip.

- Carry the strokes into the gluteus maximus. Use gliding with a compressive element and drag toward the hip. Repeat with the latissimus dorsi in relationship to hip function.
- Begin at the shoulder and carry the stroke all the way into the opposite gluteus maximus. If any area binds against the drag, working across the grain of the muscle and in the opposite direction may be beneficial.
- Any areas that redden may be housing trigger point activity. Because trigger points can cause muscles to fire out of sequence, it is important to restore as much normalcy to the tissue as possible.
- To increase circulation to the area and shift neuroresponses of trigger points, move the skin into multiple directions of ease over the suspected trigger point area and hold the ease position for up to 30 seconds.
- If this does not relieve the tenderness, positional release is the next option, followed by muscle energy methods, if necessary.
- Local lengthening of the tissue containing the trigger points is effective.
- Finish the area with kneading, making sure that the muscle tissue lifts easily off the layer underneath it.

The main muscles being addressed are portions of gluteus medius, gluteus minimus, and deep lateral hip rotators. It is helpful to place the surface layer of tissue in a slack position by passively supporting the hip in extension. This can be done either in prone or side-lying position.

- Begin at the iliac crest attachments and use a compressive gliding deep enough to address this layer of tissue. Broaden the base of contact so that the surface tissue does not tighten to guard against poking.
- Glide toward the greater trochanter. Repeat three or four times, each time slower and at a slightly different angle.
- Glide and knead slowly across the fiber direction, using enough pressure and lift to ensure that you are affecting muscle fiber in this layer. These methods address both the connective tissue and the neuromuscular elements of the muscles. Repeat three or four times, increasing the depth and drag each time, and being aware of the muscle moving with the application.
- Next, address the deep lateral hip rotators.
- With the surface layer still in a slack position, apply a broad based compression using the forearm into the space between the sacrum and the

greater trochanter. This is best accomplished in the prone position.

- Bend the client's knee and move the hip back and forth from medial to lateral rotation. This can be thought of as moving 'into the 4 and out of the 4.' The action can be active or passive.
- Repeat three or four times, slightly changing the angle. Do not put constant compression on the sciatic nerve. Lighten the compressive force at least every 30 seconds to allow for proper circulation to the area.

The sidelying position is effective for addressing the gluteus medius and tensor fasciae latae on the upper side and quadratus femoris on the opposite (closer to the table) side. Use a broad based compression with the forearm on the gluteal tissues.

Finish by gliding and kneading the entire area. Add oscillation (rocking and shaking) in various positions. As a finishing stroke, drain the area.

THIGH

Lumbar and sacral plexus impingement can cause radiating pain in the legs. The muscles that most often cause impingement are the quadratus lumborum and multifidi. Lumbar plexus impingement causes radiating pain in the thigh whereas sacral plexus impingement causes radiating pain in the back of the thigh and calf.

The thigh and leg are in closed chain function most of the time, meaning that the hip, knee, and ankle do not function independently of each other. Even in open chain function, these joints and tissues influence each other.

The muscles of the thigh primarily work at the knee. The rectus femoris, hamstring group, and sartorius cross two joints and function at both the hip and knee. Some of the muscles of the leg also cross the knee, such as the gastrocnemius.

The gait reflexes coordinate interaction between the arms and legs with a flexor, adductor, and internal rotation pattern on left arm and right leg during forward motion (concentric contraction), facilitating with antagonists that are functioning eccentrically for deceleration; and then concentric contraction transfers into the right arm and left leg, and the opposite pattern is activated. At the same time, the extensor, abductor, and external rotation pattern is facilitating in concentric contraction in the contralateral side of the body, and the antagonist pattern is functioning eccentrically. This back and forth movement of gait is necessary for postural stability, fluid motion, and agility.

Gait function can become disrupted during illness and injury, and repetitive training activities. It is often necessary to work with the arms and legs in some sort of coordinated pattern to increase effectiveness of the massage. For example, the client can actively bend the elbow back and forth in an open chain position while massage is being applied to the opposite leg, or the flow of the massage application may proceed from the left arm to the right leg and then from the right arm to the left leg. Another way to explain this would be to work with the right biceps and the left hamstring, then the right quadriceps and the left triceps, and vice versa. The sidelying position gives access for optimal body mechanics, but the supine or prone position can be used as well.

The thigh muscles are basically in two layers. In the superficial layer, the three heads of the hamstrings are thick muscles that superiorly attach in close proximity on the ischial tuberosity and can bind or get stuck together. The four heads of the quadriceps are also thick muscles, three of which have proximal attachments on the shaft of the femur, and all four have distal attachments on the tibia, which can become a source of binding if layers are stuck together. The vastus intermedius is the main second layer muscle.

The thigh also contains the large group of adductor muscles. This group is very involved in core stability and antigravity function.

The thigh can be massaged in all basic positions and is often addressed more than one time during the massage (Figs 8.26–8.29). When the client is in the prone position, the back of the thigh is accessible. With the client in the sidelying position, the adductors and IT band are accessible. With the client supine, the anterior thigh is easily reached. These muscles need to

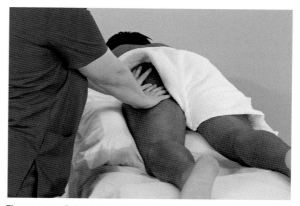

Figure 8.26 Palpation of the skin of the lower limb – assessment using skin drag, tissue bind and hot and cold.

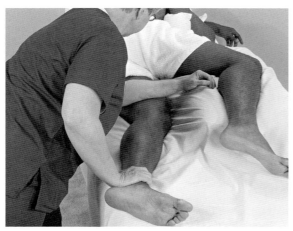

Figure 8.27 Thigh position (patient sidelying): gliding used at various pressure depths, speeds, directions, and durations for assessment and treatment.

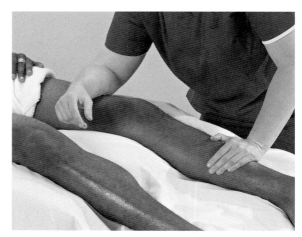

Figure 8.29 Forearm gliding to influence fluid movement: primarily venous blood or to reduce motor tone.

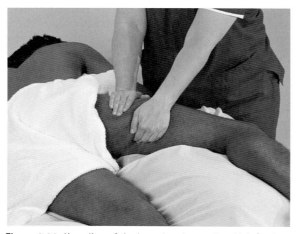

Figure 8.28 Kneading of the lateral and posterior thigh (patient sidelying).

glide over the bone, so rolling tissues over the femur is important.

Massage of the thigh naturally progresses from hip and calf. Assessment of all range of motion patterns and muscle strength will indicate which structures are short and which are long.

Like other body regions, massage begins with superficial work, progresses to deeper layers, and then finishes off with superficial work. Initial applications are palpation assessment, range of motion, strength, and neurologic assessment. Massage typically begins with the client in the prone position.

- Move the thigh and knee both actively and passively through flexion, extension, and internal

and external rotation. Compare active and passive movement of the right and left limbs.
- Gently, compress the knee joints to make sure that there is no intracapsular involvement. If there is, refer the client to the appropriate specialist. Massage can still be performed, but be aware that muscle tension patterns may be guarding to create appropriate compensation.

Any areas that are not functioning optimally should be noted and reassessed after the area is massaged.

- Systematically lightly stroke the area to assess for temperature changes, skin texture, and damp areas. Observe for skin reddening.
- Increase the pressure slightly and assess for superficial fascial bind, changes in skin pliability, and accumulation of interstitial fluid as indicated by boggy or edematous tissue and/or increased skin pressure.
- If increased fluid pressure is evident, drain the area using a combination of light pressure to drag the skin and deeper, rhythmic, broad based compression and kneading to stimulate the deeper vessels.
- Begin with lighter pressure directed toward the groin, covering the entire area.

Next, address the superficial fascia by assessing for tissue bind, always observing for involvement in adjacent areas such as the tissue leading into the hip and knee. Pay particular attention to the IT band and the junctions of the hamstring and quadriceps to this connective tissue structure.

- Move the skin to identify any areas of bind in the superficial connective tissue. Notice whether any

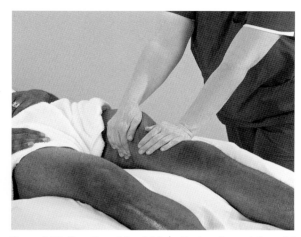

Figure 8.30 Kneading of the thigh (patient supine and therapist standing) influences fluid movement and muscle, motor, and fascial tone.

bind areas correspond to the areas of skin reddening or gooseflesh identified by the light stroking. Pay particular attention to any scars, because connective tissue bind is common at these sites.

- Treat areas of superficial fascial bind with myofascial release methods. Bending and torsion forces using kneading can be introduced, and these methods are especially effective on the IT band. Subtle changes in the lines of force serve to load and unload the tissue.
- Do not use tension force application (gliding) with deep pressure over the IT band. Compression of the nerve structures may result. Instead use kneading.
- Address muscle layers systematically, moving from superficial to deep.

It is important to make sure that muscle layers are not adhered to each other. This is particularly important in the thigh. The most common locations of adherence are at the rectus femoris on the vastus intermedius, at the edges of the two medial hamstrings (semimembranosus and semitendinosus) as they meet in the middle of the posterior thigh, and where the vastus lateralis and lateral hamstring (biceps femoris) weave into the iliotibial band near their distal insertions. In both the quadriceps and hamstrings groups, it is necessary to make sure that the heads of the muscles are not stuck together, as each part of the muscles has somewhat of a different angle of pull. One muscle layer should be sheared off the next deeper layer and from the structures next to it. It is helpful to place the client so that the surface layer is in a slack position with the attachments of the muscle close together and bolstering the client so that he/she stays relaxed (Fig. 8.30).

- Begin at the knee. Carry the strokes into the posterior hip. Reverse the direction using compression toward the knee, and then glide again toward the hip.
- Repeat three or four times, each time slower and deeper, maintaining a broad based contact to protect the more surface tissue and reduce the potential for guarding.

If any area binds against the drag, working across the grain of the muscle and in the opposite direction may be beneficial.

- Glide slowly across the fiber direction, using enough pressure to be sure that you are affecting muscle fiber. This method addresses both the connective tissue and the neuromuscular elements of the muscle.
- Repeat three or four times, increasing the depth and drag each time, being aware of the muscle moving with the application.

With the client in the sidelying position, the medial, lateral, posterior, and anterior thigh can be massaged, and range of motion is not limited by the table. This is the best position for massage of the medial and lateral thigh. The supine position is most effective for massage of the anterior thigh.

When an area is located that creates symptoms that are bothering the client, compression combined with muscle energy methods, from the least invasive positional release to integrated methods, can be used. The goal is to temporally inhibit the motor tone of the muscle bundle that is problematic so that it can be lengthened to the appropriate resting length and reduce pressure on the nerves or vessels.

When addressing deeper tissue layers, always remember to protect the more superficial muscles by applying pressure gradually and with as broad a base of contact as the area with allow.

- Finish by gliding and kneading the entire area. Add oscillation (rocking and shaking) in various positions.
- As a finishing stroke, drain the area.

LEG, ANKLE, AND FOOT

The leg muscles function at the knee, ankle, and foot. Repetitive movement is common for these muscles, as is repetitive strain illness and injury. The goal of the massage is to maintain normal tissue function so that repetitive movement does not become repetitive strain. The muscles of the leg are categorized as superficial, intermediate, and deep. The muscles can adhere to each other in their side by side positions and between

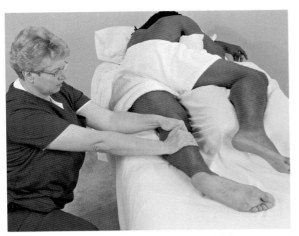

Figure 8.31 Kneading of the calf to assess and influence muscle movement, fascial tone, and movement of fluid, especially in the microvascular structures.

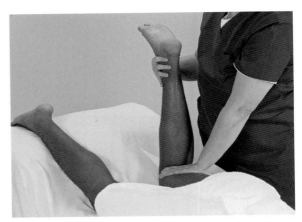

Figure 8.32 Inhibitory pressure to the gastrocnemius and hamstring attachments.

layers. It is especially important that the popliteus, soleus, and gastrocnemius are not stuck together. The superficial muscle layer primarily functions at the ankle, with some activity at the knee. The intermediate layer functions at the ankle, and the deep layer works the toes, with some activity at the ankle.

The belly of these muscles lies closer to the knee, and they taper to the tendons in the ankle and foot. It is important to gauge pressure. Deeper pressure is used in the proximal half of the lower leg where the muscle bulk is located. Connective tissue binding often occurs in the distal half of the lower leg into the foot. This is common at the Achilles tendon and plantar fascia.

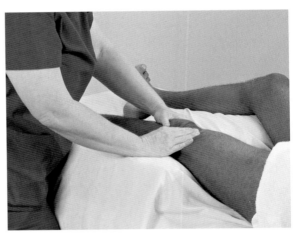

Figure 8.33 Palpation assessment of patellar mobility.

Procedures for the leg, ankle, and foot (Figs 8.31–8.34)

The knee joint is complex and should be addressed by massage of the thigh and lower leg. In addition, make gentle movements of the patella to ensure it moves freely.

The pes anserinus tendon on the medial aspect of the tibia is where the distal attachments of the sartorius, gracilis, and semitendinosus blend into one structure just below the knee. Bending can interfere with knee function. Connective tissue application is effective.

The massage pattern is very similar to those presented in other areas. All three basic positions can be used. Massage of the ankle and foot first involves working with the muscles of the lower leg in relationship to the action of the ankle, foot, and toes. Apply systematic compression to the muscles of the lower leg, beginning at the knee and working toward the ankle

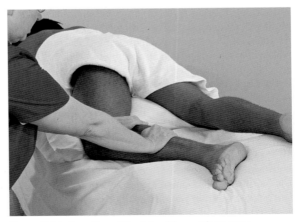

Figure 8.34 Kneading of the lateral leg: patient prone.

while the client moves the ankle and toes in circles (Fig. 8.35).

To isolate a particular muscle pain in the ankle or foot action, have the client move the ankle or foot in the way that creates the symptom; palpate the muscles to see which ones are activated and then address those muscles (Fig. 8.36).

Once this is complete, attention is giving to the range of motion of the ankle. Proper ankle mobility is necessary for knee and hip function. Often knee pain is related to disruption of ankle function. The ankle may be jammed, with a reduction in joint play. A general method to restore joint play is the 'mobilization with movement' sequence, which involves traction of a joint and moving the joint into the ease and pain free position by the therapist. The client is passive while the position is being located. The ease position is maintained by the therapist while the client actively moves the joint through a full range of motion.

The intrinsic muscles of the foot are addressed next. Sidelying is the best position.

- Systematically work using compression and gliding of the soft tissue of the sole of the foot.
- Rhythmic compression of the network of lymphatic vessels in the sole of the foot will assist lymphatic movement (Fig. 8.37).
- Direct pressure or tapping can stimulate acupuncture points at the side of each toenail. There is also a network of lymphatic vessels in the sole of the foot that, when rhythmically compressed, will assist lymphatic movement. An easy way to do this is to squeeze, release, and repeat three or four times, on the lateral and medial side of each toenail.
- When the tarsal and toe joints become jammed, joint play methods can increase mobility in this area. The toes are hinge joints and once traction is applied and the ease position found, the client moves the area back and forth.
- To finish off, use oscillation and lymphatic drain.

Thorough and specific massage of the foot is essential for clients. Awareness of reflexology is helpful and integrating it into the massage is appropriate (Figs 8.37–8.39).

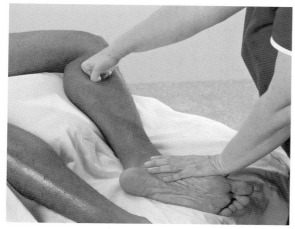

Figure 8.35 Compression and movement at knee attachment structures. Notice the position of the leg.

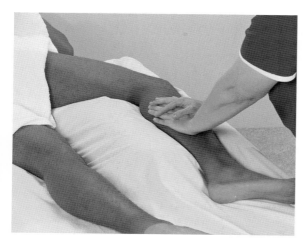

Figure 8.36 Compression with the palms to address fluid movement, particularly arterial blood flow.

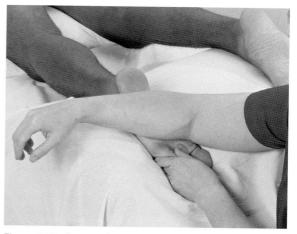

Figure 8.37 Compression of the sole of the foot with the forearm.

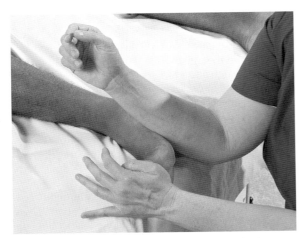

Figure 8.38 Compression and tension forces, combined loading.

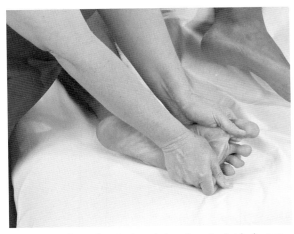

Figure 8.39 Spreading the toes to lengthen the intrinsic muscles of the foot.

Box 8.1 Just between you and me

I have performed some variation of this protocol at least 20 000 times over the last 25+ years of practice. It really is the same thing over and over, moving from one region of the body to another and only changing the names of the bones, joints, and muscles. However, there are specific cautions and suggestions for particular regions, and textbooks have a vital role as reference sources as well. I believe many readers will use specific sections of this protocol during massage, either while learning or later on, to recall details. So this is a deliberate strategy: you can find what you need about any particular region of the body as you need to, using resource material. This protocol in all its variations is what I consider my 'weekly house-cleaning massage.'

PROTOCOL FOR THE ILL, FRAGILE, OR PRE- AND POST SURGERY CLIENT

30–45 minutes – no assessment. General inhibition pleasure-based application.

Face and head

- Lightly and systematically, stroke the face. Massage in the direction of the smile.
- Address the muscle structures. Light to moderate compressive force is adequate to address the area. To increase circulation to the area and shift neuroresponses, move the skin into multiple directions of ease, and hold the ease position for up to 30–60 seconds.

A combination of compression (acupressure) on points if combined with a light rhythmic on/off pressure in about 10 repetitions against the sinus cavities encourages drainage.

To finish the face, return to the initial light stroking. Working with the face is relaxing. Therefore, if the face is done first, it can set the stage for a calming massage; if the face is done at the end of the session, it will gently finish the massage.

Place the hands on either side of the head by the ears.

- Some clients enjoy having their hair gently stroked and pulled.
- Compression to the sides of the head and to the front and back, coupled with a scratching motion to the scalp, can be very pleasant.

Neck

- Address this area with the client prone and sidelying.

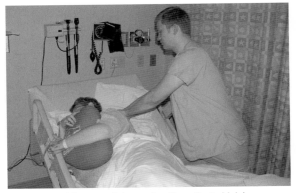

Figure 8.40 Massage of the neck with patient sidelying. (Photograph courtesy Laura Cochran.)

- Systematically, lightly stroke the skin. Increase the pressure slightly as is comfortable, while slowly moving the tissue into ease.
- Use gliding with a compressive element, beginning at the middle of the back of the head at the trapezius attachments, and slowly drag the tissue to the distal attachment of the trapezius at the acromion process and lateral third of the clavicle.
- With the client prone, begin again at the head and glide toward the acromion. Then, reverse the direction and work from distal to proximal.
- Then knead and glide across the muscle fibers, making sure that bending, shear, and torsion forces are only sufficient to create a pleasurable sensation.
- Gentle rocking rhythmic ranges of motion of the area (oscillation) may be used to continue to relax the area.

Anterior torso

- Massage begins superficially and progresses to deeper tissue layers and then finishes off with superficial work again. In general, as the massage progresses hold the tissue in ease position until release is felt, or up to 30–60 seconds.
- Use gliding with a compressive element beginning at the shoulder and work from the distal attachment of the pectoralis major at the arm toward the sternum following fiber direction. This can be done in supine or sidelying position with the client rolled. Repeat three or four times, each time increasing the drag and moving slower.
- Move to the abdomen and knead slowly across the fiber direction. The abdominal organs can be rolled to encourage peristalsis.
- Rhythmic compression to the entire anterior torso area simulates the lymphatic flow, blood circulation, and relaxed breathing.

Posterior torso

- As described previously, massage begins superficially and progresses to deeper layers and then finishes off with superficial work. It is helpful to place the client so that the surface layer is in a slack position by positioning the attachments of the muscle close together and propping the clients so that he/she can remain relaxed. In some situations, the sidelying position may be better for this.
- Use gliding with a compressive element, beginning at the iliac crest, and work diagonally along the fibers of the latissimus dorsi, ending at the axilla. Repeat three or four times, each time increasing the drag and moving slower.

- Move up to the thoracolumbar junction and repeat the same sequence on the lower trapezius.
- Then begin near the tip of the shoulder and glide toward the middle thoracic area to address the middle trapezius. Repeat three or four times, increasing drag and decreasing speed.
- Begin again near the acromion and address the upper trapezius with one or two gliding stokes to complete the surface area.
- Knead the area since it is pleasurable. To increase circulation to the area and shift neuroresponses, move the skin into multiple directions of ease, and hold the ease position for up to 30–60 seconds
- Rhythmic compression to the area stimulates various aspects of fluid movement and supports relaxed breathing.

Shoulder, arm, and hand

- The area is massaged in supine, prone, sidelying, and seated positions. Massage of the torso and neck naturally progresses to the shoulder, arm, and hand.
- Commencing with the client prone, massage begins superficially, progresses to deeper layers, and then finishes off with superficial work. Finish the area with kneading, compression, and gliding.
- To increase circulation to the area and shift neuroresponses, move the skin into multiple directions of ease, and hold the ease position for up to 30–60 seconds.
- Combine compression with passive movements of the arm. A slow circumduction tends to access all areas.
- The intrinsic muscles of the hand are addressed next. Systematically work the area, using compression and gliding of the soft tissue between the fingers, the web of the thumb, and on the palm that oppose the thumb and little finger.
- There is also a network of lymphatic vessels in the palm that when rhythmically compressed assist lymphatic movement.

Hip

- The hip is massaged in prone and sidelying positions. Massage of the torso naturally progresses to the hip.
- Massage begins superficially and progresses to deeper layers and then finishes off with superficial work.
- Systematically, lightly stroke the area. To increase circulation to the area and shift neuroresponses,

move the skin into multiple directions of ease, and holding the ease position for up to 30–60 seconds.

- Increase the pressure slightly. Begin on the posterior to address the lumbar region that connects with the hip. This area was addressed while massaging the torso but now is massaged in relationship to the hip. Carry the strokes into the gluteus maximus. Use gliding with a compressive element and glide toward the hip. Repeat with the latissimus dorsi again in relationship to hip function. Begin at the shoulder and carry the stroke all the way into the opposite gluteus maximus.
- Finish by gliding and kneading the entire area. Add oscillation in various positions.

Thighs, legs, and feet

- These areas can be massaged in all basic positions.
- Massage of the area naturally progresses from the hip.
- Like other body regions, massage begins superficial, progresses to deeper layers, and then finishes off with superficial work.
- To increase circulation to the area and shift neuro-responses, move the skin into multiple directions

of ease, and hold the ease position for up to 30–60 seconds.

- Move the hip and knee passively through flexion, extension, and internal and external rotation **if comfortable.**
- Increase the pressure slightly and again use gliding and kneading to the entire area. Add gentle shaking and oscillation in various positions.
- The intrinsic muscles of the foot are addressed next. Sidelying is the best position. Systematically work using compression and gliding of the soft tissue of the sole of the foot.
- There is also a network of lymphatic vessels in the sole of the foot that, when rhythmically compressed, will assist lymphatic movement.
- There are acupuncture points at the side of each nail and direct pressure or tapping can stimulate these points. An easy way to do this is to squeeze, release, and repeat three or four times, on the lateral and medial side of each toenail.
- To finish off, use gentle shaking and oscillation and compression and passive movement.

KEY POINTS

- The general massage sequence uses a comprehensive and repetitive approach.
- The principles of the general massage sequence do not change. However, the client's goals, initial client positioning, and other contributing factors will be the differentiating factors.

- Modification to massage application consists of variation in depth of pressure, duration of massage application, speed, drag, and location.
- Massage as part of palliative care is pleasurable and does not strain adaptive capacity.

CHAPTER NINE

Adjunctive approaches and understanding and addressing breathing disorders

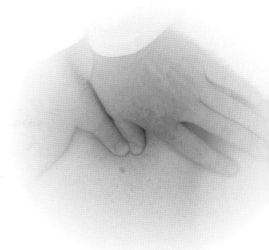

ADJUNCTIVE APPROACHES

This chapter will focus on adjunctive approaches that may prove useful in management of the symptoms of pain. A specific emphasis will be placed on understanding the role of breathing as a pain management tool with guidelines for addressing dysfunctional breathing during the massage. The adjunctive approaches can either be directly integrated into massage application or provided as self-care.

Remember that the objective is to 'lighten the adaptive load' and to enhance functionality – better mobility, flexibility, stability, balance – and of course to relieve or remove unpleasant symptoms.

Focusing on the topics that fill the remainder of this chapter will help to achieve those ends, working alongside direct manual interventions.

Also remember that because a form of treatment, or an exercise, is useful, it does not mean that there may not be 'reactions' to the inevitable changes that result from it. The more fragile and sensitive the person, the less that should be done at any time, allowing for the adaptive changes resulting from treatment to be processed by the tissues and the mind.

Another useful reminder is that not everything is fixable. Although we are always working with the aim of enhancing self-regulation, some changes – osteoarthritis, for example – or the circulatory or soft-tissue effects of old age, may involve such chronic change that the best we can hope for is a modest improvement, or a slowing of what may be inevitable decline. In such instances maintenance of the present state may be a realistic therapeutic objective.

Acupuncture (what you should know about this)

Acupuncture for pain relief is now widely used by physiotherapists, doctors of manual medicine, and of course acupuncturists. The methods used include the insertion (usually quite painlessly) of very fine, disposable, stainless steel needles, into specific 'points' on the body. The depth of insertion may be very shallow or quite deep, depending on which part of the body is involved. Some (traditional) acupuncturists manipulate the needles (rotating them) to produce a sense of heaviness in the tissues. A similar effect is achieved by other (modern) acupuncturists, who attach clamps to the needles and pass mild electrical currents through them.

Other methods of influencing the painful tissues include heating the needles (known as moxibustion). Needles may stay inserted for a matter of seconds, or for 20 minutes or more, depending on what the acupuncturist is trying to achieve.

Western medicine believes that acupuncture has its main effect on pain by blocking pain messages to the brain. Eastern concepts are that energy rebalancing is being achieved. Despite the variations in belief and in application, all acupuncturists report (and research confirms) that this is one of the most effective methods for achieving pain relief, albeit temporarily if the causes are not also dealt with.

Acupressure methods, as used in shiatsu and Thai massage (Palanjian 2004), have very similar effects to those achieved by acupuncture.

Aromatherapy

A clinical placebo controlled trial involving individuals with depression as a major feature, but with secondary symptoms of sleep disturbance and chronic headaches, were treated with massage and essential oils (selected from bergamot, clary sage, lemon, lavender, Roman chamomile, geranium, rose, sandalwood, and jasmine) in a hospital setting (Lemon 2004).

The control group received massage using grape seed oil. The essential oils selected for the treatment group had been previously shown to offer benefit in the conditions presented (Lawless 1994).

In the hospital study it was found that:

...the use of essential oils, prescribed for the relief of depression and anxiety, but also blended specifically for the client, addressed other issues such as sleep disturbance and headaches. It was concluded that this study has statistically proven that the holistic use of aromatherapy had a beneficial therapeutic effect on clients who were more than mildly depressed or anxious.

Emotion/stress management and relaxation methods

Stress management may play a part in easing the adaptation load in conditions such as recurrent or chronic head/neck pain, and this may call for specialized professional advice and/or treatment. However, in order to defuse, reduce, and minimize the effects of chronic emotional stress, a wide range of simple strategies exist, that can do no harm, and which might be extremely helpful, even though they are not addressing the primary features of the problem.

The methods described below – neutral bath, progressive muscular relaxation, and autogenic training exercises – can all be used at home without any risk, and with potentially beneficial effects.

Note: Clearly these methods do not address the underlying causes of emotional distress, but appear to offer relief from its effects in a safe manner. Ideally individuals where chronic anxiety, for example, is a feature of life, should seek appropriate professional advice and help.

The neutral bath: for inducing deep relaxation/sleep enhancement

A neutral bath is one in which the body temperature is the same as that of the water. This produces a relaxing influence on the nervous system (this was the main method of calming violent and disturbed patients in mental asylums in the 19th century).

Indications In all cases of anxiety, feelings of 'being stressed,' and for relieving chronic pain and/or insomnia.

Materials required Bathtub, water, bath thermometer.

Method Run a bath as full as possible, and with the water as close to 97°F (36.1°C) as possible, and certainly not higher. (The bath has its effect because the water is close to body temperature. Immersion in water at this neutral temperature has a profoundly relaxing, sedating effect.)

Instructions
- Lie down in the bath so that, if possible, water covers your shoulders.
- Rest your head on a towel or sponge.
- A bath thermometer should be in the water and the temperature should not be allowed to drop below 92°F/33.3°C.
- It can be topped up periodically, but must not exceed the 97°F/36.1°C limit.

- The duration of the bath should be anything from 30 minutes to 2 hours – the longer the better as far as relaxation effects are concerned.
- After the bath, pat dry quickly and get into bed.

Caution: Neutral baths are suitable for most people but contraindicated where there are skin conditions which react badly to water, or if there is serious cardiac disease.

Progressive muscular relaxation exercise (time required approximately 20 minutes) (Carroll & Seers 1998)
Autogenic training and (Erickson's) progressive muscular relaxation were evaluated for its benefits in patients with fibromyalgia (Rucco et al 1995). The researchers reported that:

> This auto-hypnotic technique (autogenics) was compared to Erickson's relaxation training in a randomized controlled trial, with 53 fibromyalgia patients. The authors found that the latter approach was more suited to FM patients and led to a faster relief of symptoms.

Instructions
- Lie comfortably on a draft-free carpeted floor, arms and legs outstretched.
- Tense the fist of your dominant hand and hold tight for 10 seconds.
- Let go the tense fist and enjoy the sense of release for 10 seconds.
- Repeat this, and then do the same with the other hand.
- Go to your dominant side foot and draw the toes upwards towards the knee, tightening the muscles. Hold this for 10 seconds.
- Release and relax for 10–15 seconds, then repeat once before going to the other foot.
- Perform a similar sequence in at least 5 other sites (each on both sides of the body, making 10 more sites) such as:
  – back of lower legs, but this time point the toes
  – upper leg – by 'pulling' the kneecap towards the hip
  – squeeze the buttocks together
  – hold an inhaled breath and at the same time draw the shoulder blades together
  – pull the abdominal area in strongly
  – draw the upper arm into the shoulder, strongly
  – tighten the face muscles around the eyes and mouth, or frown strongly.

Other muscles can also be contracted by working out just what tightens them.

Holding extreme tightness, followed by release, gives you awareness of the contrast between tension and relaxation, and this lets you recognize muscular tension as it builds up, allowing you to stop it early.

After a week or so of doing this once or twice daily, start to combine muscle groups, so that the entire hand/arm on both sides can be tensed and then relaxed together, followed by the face and neck, then the chest, shoulders and back, and finally the legs and feet.

After another week, abandon the tension element of the exercise and you should be able to simply lie down and focus on the different regions, and note whether they are tense or not, and instruct them to relax. By doing this in the head/neck region you should be able to modify tension headache symptoms.

Results should come quickly but only if the exercise is performed regularly!

Autogenic training (Rucco et al 1995)
Every day, for ten minutes do the following:
- Lie comfortably, a cushion under the head, knees bent, eyes closed.
- Focus attention on your dominant (say, right) hand/arm and silently say, 'My right arm (or hand) feels heavy.'
- Sense the arm relaxed and heavy. Feel its weight. For about a minute repeat the affirmation, 'My arm/hand feels heavy,' several times, and try to stay focused on its heaviness.
- You may lose focus as your mind wanders periodically. This is normal, so don't be upset, just return to your arm and its heaviness.
- Try to enjoy the sense of release – of letting go – that comes with this heavy feeling.
- Next focus on your left hand/arm and do exactly the same thing for about a minute.
- Move to the left leg, and then the right leg, for about a minute each, with similar messages, focusing attention for about 1 minute each.
- Return to your right hand/arm and this time affirm a message which says, 'My hand is feeling warm (or hot).'
- After a minute go to the left hand/arm, then the left leg, and then finally the right leg, each time with the 'warming' message and focused attention. If warmth is sensed, feel it spread, and enjoy it.
- Finally focus on your forehead and affirm that it feels cool and refreshed. Hold this thought for about 1 minute.
- Finish by clenching your fists, bending your elbows and stretching out your arms. The exercise is complete.

Repeat the whole exercise at least once a day and you will gradually be able to stay focused on each region and sensation.

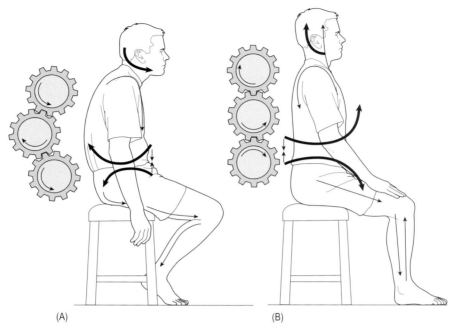

Figure 9.1 Seated posture. A: Poor positioning resulting in biomechanical strain. B: Ergonomically and biomechanically efficient.

Using autogenics to ease pain

Once you have learned to stay focused, if there is pain relating to muscle tension (e.g. headache), these methods can be used to reduce tension by focusing thoughts of 'heaviness,' or 'lightness,' or 'warmth' into the region.

- If pain relates to poor circulation, a 'warmth' instruction can be used to improve it.
- If there is inflammation, this can be eased by 'thinking' the area 'cool.'
- You can focus on any area – for example, visualizing a stiff joint easing and moving, or a congested swollen area returning to normality.

Breathing for pain relief

By practicing the *pursed lip breathing* described later in this chapter, a sense of calm and ease should emerge after some minutes of repeating the pattern of slow exhalation through pursed lips–pause–inhalation through the nose.

Ergonomics

The concept of specific adaptation to imposed demands is essential in understanding how the human biomechanical design evolved, and what interventions can be made to enhance biomechanics – whether through treatment, stretching programs, or corrective or performance based exercise (Figs 9.1 and 9.2).

It may be possible, for example, to minimize the pain and discomfort of sitting in one position for several hours/day by offering advice regarding supports (lumbar supports, foot rests, wrist supports, head rests, etc.).

Questions should be asked about work and recreation positions and activities. In addition, sleeping, driving, and standing postures should be evaluated, and advice offered, or referral made to suitably trained and licensed professionals for such advice. Figure 9.2 shows a possibly unavoidable posture for someone playing the guitar. Treatment of the stressed and distressed tissues, along with home stretching advice, should effectively reduce the soft tissue changes resulting from being in such a position for lengthy periods.

High velocity manipulation (what you should know about this)

Chiropractors, osteopaths, and some physical therapists utilize manipulation described as high velocity, low amplitude (HVLA). Licensing is required, demonstrating that appropriate training has been received in the use of these usually safe, but potentially dangerous methods, if used inappropriately.

The therapeutic effects of HVLA are summarized in Figure 9.3.

Safety

Most issues of safety in relation to the use of HVLA involve the cervical spine. While practitioners using

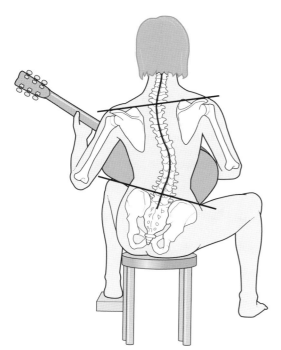

Figure 9.2 An example of specific adaptation to imposed demands caused by playing the guitar.

HVLA report that minor side effects (local discomfort, headache, tiredness, radiating discomfort) occur after approximately 33% of visits, these are usually no longer present after 24 hours (Malone et al 2002).

Major complications from cervical manipulation are rare (between 1 in 400 000 and 1 in 10 million; Shekelle et al 1992) but can be serious (Coulter et al 1996).

It is worth acknowledging that complications resulting from most other forms of treatment of neck pain, for which data are available, are estimated to be higher than those for manipulation. Haldeman et al (2002) note that in reviewing nearly 400 cases of vertebrobasilar artery dissection, it was not possible to identify a specific neck movement, type of manipulation, or trauma that would be considered the offending activity in the majority of cases.

An editorial (Hill 2003) in the *Canadian Journal of Neurological Sciences* stated:

> Despite strong circumstantial reports and opinions, the quality of evidence that minor neck trauma including chiropractic neck manipulation causes vertebral or carotid artery dissection remains weak. A majority of papers are case reports or series only representing the weakest tier of clinical evidence.

Conclusion: If an appropriately trained and licensed practitioner performs HVLA manipulation after full assessment and observation of standard precautions, the evidence suggests that the procedure is safe.

Hydrotherapy
See also 'neutral bath' methods under subheading 'Emotion/stress management and relaxation methods' earlier in this chapter.

Constitutional hydrotherapy (Watrous 1996, Blake 2006)
Constitutional hydrotherapy (CH) has a nonspecific 'balancing' effect, inducing relaxation, reducing chronic pain, enhancing immune function, and promoting healing when it is used daily for some weeks.

Because effects are general, CH is ideal for treatment (and self-treatment) where a clear diagnosis is absent, since its effects are universally helpful, with no obvious contraindications.

The method described below is adapted for home use. (*Note:* Help is required to apply HC.)

Materials required
- A full-sized sheet folded in two, or two single sheets.
- Two blankets (wool if possible).
- Three bath towels (when folded in two each should be able to reach side to side and from shoulders to hips).
- One hand towel (each should, as a single layer, be the same size as the large towel folded in two).
- Hot and cold water.

Method
- Undress and lie face up between the sheets and under the blanket.
- Whoever is assisting you should place two hot folded bath towels (i.e. four layers of damp/hot toweling) to cover the trunk, shoulders to hips.
- Cover the towels with a sheet and blanket and leave for 5 minutes.
- Your helper then returns with a single layer (small) hot towel and a single layer cold towel.
- The 'new' hot towel is placed on top of the four 'old' hot towels, and these are 'flipped over' so that the new hot towel is on the skin. The used/old towels are discarded.
- Immediately place the cold towel onto new hot towel, and flip again, so that the cold towel is on the skin. Remove and discard the single hot towel.
- Cover the whole body with a sheet and leave for 10 minutes or until the cold towel warms up.
- Remove the previously cold, now warm, towel and turn onto stomach.
- Repeat steps 2–8 to the back.

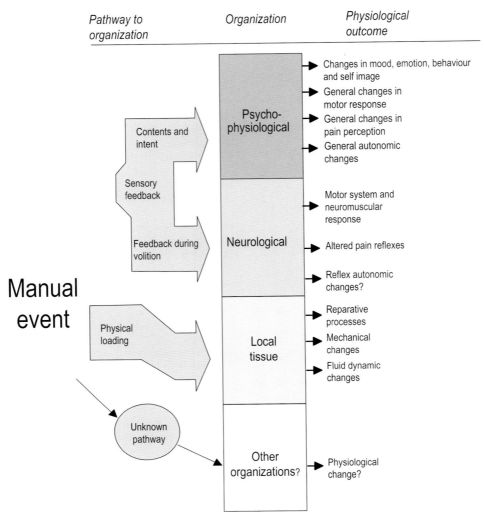

Figure 9.3 The physiological model of manipulation.

Suggestions and notes

- If using a bed take precautions not to get this wet.
- 'Hot' water in this context is a temperature high enough to prevent you leaving your hand in it for more than 5 seconds.
- The coldest water from a running tap is adequate for the 'cold' towel. On hot days, adding ice to the water in which this towel is rung out is acceptable if the temperature contrast is acceptable to the patient.
- If the person being treated feels cold after the cold towel is placed, use back massage, foot, or hand massage (through the blanket and towel) to warm up.
- *Apply daily or twice daily if pain is chronic.*
- There are no contraindications to constitutional hydrotherapy.

Hot mustard foot bath

The hydrostatic effect in hydrotherapy involves the shifting of fluid from one part of the body to another. The hydrostatic effect can be used clinically in the treatment of conditions in which it is suspected that there is a locally congested area which is giving rise to symptoms, such as congestive headache or sinusitis. Dilation of the blood vessels of the skin at some area distal and inferior (e.g. feet) to the area affected (e.g. head) can be effective in relieving congested tissues (Blake 2008).

Self-help instructions for tension headache home hydrotherapy method

This is a traditional naturopathic hydrotherapy method for tension headaches.

Note: this method is likely to help tension type headaches if started early on, not when the pain is well established.

- Place 9 liters (2 gallons) of hot water (not scalding!) into a bowl large enough for both feet to rest in.
- Stir 1–2 teaspoons of mustard powder into this and put your feet, up to the ankles, in the water.
- Wrap a large bag of frozen peas in a towel and place this behind your neck (if you use an upright chair and place this against a wall, you can lean back onto the towel containing the peas), or
- Wrap a damp (not dripping) cold towel around your head.
- Spend at least 10 minutes in this position and then lie down and rest.

Lifestyle changes, including nutrition and exercise

Lifestyle includes the activities of work and leisure; how much exercise and sleep we get; what, how much, and how often we eat and drink; and pretty much everything else we do.

Lifestyle is – economic considerations excluded – to a very large degree, a matter of choice. Unless the following choices are dictated by circumstances out of our control (working environment, economic status), we choose what we wear (high heels, tight, constricting undergarments, etc.). We choose what and how often we eat and drink, and whether we do so slowly or quickly; and whether we follow a diet high in saturated fat and sugar, or one more in tune with healthy outcomes. We choose whether we drink alcohol, caffeine rich liquids, and fizzy, chemical laden fluids, or pure water. We choose whether we exercise or not. Even our posture and breathing patterns are largely a result of habitual choices.

Some 30 years ago Boris Chaitow ND DC wrote the following, which summarizes much of the problem highlighted in the previous paragraph:

> When humans were evolving, nutrition consisted of fruits, nuts, whole cereals, vegetation, roots, herbs, possibly small living creatures, all nutritionally whole, all rich in the essential factors that the body requires for high efficiency, energy and freedom from disease – especially in amino acids, trace elements, vitamins, enzymes etc.
>
> Western man's diet today is excessive in high animal proteins, cooked, rich and fatty – high level of carbohydrates, largely derived from refined ingredients such as white bread, buns, cakes, biscuits, pastries, puddings, pies, as well as white sugar, sweets, chocolates, preserves and jams; cooked

> refined porridge, processed cereals, white rice, ice-cream etc., fluids from tea, coffee, cocoa, alcohol and synthetic and artificially sweetened, bottled drinks – fried, pickled, preserved, cured, smoked, salted and tinned meats and fish; dairy products that are pasteurized and distorted – all of which contribute to the noxious encumbrances and the deficiencies contributing to today's tragic state of ill-health. And on top of that, many other items of civilized foods are 'doctored' by colouring, flavouring, preserving, sweetening, salting, chemicalizing and generally overcooking, to create 'foodless' material, that in laboratory experiments causes rats to lose their hair and teeth, to abort their young, to become irritable, pugnacious and cannibalistic – and in ludicrous seriousness causes pain-ridden humans to become pouchy, grouchy, with falling hair, rotting teeth, poached-egg eyes, pickled livers, bleeding piles, and no idea what eating is all about. (Chaitow 1980)

If a patient/client has any chronic health problem, such as musculoskeletal pain, these issues may be contributing to the adaptive load to which the individual is reacting. Appropriate nutritional and lifestyle advice should be offered (exercise, sleep, ergonomics, diet, etc.), or the person should be referred to health care providers who can offer such advice.

Posture

Experts in postural dysfunction, such as Janda (1982) and Lewit (1999), identified patterns of posture that were described as 'crossed pattern syndromes,' as well as a 'layered syndrome.' These crossed patterns demonstrate the imbalances that occur as antagonists become inhibited due to the overactivity of specific postural muscles. The effect would be to create an environment conducive to pain and dysfunction.

One of the main tasks in rehabilitation of such pain and dysfunction (see below in this chapter) is to normalize (as far as is possible) these imbalances, to release and stretch whatever is over-short and tight, and to encourage tone in those muscles that have become inhibited and weakened.

Upper crossed syndrome (see Chapter 5, Fig. 5.8)
The muscular changes here include:
- *Shortened:* cervical extensors, suboccipitals, rotator cuff muscles, upper trapezius, levator scapulae, pectorals.
- *Lengthened/weakened/inhibited:* deep neck flexors, serratus anterior, lower and middle trapezius.

Lower crossed syndrome (see Chapter 5, Fig. 5.9)
The muscular changes here include:

- *Shortened:* psoas, erector spinae, tensor fasciae latae, piriformis, quadratus lumborum, hamstrings, latissimus dorsi.
- *Lengthened/weakened/inhibited*: abdominal muscles, gluteals.

Layered syndrome (see Fig. 9.4)
The muscular changes here include:

- *Shortened:* hamstrings, thoracolumbar erectors, upper fibers of trapezius, levator scapulae, suboccipitals, hip flexors (rectus femoris and iliopsoas).

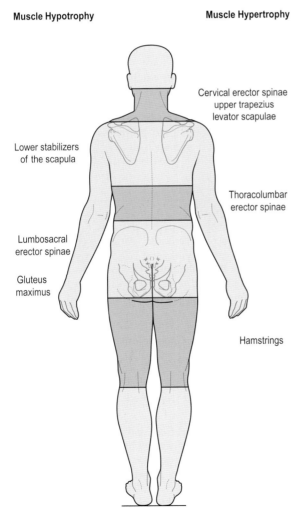

Muscle Hypotrophy   **Muscle Hypertrophy**

Lower stabilizers of the scapula

Lumbosacral erector spinae

Gluteus maximus

Cervical erector spinae
upper trapezius
levator scapulae

Thoracolumbar erector spinae

Hamstrings

Figure 9.4 The layered syndrome.

– *Lengthened/weakened/inhibited:* gluteus maximus, upper thoracic erectors, lower/middle fibers of trapezius.

Postural rehabilitation
Postural rehabilitation implies returning the individual toward a state of normality that has been lost through trauma, poor habits of use, or ill health. Among the many interlocking rehabilitation features involved in any particular case are the following:

- Normalization of soft tissue dysfunction, including abnormal tension and fibrosis. Treatment methods might include massage, neuromuscular techniques, muscle energy techniques, myofascial release, positional release techniques and/or articulation/mobilization, and/or other stretching procedures, such as yoga.
- Deactivation of active myofascial trigger points, possibly involving massage, neuromuscular techniques, muscle energy techniques, myofascial release, positional release techniques, or spray-and-stretch. Appropriately trained and licensed practitioners might also use injection, dry needling, or acupuncture in order to deactivate trigger points.
- Strengthening weakened structures, involving exercise and rehabilitation methods, such as Pilates.
- Proprioceptive reeducation, utilizing manual therapy methods (e.g. balance retraining – see below – and/or use of balance sandals or a wobble board) as well as spinal stabilization exercises and methods such as those devised by Feldenkrais, Hanna, Pilates, Trager, and others.
- Postural retraining using Alexander technique (referral to specialized teachers of this method is recommended) as well as a breathing reeducation (see notes below) as well as yoga, tai chi, and similar systems.
- Ergonomic, nutritional, and stress management strategies (see below).
- Psychotherapy, counseling, or pain management techniques, such as cognitive behavior therapy, that may require specific referral to trained and licensed experts.
- Occupational therapy that specializes in activating healthy coping mechanisms, determining functional capacity, and increasing activity that will help return the individual to a greater level of self-reliance and quality of life (Lewthwaite 1990).
- Appropriate exercise strategies to overcome deconditioning (Liebenson 1996).

A team approach to postural rehabilitation is called for where referral and cooperation allow the best outcome to be achieved.

Self-care (including balance training)

Single leg stance balance test (Bohannon et al 1984)
Posture and general stability are enhanced by ensuring that balance is optimal. When balance is not optimal postural adaptations are likely, placing stress on the entire musculoskeletal system.

A reliable procedure for information regarding balance/stability as well as being useful for retraining if necessary that requires no equipment other than a timer is described below (see Fig. 9.5).

Procedure

- The person is asked to stand, barefoot, and to raise one foot up without touching it to the support leg.
- The knee can be raised to any comfortable height.
- The person is then asked to balance on one leg for up to 30 seconds with eyes open.
- After standing on one leg in this way, standing on the other should be tested.
- When single leg, standing with eyes open, is successful for 30 seconds the person is asked to identify a feature/spot on a wall opposite, and to then close the eyes while visualizing that spot.
- An attempt should be made to balance for 30 seconds, before switching legs and repeating the exercise.

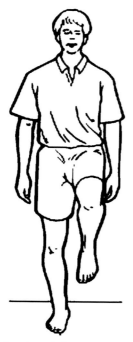

Figure 9.5 Single leg stance balance test.

Scoring The time is recorded when any of the following occurs:

- The raised foot touches the ground or more than lightly touches the other leg.
- The stance foot changes (shifts) position or toes rise.
- There is hopping on the stance leg.
- The hands touch anything other than the person's own body.

By regularly (daily) practicing this balance exercise the time achieved in balance with eyes closed will increase.

Over time more challenging balance exercises can be introduced, including use of wobble boards and balance sandals.

It is important to give people home exercises to improve the self-management of their musculoskeletal conditions. Balance training is very simple to use and requires very little, if any, equipment so it is ideal for self-care.

Regular attendance at tai chi classes/practice will help achieve similar enhanced balance and stability.

BREATHING

Research on breathing as a pain intervention

Many studies of pain control are performed with experimentally induced pain, on normal subjects. This temporary, induced pain differs from natural chronic pain in that is introduced to a noncompromised nervous system; research subjects are usually screened out if they have a chronic pain condition. In such cases, phenomena such as central and peripheral sensitization, kindling, windup, hyperalgesia, and allodynia typically develop, amplifying and complicating the pain sensations. All this constitutes malfunction of the pain detection system, and studies using acute, experimental pain do not address the extra factors that chronic pain presents.

Heart rate variability (HRV) is an emerging variable in the study of pain. It is a measure of cardiac activity sensitive to balance between sympathetic and parasympathetic influence, and can also be used as a biofeedback signal to help the patient regulate and balance the autonomic nervous system (ANS) by altering breathing. ANS imbalance is implicated in irritable bowel syndrome, for example (Mazur 2007). A study by Appelhans (2008), using an applied thermal pain stimulus and frequency domain based spectral analysis with 59 normal subjects, found an inverse relationship between greater low frequency HRV and pain intensity, including unpleasantness ratings. The low frequency band (0.04–0.15 Hz) increases with both regular breathing and emotional calmness, and generally correlates with ANS balance and cardiovascular health.

An experimental pain stimulus such as heat or intra-muscular hypertonic saline infusions can be adjusted and administered in order to measure pain thresholds. For example (Chalaye et al 2009), to study variability of pain tolerance and thresholds, the researchers applied thermal pain stimuli to subjects under two breathing conditions, distraction and feedback of HRV. Compared with a 16/min breathing rate, slow deep breathing at a rate of 6/min resulted in better pain tolerance and higher pain thresholds. Increase in HRV correlates with increased vagal tone and general lowering of arousal.

Tan et al (2009), using data from US war veterans suffering from chronic pain and other injuries, used a time domain analysis of HRV. A −0.46 correlation was found between HRV (in this case, SDNN, a time measure of variability) and presence of pain. So in these two samples, a variable associated with breathing quality was also associated with presence of pain or sensitivity to pain. This is significant because HRV is a widely used biofeedback modality, and learning to raise low frequency HRV by regulating breathing may have favorable effects on pain and homoeostasis in general.

A study of experienced Zen meditators found that breathing pattern correlated with a significantly higher pain threshold to an applied heat stimulus. Better control over pain sensitivity was attributed to both attentional regulation and breathing regulation. The breathing pattern, being subject to disruptions in calmness and predictability, may be a good general index of peace of mind, which raises the threshold for pain of any sort.

Zautra et al (2010), comparing fibromyalgia patients with healthy controls, assigned slow breathing to volunteers subjected to controlled thermal stimuli. 'Slow breathing' was defined as breathing at one-half their normal rate. In general, slow breathing reduced pain intensity and unpleasantness more than normal breathing. The authors cited these results as support for Zen meditation and yogic breathing as a way to combat pain.

Pain may seem like a simple unitary sensation, but it has several facets, some mainly psychological. Using a brief intervention, Downey and Zun (2009) instructed patients in an emergency department to handle their pain by slow deep breathing. By self-report, no significant reduction in pain resulted, but the patients reported significant improvements in rapport with treating physicians, greater willingness to follow the medical recommendations, and conclusions that the intervention was useful.

Another study (Flink et al 2009) of back pain patients showed that the effect of practicing breathing exercises for 3 weeks was not so much on reducing pain levels as lowering catastrophizing and pain related distress, along with greater acceptance of the pain condition.

Stress and breathing

Under stress of many sorts, the breathing pattern is likely to be disrupted. Breath holding may occur as part of a state of suspense, becoming extra vigilant, as in trying to detect a slight movement or sound. Gasping and sighing are more likely to occur during emotional instability, intense emotion, or preparation for exertion. Mouth breathing can also be part of the preparation for heavy effort, since a larger volume of air can be inhaled quickly. Rate of breathing is sensitive to mental confusion or conflict, because thoughts and feelings carry various emotional loads which put conflicting demands on the respiratory system: freeze and remain concealed, get ready to run, prepare for attack, express anger, etc. Rapid breathing is common in anticipatory anxiety. Breathing changes may function like facial expressions, displaying emotional states to those nearby. In the same way that a scowl can be intimidating to humans or primates, breathing that shows aggression or preparation for action can convey it to others so they can act accordingly.

The human capacity for imagination allows us to create any scenario at any time, often in enough detail to initiate body responses as if the scene were real. Simply thinking about situations that require concealment, action, vigilance, or emotional expression is likely to cause corresponding changes in the breathing pattern.

Another aspect of the interaction between breathing and emotion is the location of breathing in the body. Optimal breathing most often involves the diaphragm flattening on inhalation and the lower ribcage expanding outward, with the abdomen also expanding forward and laterally. Chest breathing, by contrast, minimizes the diaphragm action and substitutes pectoral, scalene, trapezius, SCM, and upper intercostal muscles. This latter type of breathing is more prevalent during emotional stress and preparation for action. Thoracic breathing actually produces increases in cardiac output and heart rate (Hurwitz 1981). During emergency action, this kind of breathing would provide an advantage. The diaphragm also contributes to spinal stabilization, so during action preparation it is likely to be diverted from breathing duties.

Conditioned breathing responses

Breathing can be disrupted not only by current situations, but also by conditioned associations. A disturbing experience, whether traumatic or less so, can affect the breathing pattern in one of the ways described above. But unconscious memory processes link the experience with the body response in a way that preserves it, in case the experience, or something resembling it, occurs again. Reminders of the experience can be sufficient to reenact the original physiological responses; for instance, the screech of brakes or a car horn reminding someone of an automobile crash.

This associative mechanism is activated not only for negative, disturbing experiences; recalling a pleasant, satisfying experience will activate the corresponding breathing pattern, in this case toward lower arousal and emotional calm. Using controlled breathing to calm down, take time out to think, and restore emotional balance is a fairly universal human strategy, and takes advantage of the conditioned link between, for example, visiting a peaceful lake and feeling the breathing become slow and full. If instructing someone in the details of breathing more abdominally (reducing the rate, keeping it more regular, breathing through the nose, etc.) seems too difficult, suggesting recall of a pleasant relaxing scene from the individual's personal past may do as well.

Repercussions of breathing pattern disorders

Breathing pattern disorders (BPD) have been shown to potentially have multiple, bodywide, influences, summarized below. For example, Nixon and Andrews (1996) vividly summarize a common situation applying to the individual with BPD tendencies:

> Muscular aching at low levels of effort; restlessness and heightened sympathetic activity; increased neuronal sensitivity; and, constriction of smooth muscle tubes (e.g. the vascular, respiratory and gastrointestinal) can accompany the basic symptom of inability to make and sustain normal levels of effort.

BPD (with hyperventilation as the extreme of this) may influence health by:

- altering blood pH, creating respiratory alkalosis (Pryor & Prasad 2002, Celotto et al 2008)
- inducing increased sympathetic arousal, altering neuronal function – including motor control (Dempsey et al 2002, Brotto et al 2009)
- encouraging a sense of apprehension and anxiety, affecting balance, muscle tone, and motor control (Rhudy & Meagher 2000, Balaban & Thayer 2001, Van Dieën et al 2003)

- depleting Ca and Mg ions, enhancing sensitization, and encouraging reduced pain threshold and the evolution of myofascial trigger points (Gardner 1996, Travell & Simons 1999, Cimino et al 2000, Schleifer et al 2002)
- triggering smooth muscle cell constriction, leading to vasoconstriction and/or spasm – including colon spasm (Ford et al 1995, Yokoyama et al 2008, Debreczeni et al 2009) or pseudoangina (Evans 1980, Wilke et al 1999)
- reducing oxygen release to cells, tissues, and brain (Bohr effect) so encouraging ischemia, fatigue, pain, and the evolution of myofascial trigger points (Freeman & Nixon 1985, Suwa 1995)
- creating biomechanical overuse stresses and compromising core stability and posture (Lewit 1980, 1999, Haugstad et al 2006b, Hodges et al 2007).

Varieties of BPD

Courtney et al (2008, 2009a) suggest a distinction can be made between those BPD that appear to have a predominately biomechanical nature – where the patient may have a 'perception of inappropriate, or restricted, breathing,' as distinguished from BPDs where a chemoreceptor etiology may exist, for example linked to reported sensations such as there being a 'lack of air.' Courtney et al (2008) note that the sensory quality of 'air hunger' or 'urge to breathe' is most strongly linked to changes in blood gases, such as CO_2, or changes in the respiratory drive deriving from central and peripheral afferent input. These sensations may be distinguishable from breathing sensations related to the effort of breathing, which are biomechanical in nature (Simon et al 1989, Banzett et al 1990, Lansing 2000, Chaitow et al 2002).

Questionnaires exist for assessment of these BPD variations – with the Nijmegen Questionnaire (NQ; see Box 9.4) (van Dixhoorn & Duivenvoorden 1985) having greater relevance for hyperventilation, and the Self-Evaluation Breathing Questionnaire (SEBQ) (Courtney 2009b) discriminating between the chemoreceptor and the biomechanical variations of BPD.

Irrespective of the major etiological features (see above and listed below), chronic BPD results in altered function and, in time, structure, of accessory and obligatory respiratory muscles. It is suggested that these should attract therapeutic attention in any attempt to normalize breathing, or the distant effects of BPD on pelvic function (Chaitow 2004). The general massage protocol presented in Chapter 8 can be modified to specifically address breathing function.

Etiological features in BPD
Beyond these distinctions – which have implications in rehabilitation/retraining choices – a variety of factors may lead to individuals experiencing changes in their breathing patterns:

Acidosis Hyperventilation may represent a homeostatic response to acidosis. Chaulier et al (2007) note that acidosis may result from iaterogenic sources, major hypoxemia, cardiovascular collapse, or sepsis.

Atmosphere/altitude 'During expeditions...mountaineers have extremely low values of arterial oxygen saturation (SaO_2), similar to those of patients with severe respiratory failure.' Hyperventilation would be the physiological response to this (Botella De Maglia et al 2008). Altitude implications are not confined to mountaineers. Travelers to, for example, Johannesburg, Mexico City, or Denver would find themselves at altitude and potentially hyperventilating for some days, or weeks, before acclimatizing.

Allergies/intolerances Haahtela et al (2008) report that airway inflammation commonly affects swimmers, ice hockey players, and cross-country skiers, which suggests multifactorial features in which both allergic and irritant mechanisms play a role in resultant overbreathing.

Deconditioning Nixon and Andrews (1996) suggest that deconditioned individuals utilize anaerobic glycolysis to generate energy, resulting in relative lowering of pH and consequent homoeostatic hyperventilation.
    This is contradicted by Troosters et al (1999), who suggest that research indicates that physical deconditioning is more a consequence, than a cause, of the response to exercise, possibly explained by psychological conditioning.

Diabetic ketoacidosis (DKA) Patients with DKA generally present with classic clinical findings of hyperventilation, altered mental status, weakness, dehydration, vomiting, and polyuria (Bernardon et al 2009; see also Kitabchi et al 2006).

Emotional states Stress or fear can '*completely overwhelm*' the reflex centers, causing an increase in ventilation (Levitsky 2003).
    A wide range of symptoms have been shown to be related to stress induced hyperventilation (Schleifer et al 2002), frequently leading to:

> disruption in the acid–base equilibrium [which] triggers a chain of systemic physiological reactions that have adverse implications for musculoskeletal

health, including increased muscle tension, muscle spasm, amplified response to catecholamines, and muscle ischemia and hypoxia.

Habit According to Brashear (1983) the causes of hyperventilation are: 1) organic and physiologic, and 2) psychogenic (emotional/habit) – and hyperventilation and respiratory alkalosis, accompanied by various signs and symptoms, occur in about 6–11% of the general patient population.
    Lum (1984) discusses the reasons for people becoming hyperventilators:

> Neurological considerations leave little doubt that habitually unstable breathing is the prime cause of symptoms. Why people breathe in this way must be a matter for speculation, but manifestly the salient characteristics are pure habit.

Hormonal (progesterone, estrodiol) Slatkovska et al (2006) demonstrated that phasic menstrual cycle changes in PaO_2 may be partially due to stimulatory effects of progesterone and estrodiol on ventilatory drive. (See also Damas-Mora et al 1980.)

Pain Kapreli et al (2008) suggest that the connection between neck pain and respiratory function could impact on patient assessment, rehabilitation, and pharmacological prescription.
    Nishino et al (1999) found that pain intensifies dyspneic sensation (commonly linked with BPD), presumably by increasing the respiratory drive.
    Perri and Halford (2004), in a survey of a convenience sample of 111 consecutive patients attending a chiropractic clinic, reported that neck pain had a significant relationship with dysfunctional breathing patterns.

Pregnancy Jensen et al (2008) suggest that hyperventilation and attendant hypocapnia/alkalosis during pregnancy results from an interaction of pregnancy induced changes in central chemoreflex drives to breathe and wakefulness, acid–base balance, metabolic rate, and cerebral blood flow.

Pseudoasthma A high proportion of individuals diagnosed as asthmatics have been shown to in fact be hyperventilators.
    Weinberger and Abu-Hasan (2006) note that the perception of dyspnea is a prominent symptom of hyperventilation attacks that can occur in those with or without asthma, and that patients with asthma may not readily be able to distinguish the perceived dyspnea of a hyperventilation attack from asthma.
    Ternesten-Hasséus et al (2008) report that exercise induced dyspnea may be associated with

hypocapnia, resulting from hyperventilation, and that the diagnosis of exercise induced asthma should be questioned when there are no signs of bronchoconstriction.

Sleep disorders There is an direct temporal, and possibly etiological, connection between sleep disorders and overbreathing – including sleep apnea and cardiorespiratory fitness (Vanhecke et al 2008).

Anatomy of breathing

The pelvic floor (PF) and the respiratory diaphragm are structurally and functionally bound together by fascial and muscular connections (Fig. 9.6). The abdominal canister has been described as a functional unit that involves the diaphragm, including its crura; psoas; obturator internus; deep abdominal wall and its associated fascial connections; deep fibers of multifidus; intercostals; quadratus lumborum; thoracolumbar vertebral column *(T6–12 and associated ribs, L1–L5)*; and osseus components of the pelvic girdle (Gibbons 2001, Jones 2001, Newell 2005, Lee, Lee & McLaughlin 2008). Gibbons (2001) has described the anatomical link between the diaphragm, psoas, and the PF: 'The diaphragm's medial arcuate ligament

is a tendinous arch in the fascia of the psoas major. Distally, the psoas fascia is continuous with the PF fascia, especially the pubococcygeus.'

Newell (2005) has further detailed the relationship between psoas and quadratus lumborum with the diaphragm and thoracic structures, observing that the posterior edge of the diaphragm crosses the psoas muscles medially, forming the medial arcuate ligaments, and the quadratus lumborum muscles laterally, forming the lateral arcuate ligaments.

The skeletal attachments of the lateral arcuate ligaments are the first lumbar transverse process and the midpoint of the 12th rib. The costal origins include the lower six ribs and costal cartilages, the fibers of the diaphragm interdigitating with those of transversus abdominis.

The medial arcuate ligament is continuous medially with the lateral margin of the crus, and is attached to the side of the body of the first or second lumbar vertebra. Laterally, it is fixed to the front of the transverse process of T12 and arches over the psoas muscle. Abnormal tensions in this ligament may irritate psoas, resulting in pain and spasm. Conversely, psoas spasm may influence diaphragmatic mechanics (Burkill & Healy 2000, Carriere 2006).

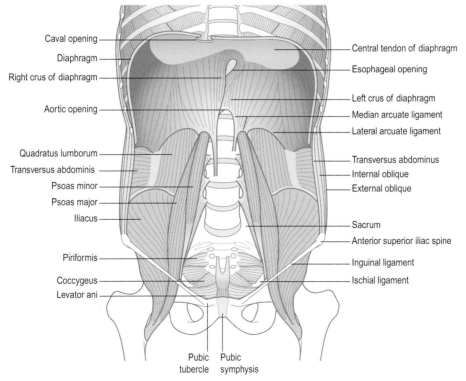

Figure 9.6 The lumbopelvic cylinder.

Furthermore, lying between the posterior parietal peritoneum and the transversalis fascia is the retroperitoneal space, an anatomical region seldom discussed in relationship to chronic pelvic pain (Burkill & Healy 2000). This space houses (in whole or in part): the adrenal glands, kidneys, ureters, bladder, aorta, inferior vena cava, esophagus (part), and superior two-thirds of the rectum; as well as parts of the pancreas, duodenum, and colon (Ryan et al 2004). This area involves vital connections that intimately bind pelvic and thoracic structures. The anterior pararenal space extends superiorly to the dome of the diaphragm, and hence to the mediastinum. Inferiorly it communicates with the pelvis and below the inferior renal cone with the posterior pararenal space. The posterior pararenal opens inferiorly towards the pelvis but fuses superiorly with the posterior perirenal fascia, the fascia of the quadratus lumborum (QL) and psoas muscles (Burkill & Healy 2000).

With structural and functional continuity between the diaphragm, pelvis, pelvic floor muscles, quadratus lumborum, psoas, and organs of the retroperitoneal space, it suggests that structures of the abdominal canister require assessment and, if appropriate, treatment, in relation to pelvic dysfunction.

Grewar and McLean (2008) indicate that respiratory dysfunctions are commonly seen in patients with low back pain, PF dysfunction, and poor posture. Additional evidence exists connecting diaphragmatic and breathing pattern disorders with various forms of pelvic girdle dysfunction (including sacroiliac pain) (O'Sullivan et al 2002, O'Sullivan & Beales 2007) as well as with chronic pelvic pain and associated symptoms, such as stress incontinence (Hodges et al 2007). Similarly, Carrière (2006) noted that disrupted function of either the diaphragm or the PFM may alter the normal mechanisms for regulating intra-abdominal pressure.

With structural and functional continuity between the diaphragm, the pelvis, the pelvic floor and organs of the retroperitoneal space it suggests that structures such as psoas and QL require assessment and, if appropriate, treatment, in relation to pelvic dysfunction.

Key (2010) suggests that:

Clinicians should keep in mind: the continuous, largely internal three-dimensional myofascial web, providing a scaffold of tensile inner support and stability...contributing to a structural and functional bridge between the lower torso and legs.

Key also notes that:

This includes the obvious contractile elements for which there is accumulating evidence of deficient function in subjects with low back and/or pelvic pain – the transversus abdominis (Hodges and Richardson 1996, 1998, 1999), multifidus (Hides et al 1996), the diaphragm and PFM. Impressions from clinical practice suggest inclusion also of the *obturators*, iliacus, *psoas*, and all their related and interconnecting fascial sheaths. Sound activity within this myofascial 'inner stocking' sustains many functional roles: – providing deep anterior support to the lower half of the spinal column; with the spinal intrinsics it contributes to lumbopelvic control (Hodges, 2004); while also contributing to the generation of IAP (Cresswell et al 1994), continence and respiration.

The lack of normal diaphragmatic movement in individuals with BPD deprives the viscera and abdominal cavity of rhythmic stimulation (internal 'massage') which may be important for maintaining normal pelvic circulation. Pelvic pain and congestion have been correlated with chronic muscle tension, chronic hypoxia, as well as accumulation of metabolites such as lactic acid and potassium (Kuligowska 2005).

Hodges et al (2001) have demonstrated that, after approximately 60 seconds of overbreathing (hyperventilation), the postural (tonic) and phasic functions of both the diaphragm and transversus abdominis are reduced or absent, with major implications for spinal and sacroiliac stability. As major hip flexors the psoas muscles have the potential to influence pelvic girdle position and function. They should therefore attract therapeutic attention (along with the accessory breathing muscles) in any attempt to rehabilitate respiratory or pelvic function.

Ford et al (1995) have reported on the high incidence of increased colonic tone and dysfunction in hyperventilating individuals. Hypocapnic hyperventilation (low CO_2 blood levels) produces an increase in colonic tone and phasic contractility in the transverse and sigmoid regions. These findings are consistent with either inhibition of sympathetic innervation to the colon, or the direct effects of hypocapnia on colonic smooth muscle contractility, or both.

It has also been observed – based on rectal and anal sphincter recordings – that during defecation the respiratory diaphragm and abdominal wall contract together, which results in an increase in intra-abdominal and rectal pressure (Olsen & Rao 2001).

Additionally, PF contraction during exhalation allows for synergy between the pelvic and respiratory diaphragms (Prather et al 2009), suggesting that when normal, respiratory function and the PF can be seen to synchronize intimately.

The anatomical location and innervation of both bladder and colon mean that they share similar vital functions, so that malfunction of one organ may result in a functional disturbance in the other. Furthermore the concepts of organ cross-talk and organ cross-sensitization between the bladder and the colon are important in the understanding of complex chronic pelvic pain syndromes (Watier 2009).

BPD: the postural connection

Carrière (2006) has reported that respiratory dysfunction is commonly observed in patients with low back pain and PF dysfunction.

Key et al (2007) have observed and catalogued a number of variations within the patterns of compensation/adaptation associated with chronic postural realignment involved in crossed syndromes – commonly associated with pelvic deviation.

In Figure 9.7A the major features include:

- trunk extensors shortened
- thoracolumbar region hyperstabilized in extension
- poor pelvic control
- decreased hip extension
- abnormal axial rotation.

In Figure 9.7B the major features include:

- flexors tend to dominate
- loss of extension throughout spine
- thoracolumbar junction hyperstabilized in flexion.

The likely outcome of such postural distress, Key et al (2007) suggest, would include dysfunctional breathing patterns and pelvic floor dysfunction.

BPD and hyperventilation: physical features

Deep and rapid breathing (hyperpnoea) results in progressive muscular fatigue and increasing sensations of distress, to the point of breathlessness. For example, Renggli et al (2008) report that during normocapnic hyperpnoea (involving partial rebreathing of CO_2), contractile fatigue of the diaphragm and abdominal muscles develops, long before task failure, triggering an increased recruitment of ribcage muscles. Since the diaphragm and abdominal muscles are key features of low back and pelvic stability, the implications for core instability of chronic, habitual overbreathing – where normocapnic hyperpnoea would be unlikely – is clear. Respiratory alkalosis, and its numerous effects as described earlier in this chapter, would then accompany reduced pelvic and low back stability.

The implication is that methods to help avoidance of hyperpnoea should be a feature of breathing retraining.

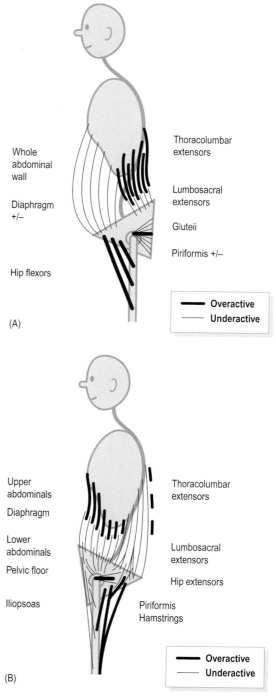

Figure 9.7 A: Schematic view: anterior pelvic crossed syndrome. B: Schematic view: posterior pelvic crossed syndrome.

Implications of breathing retraining for pain management

Hudson et al (2007) observe that human scalenes are *obligatory* inspiratory muscles that have a greater mechanical advantage than sternocleidomastoid (SCM) muscles, which are *accessory* respiratory muscles. They found that irrespective of respiratory tasks these muscles are recruited in the order of their mechanical advantages – with scalenes starting to operate earlier than SCM, involving what they term to be an 'efficient, fail-safe, system of neural control.'

The implication in breathing rehabilitation is to ensure that these muscles receive focused attention as to their functionality.

Schleifer et al (2002) recapitulate the known effects of overbreathing which they have identified as occurring in stress related work settings:

Hyperventilation (overbreathing) refers to a drop in arterial CO_2, caused by ventilation that exceeds metabolic demands for O_2. Excessive loss of CO_2 that results from hyperventilation produces a rise in blood pH (i.e. respiratory alkalosis). This disruption in the acid–base equilibrium triggers a chain of systemic physiological reactions that have adverse implications for musculoskeletal health, including increased muscle tension, muscle spasm, amplified response to catecholamines, and muscle ischemia and hypoxia. Hyperventilation is often characterized by a shift from a diaphragmatic to a thoracic breathing pattern, which imposes biomechanical stress on the neck/shoulder region due to the ancillary recruitment of sternocleidomastoid, scalene, and trapezius muscles in support of thoracic breathing.

The implications suggest that these changes: 'provide a unique rationale for coping with job stress and musculoskeletal discomfort through breathing training, light physical exercise, and rest breaks.'

Masubuchi et al (2001) used fine wire electrodes inserted into muscles, and high resolution ultrasound, to identify the activity of three muscle groups, in response to various respiratory and postural maneuvers. They concluded that the scalenes are the most active, and trapezius the least active, cervical accessory inspiratory muscles, while SCM is intermediate.

This confirms what has long been suspected by observation and palpation – that the scalenes are the most important respiratory muscle group lying superior to the thorax.

Scalene dysfunction and the presence of trigger points ('functional pathology') were identified in excess of 50% of individuals, in a series of 46 hospitalized patients who demonstrated paradoxical patterns of respiration. A combination of muscle energy technique ('post-isometric relaxation') and self-stretching of the scalenes, was used during rehabilitation (Pleidelová et al 2002).

The implication is that these key respiratory muscles require focused attention via palpation and appropriate therapeutic interventions, as part of breathing rehabilitation.

Renggli et al (2008) showed (see above) that the progressive fatigue of the diaphragm and abdominal muscles, during overbreathing, results in recruitment of the muscles of the ribcage (intercostals).

Han et al (1993) described the action and interaction of these ribcage muscles during ventilation, noting that the parasternal intercostal muscles act in concert with the scalenes to expand the upper ribcage, and/or to prevent it from being drawn inward by the action of the diaphragm, during quiet breathing. The respiratory activity of the external intercostals, however, appears to constitute a reserve system, only to be recruited when increased expansion of the ribcage is required.

The implications of this information points to the need for attention to the often neglected intercostal muscles, during breathing rehabilitation.

'Biologically unsustainable patterns' (Garland 1994)

Garland has summarized the structural modifications that are likely to inhibit successful breathing rehabilitation, as well as psychological intervention, until they are at least in part normalized.

He describes a series of changes including:

- visceral stasis/PF weakness
- abdominal and erector spinae muscle imbalance
- fascial restrictions from the central tendon via the pericardial fascia to the basiocciput
- upper rib elevation with increased costal cartilage tension
- thoracic spine dysfunction and possible sympathetic disturbance, accessory breathing muscle hypertonia and fibrosis
- evolution of myofascial trigger points in hypertonic and ischemic tissues
- promotion of rigidity in the cervical spine with possibility of fixed lordosis
- reduction in mobility of 2nd cervical segment and disturbance of vagal outflow.

These changes, Garland states:

Run physically and physiologically against biologically sustainable patterns, and in a vicious circle, promote abnormal function, which alters structure, which then disallows a return to normal function.

Myofascial trigger points

Within the patterns of overuse and misuse that characterize postural and respiratory insults to the body as described above, the evolution of myofascial trigger points is a common feature (Lewit 1999, Travell & Simons 1999, Schleifer et al 2002, Anderson 2009, Key 2010).

BREATHING RETRAINING ASSESSMENT AND INTERVENTION

Breathing retraining appears to require a combination of elements for best results:

- Understanding the processes – a cognitive, intellectual awareness of the mechanisms and issues involved in breathing pattern disorders.
- Retraining exercises that include aspects that operate subcortically, allowing replacement of currently habituated patterns with more appropriate ones.

- Biomechanical structural modifications that remove obstacles to desirable and necessary functional changes.
- Time for these elements to merge and become incorporated into moment-to-moment use patterns.

Box 9.1 offers a summary of physical medicine approaches as utilized by one of this chapter's authors (LC).

Functional examination: identifying the locus of motion

An initial assessment is required to determine whether the breathing pattern is paradoxical, upper chest or diaphragmatic/abdominal (Lewit 1980). Two validated methods are described below – the so-called Hi-lo test (Bradley 1998, Courtney et al 2009), and the MARM (manual assessment of respiratory motion) method (Courtney et al 2008, Courtney et al 2009).

Box 9.1 Phases of breathing intervention

Assessment
- Identify symptoms related to poor breathing chemistry and biomechanics
- Observe breathing pattern, e.g. paradoxical pattern/upper chest (Courtney et al 2008, 2009)
- Observe posture – particularly crossed patterns (Key et al 2006)
- Assess spinal, rib mobility/restriction, form/force closure (active straight leg raise test), shortness and/or weakness of key muscles, as well as assessing for active trigger points (Lee & Lee 2004, Lee 2007, Lee et al 2008)
- Identify BPD triggers (pain, stress, situations, thoughts, emotions, etc.)
- Identify faulty breathing behaviors (upper chest, no pause between breaths, etc.)
- Utilize questionnaires (Nijmegen, SEBQ – see below)
- Utilize palpation assessments such as hi-lo and MARM (see below).

Education
- Inform as to role altered breathing can play in symptom production
- Discuss assessment findings
- Teach elements of appropriate breathing
- Discuss symptoms of breathing pattern disorders
- Help with understanding of external situations and internal states (thoughts, emotions) that may trigger altered breathing.

Retraining
- Teach smooth and rhythmic breathing methods in which ratio of inhalation to exhalation is roughly 1:2 (i.e. exhale should take longer). A key to changing breathing behavior is to focus on long, slow exhalation, informing patient that if this is adequate: 'inhalation takes care of itself'
- Consider home use of a capnograph designed for biofeedback, which can help skill acquisition.

Behavior modification
- Modify poor breathing in response to subtler and subtler cues through increased awareness of the symptoms and mechanics of both poor and good breathing
- Teach basic strategies to inhibit habitual overuse of accessory breathing muscles on inhalation (see below)
- Encourage daily practice, morning and evening, of breathing exercises, to reinforce new learning.

(Continued)

Box 9.1 (Continued)

Manual therapy
- If restrictions are identified in the articular or myofascial tissues of the trunk or cervical spine, use manual therapy to free the tightness and provide extensibility, particularly of key muscles: psoas, QL, scalenes, intercostals, diaphragm attachment region
- If pelvic girdle structures are restricted, these should be mobilized
- If poor motor control is identified in the trunk or cervical spine, add an appropriate exercise program
- Postural correction may be required to optimize ventilation mechanics.

Time
- Depending on chronicity, evidence suggests 6 weeks to 6 months may be required to normalize breathing habits (Lum 1996).

Modified from McLaughlin 2009.

Hi-lo test (Fig. 9.8)

Courtney (2009) notes that:

> The Hi Lo test can be used to assess the motion of the upper rib cage and lower rib cage/abdomen and determine aspects of breathing such as rate, rhythm, relative motion and phase relation of upper and lower breathing compartments.

The client/patient is requested to place one hand on the sternum, and one hand on the upper abdomen. The practitioner/observer stands in front and to one side of the client/patient, so that a clear view is possible of the abdomen, thorax, and hands. By observing the direction and degree of hand movement, the observer determines whether thoracic or abdominal motion is dominant, during inhalation, or whether it is balanced.

If the abdomen moves in a direction opposite to the direction of movement of the thorax during inhalation or exhalation, this is regarded as a paradoxical pattern (for example, if during inhalation the abdomen moves toward the spine, and/or if during exhalation the abdomen moves in an outward direction, paradoxical breathing is taking place).

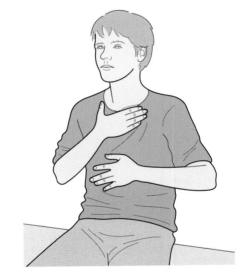

Figure 9.8 Hi-lo upper breathing pattern test.

Manual assessment of respiratory motion (MARM) (Fig. 9.9)

The examiner sits behind the subject with hands resting lightly on the lower lateral rib cage, so as to not inhibit breathing motion.

The hands should be placed so that the little fingers are oriented horizontally, with the thumbs more or less vertical. The lower fingers should be inferior to the lower ribs to allow assessment of abdominal expansion.

An attempt should be made to assess the overall vertical motion relative to the overall lateral motion. Judgement is exercised as to the degree that motion is taking place predominantly in the upper ribcage, or in the lower ribcage/abdomen.

Charting is possible by means of two lines being drawn relative to a horizontal line representing the lumbodorsal junction (see the line marked 'C' on Fig. 9.10). The upper line (A) represents the degree of vertical and upper thoracic motion, while the lower line (B) represents the degree of lower rib and abdominal motion. Calculations are made for thoracic diaphragm 'balance' and percentage of ribcage motion (see Fig. 9.10).

Current thoracic excursion

For the purpose of subsequent reassessment, a record of the current excursion at various levels of the thorax should be recorded. Pryor and Prasad (2002)

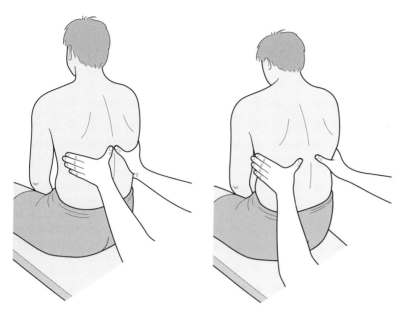

Figure 9.9 Manual assessment of respiratory motion.

report that normal total lateral rib excursion in the lower thorax is between 3 and 5 cm – ideally with an equal excursion bilaterally. Assessment is accurately achieved by means of a cloth tape measure.

The reliability of measuring thoracic excursion has been established, ideally using a standard cloth tape measure. It is suggested that upper thoracic excursion measurements should be taken at the level of the 5th thoracic spinous process and the 3rd intercostal space at the midclavicular line. Lower thoracic excursion measurements should be taken at the level of the 10th thoracic spinous process and the xiphoid process (Bockenhauer et al 2007).

Breath-holding tests

There is no agreed 'normal' breath-holding time, but it can be a useful clinical point of reference; Gardner (1996) reports that HVS patients seldom hold beyond 10–12 seconds. In the Buteyko (1996) system, a control pause is practiced regularly to encourage increased CO_2 tolerance:

Control pause: normal exhalation is held until 'a need to breathe again' is experienced.

'Normal' is between 25 and 30 seconds. Less than 15 seconds, it is suggested, represents low tolerance to CO_2.

Courtney (2010) has suggested that two breath-holding tests may usefully be performed:

1. The participant exhales and holds the breath until experiencing a definite sensation of discomfort

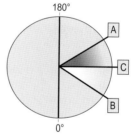

Variable	Description	Calculation
Area of breathing	Angle formed between upper line and lower line	Angle AB
Balance	Difference between angle made by horizontal axis (C) and upper line (A) and horizontal line (C) and lower line (B)	AC − CB
Percent ribcage motion	Area above horizontal/ total area between upper line and lower line × 100	AC/AB × 100

Variables calculated from MARM graphic notation

Figure 9.10 Thoracic diaphragm calculations.

or recognizable difficulty in holding the breath (BHT-DD).

2. The time may be measured until the first involuntary movement of respiratory muscles (BHT-IRM).

Courtney et al (2008, 2009) found that where MARM assessment demonstrated thoracic dominance, this correlated with diminished breath-holding time until first involuntary movement (BHT-IRM).

They hypothesize that this may be because both measures reflect respiratory drive, with increased respiratory drive increasing extent of thoracic breathing and decreasing breath-holding time.

Advantages of controlled breathing:

- Promotes general calming, reduction of emotional arousal, and feeling of control.
- Ensures that the level of CO_2 in the bloodstream is optimal, so that pH stays in the normal range, muscle tension and myofascial trigger points are not stimulated, smooth muscle is less likely to constrict, and cerebral circulation remains stable.
- Abdominal circulation of both the blood and the lymph is stimulated by regular diaphragm action.
- PF muscles are 'entrained' by diaphragmatic action and participate in the rhythmic contraction and relaxation.
- HRV is enhanced by breathing at a particular frequency. This also helps stabilize the ANS.
- The PNS becomes stronger relative to the SNS because of prolonged exhalation. Imbalance of SNS relative to PNS is minimized.

Teaching individuals to alter their breathing patterns is more complicated if the goal goes beyond producing a temporary change to revising faulty breathing habits. Some suggestions for this procedure, using generally accepted guidelines from physiotherapy, respiratory therapy, and psychology, are presented in Box 9.2.

These are brief instructions and practice procedures for teaching relaxed breathing, first for quick intervention with full consciousness, and eventually for forming habits of better breathing. Fuller coverage of breathing improvement can be found in Dinah Bradley's *Hyperventilation syndrome* (2001), Ley and Timmons *Behavioral and psychological approaches to breathing disorders* (1994), and the work of J. van Dixhoorn.

In breathing training (some say 'retraining') the goal is to simulate natural, optimal breathing, which would occur in most individuals under ideal conditions of calm, low stress, and no pain. Distressed breathing deviates from this ideal pattern toward an action preparation or 'freeze' mode which includes upper chest breathing rather than abdominal, a faster, usually shallower breathing rate; irregular rhythm from one breath to the next with more frequent sighs or gasps; and breathing through the mouth (see Box 9.2 & 9.3).

Natural relaxed breathing, when at rest physically and emotionally, will normally be more abdominal, with the external abdominal muscles relaxed and able to expand; more diaphragmatic movement; lips closed; minimal chest expansion; slower rate; regular rate (usually 12–14); fewer sighs; and sometimes prolonged exhalation. Unless using pursed lips to slow the exhale, breathing should be done through the nose, both in and out. Simulating the breathing style of a relaxed person will begin to create the desired state, to a degree, with some or all of the benefits listed above. (See pursed lip breathing instructions below.)

Dinah Bradley, a New Zealand physiotherapist and author of *Self-help for hyperventilation syndrome* (2001), recommends to patients the phrase 'low and slow' to encapsulate good breathing. This means breathing low down in the upper body, expanding the abdomen during inhalation, and reducing the breathing rate.

A more detailed approach might list specific goals and encourage practice of each control procedure separately:

1. Practice slowing the breathing rate to 20–30% below whatever it is at that moment. Tidal volume should automatically enlarge to compensate for the reduced rate. If that goes well, try for even slower, down to 6 breaths per minute without straining or gasping.
2. Practice abdominal breathing, including lateral expansion of lower ribs. Stand before a mirror or use your hands to note where the body is expanding. This will usually help regain a natural breathing style and relieve overuse of chest and neck accessory breathing muscles.
3. Practice shifting between abdominal and 'paradoxical breathing' – meaning drawing in the abdomen and expanding the chest on the inhale. Alternating between one and the other, and comparing the two, accentuates the contrast between the two styles and strengthens the ability to shift into abdominal breathing.
4. Prolong the exhale to a maximum of twice as long as the inhale. This can be done either with diaphragm control or with pursed lips exhalation.
5. Imagine breathing as an internal downward expansion, feel the sensations of this action, and imagine the abdominal and pelvic organs being gently massaged by this breathing.

Each of the steps above can be expanded in sensory and motor detail and practiced so that they are available when needed during pain flares. With practice, relaxed breathing becomes more the default, easier to access and easier to sustain when needed.

Box 9.2 Example of breathing rehabilitation exercise (morning and evening, 30–40 cycles each session)

Pursed lip breathing, combined with diaphragmatic breathing, enhances pulmonary efficiency (Tiep 1986, Faling 1995). One study (Hochstetter et al 2005) found that pursed lip breathing has the potential to help the individual control breathing and improve functional activity during episodes of breathlessness associated with BPD as well as chronic obstructive lung disease. In addition, both anxiety and pain should reduce (Cappo & Holmes 1984, Grossman 1985).

- The client/patient is seated or supine with the dominant hand on the abdomen and the other hand on the chest.
- The client/patient is asked to breathe in through the nose, and out through the mouth, with pursed lips, ensuring diaphragmatic involvement by means of movement of the abdomen against the hand, on inhalation.
- Exhalation through the pursed lips is performed slowly, and has been shown to relieve dyspnoea, to slow the respiratory rate, increase tidal volume, and to help restore diaphragmatic function (Tiep 1986, Faling 1995).
- The client/patient is asked to imagine blowing a thin stream of air at a candle flame about 6 in from the mouth. Exhalation should be slow and continuous.
- After exhaling fully, *without strain*, a pause for a count of one is introduced, followed by inhalation through the nose.
- Without pausing to hold the breath after inhalation, the patient is asked to again exhale slowly and fully, through pursed lips, blowing the air in a thin stream, and to then pause for a count of one.
- The inhalation and exhalation should be repeated for not less than 30 cycles.
- After some weeks of daily practice, an inhalation phase which lasts 2–3 seconds and an exhalation phase of 6–7 seconds should be achieved, without strain.
- The patient is asked to practice twice daily, and to repeat the exercise for a few minutes (6 cycles takes about a minute) every hour if anxious, or when stress levels increase.

Box 9.3 Instructions to patient to minimize overuse of accessory breathing muscles during retraining – using Brügger's Relief Position (Lewit 1999, Brügger 2000, Liebenson 2006)

- Perch on chair edge, arms hanging down, feet below knees, slightly apart and turned outward
- Let arms hang loose, so that palms face forward
- Roll pelvis forward to produce *slight* low back arching
- Ease sternum *slightly* forward and up
- Tuck chin in
- Practice slow, pursed lip breathing, turning arms further outward until thumbs face slightly back, *on inhalation*
- Relax arms to neutral, *on exhalation*.

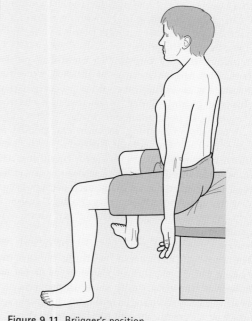

Figure 9.11 Brügger's position.

In the case of pelvic pain, positive changes in breathing and emotion interact with pelvic physiology and can affect pain mechanisms in both general and specific ways (inhibiting pain through descending inhibitory tracts, raising endorphins and dopamine, interrupting cycles of worry and suffering, lowering CCK and adrenaline, reducing sympathetic output to trigger points, and resuming rhythmic stimulation of viscera and PFMs) (Scott et al 2007, Wager et al 2007, Zubieta & Stohler 2009).

A basic sketch is as follows: breathing that is primarily thoracic deprives the viscera and abdominal cavity of rhythmic stimulation, normally provided by the push–pull vertical movement of the pulmonary diaphragm. In addition, excessive breathing in relation to oxygen demand excretes more CO_2 from the body than is being replaced, creating hypocapnic, high pH conditions. The systemic effect of the combined low CO_2 and alkalinity is to interfere with circulation throughout the body, constricting critical blood vessels. In addition, visceral and pelvic smooth muscle suffers from the same constriction. The Bohr effect reduces oxygen available to tissues. The skeletal muscles of the pelvic floor are subject to the same tension increase as other muscles, plus they are deprived of the rhythmic diaphragm movement which may stimulate circulation. In this impoverished environment trigger points may develop, becoming another source of pain.

Pelvic and abdominal pain from trigger points or other pain sources can be aggravated by full abdominal breathing, so downward expansion may be avoided, consciously or not. Shallow thoracic breathing is substituted, but this compounds the problem. The thoracic breathing is consistent with excessive emotional arousal, which may further the dysfunctional breathing pattern. Lewit (1999, described in Carrière 2006) describes how trigger points in either the diaphragm or the PF can make full abdominal breathing painful, and also that manually releasing trigger points in one region can relieve them in the other.

Psychology is very relevant to breathing pattern problems. The original source of thoracic breathing and chronic hyperventilation could be in early experience, trauma, chronic abuse, or an insecure environment fostering hypervigilance (Conway 1988, Gilbert 1998). A transient breathing reaction can persist for years and become the default breathing style, even if the formative context has changed; breathing habits can be embedded through repetition. Lum (1975) observed that regardless of the source of hyperventilation, it could become habitual, persistent, but amenable to reversal through breathing retraining with therapeutic guidance.

Changing the emotional and psychological context maintaining the thoracic breathing pattern may seem like a large task, but assessments of mood and psychological comfort usually show improvement as the breathing pattern changes and pain diminishes, so there may be a synergy among the factors involved.

Manual treatment of selected key structures associated with respiration

Therapeutically, it is suggested that rehabilitation of the pelvic girdle and pelvic floor will be enhanced by more normal physiological breathing patterns, while enhancing these patterns will be aided by pelvic functionality, whether achieved through exercise, breathing retraining, manual therapy, or other means (Mehling et al 2005, Chaitow 2007, McLaughlin 2009).

Lewit (1999), Gibbons (2001), Pleidelová et al (2002), Cox (2005), Newell (2005), Janda and Liebenson (2007), Fitzgerald (2009), Prather (2009), and many others have implicated (in particular) psoas, iliacus, quadratus lumborum, piriformis, the adductors, rectus abdominis, abdominal obliques, scalenes, and intercostals.

The muscles associated with respiratory function can be grouped as either inspiratory or expiratory, and are either primary in that capacity or provide accessory support.

It should be kept in mind that the role which these muscles might play in inhibiting respiratory function (due to trigger points, ischemia, etc.) has not yet been clearly established and that their overload, due to dysfunctional breathing patterns, is likely to impact on cervical, shoulder, lower back, and other body regions.

- The primary inspiratory muscles are the diaphragm, the more lateral external intercostals, parasternal internal intercostals, scalene group, and the levator costarum, with the diaphragm providing 70–80% of the inhalation force (Simons et al 1999).
- These muscles are supported by the accessory muscles during increased demand (or dysfunctional breathing patterns): SCM, upper trapezius, pectoralis major and minor, serratus anterior, latissimus dorsi, serratus posterior superior, iliocostalis, thoracis, subclavius, and omohyoid (Kapandji 1974, Simons et al 1999).

Trigger point release

Travell and Simons (1983, 1999) described variations on their basic trigger point release approach:

- *Ischemic compression (1983):* pressure is applied to the point lying in a fully lengthened muscle. The pressure should be sufficient to maintain pain at a level of between 5 and 7 – where 10 is the maximum that can be tolerated – until pain eases by around 50–75%, or until 90 seconds have passed.
- *Trigger point release (1999):* In this version the muscle is partially lengthened and pressure is to the first perception of a tissue barrier, ideally with no sign of discomfort. Pressure is maintained until a sense of a release of the characteristic taut band is noted, or until 90 seconds have passed.

Other versions exist including pulsed ischemic compression (Chaitow 1994) in which a trigger point in partially lengthened muscles receives 5 seconds of compression, sufficient to induce pain at level 7 (numerical pain rating scale), followed by 2 seconds of no pressure, repeated for up to 90 seconds or until local or referred pain changes are reported or palpated.

In these, and all other variants, it is considered essential to stretch the muscle housing the trigger point towards, or to, its normal resting length, subsequent to the pressure deactivation.

Diaphragm

Two manual methods to encourage release of excessive tone in the diaphragm are described here. One is based on neuromuscular technique methodology and the other on positional release methods.

NMT for diaphragm (Chaitow 2007, Chaitow & DeLany 2008)

- The patient is supine with the knees flexed and feet resting flat on the table. This position will relax the overlying abdominal fibers and allow better access to the diaphragm attachments.
- It is suggested that the upper rectus abdominis fibers should be treated before the diaphragm. This treatment of the diaphragm is contraindicated for patients with liver and gallbladder disease or if the area is significantly tender or swollen.
- The practitioner stands at the level of the abdomen contralateral to the side being treated.
- The fingers, thumbs, or a combination of thumb of one hand and fingers of the other may be used to extremely gently insinuate contact beneath the lower border of the ribcage, directed partly cephalad and obliquely laterally, until a barrier is noted.
- As the patient exhales, the fingers penetrate further.
- As the patient inhales, the diaphragm attachments press against the treating digit(s), forcing these caudally, unless this pressure is resisted – which it should be.
- When penetration appears to be as far as possible, the finger (thumb) tips are directed toward the inner surface of the ribs where static pressure or gentle friction is applied to the diaphragm's attachment.
- The treatment may be applied on full exhalation or at half-breath and is repeated to as much of the internal costal margins as can be reached.

While it is uncertain as to the degree to which the diaphragm's fibers can be reached by this exercise, the connective tissue associated with its costal attachment is probably influenced.

Simons et al (1999) describe a similar procedure, which ends in an anterior lifting of the ribcage (instead of friction or static pressure) to stretch the fibers of the diaphragm.

PRT for diaphragm

- The patient is supine and the practitioner stands at waist level facing cephalad and places the hands over the lower thoracic structures with the fingers along the lower rib shafts.
- Treating the structure being palpated as a cylinder, the hands test the preference this cylinder has to rotate around its central axis, one way and then the other. 'Does the lower thorax rotate more easily to the right or the left?'
- Once the rotational preference has been established, with the lower thorax held in its preferred rotation direction, the preference to sidebend one way or the other is evaluated. 'Does the lower thorax sideflex more easily to the right or the left?'
- Once these two pieces of information have been established, the combined positions of ease (rotation and sideflexion) are introduced, and maintained for between 30 and 90 seconds before slowly restoring the structures to neutral.
- Reevaluation should demonstrate a marked change in previously restricted motion.

Intercostals

There are many manual therapy approaches to release of excessive tone in the intercostal muscles. One, based on neuromuscular technique methodology, is described here.

NMT for the intercostal muscles

- Fingertip or thumb glides, as described below, are applied to the intercostal spaces of the posterior, lateral, and anterior thorax for initial examination as to tenderness and rib alignment. On the anterior thorax, all breast tissue (including the nipple area on men) is avoided with the intercostal treatment.
- The intercostal areas are commonly extremely sensitive and care must be taken not to distress the patient by using inappropriate pressure.
- In most instances the intercostal spaces on the contralateral side will be treated using the finger stroke.
- The (well trimmed) thumb tip or a finger tip should be run along both surfaces of the rib margins, as well as along the muscle tissue itself.
- In this way the fibers of the internal and external intercostal muscles will receive adequate assessment contacts.
- When there is overapproximation of the ribs, a simple stroke along the intercostal space may be all that is possible until a degree of rib and thoracic normalization has taken place, allowing greater access.
- The tip of a finger (supported by a neighboring digit) is placed in one intercostal space at a time, close to the midaxillary line (patient prone or supine), and gently but firmly brought around the curve of the trunk toward the midline, combing for signs of dysfunction.
- The probing digit feels for contracted or congested tissues, in which trigger points might be located.

- When an area of contraction is noted, firm pressure toward the center of the body is applied to elicit a response from the patient ('Does it hurt? Does it radiate or refer? If so, to where?').
- Trigger points noted during the assessment may be treated using standard manual protocols.

Caution: Dry needling or acupuncture to deactivate trigger points in the intercostal spaces is not recommended due to high risk of penetration of the lungs.

Psoas

There are a variety of alternative measures and strategies for reducing excessive tone and deactivating trigger points in the psoas. A muscle energy procedure, is described here.

MET for psoas (Grieve 1994, Chaitow 2006)
- The client/patient is supine with the buttocks at the very end of the table, nontreated leg fully flexed at hip and knee, and held in that state by either the client/patient or the practitioner.
- The practitioner stands at the foot of the table and the leg on the affected side (shortened/hypertonic psoas) is placed so that the medioplantar aspect of the foot rests on the practitioner's knee or shin (see Fig. 9.12).
- The leg should be placed so that the hip flexors, including psoas, are in a midrange position, not at their barrier.
- The practitioner should request the client/patient to use *a small degree of effort* to *externally rotate the leg* and, at the same time, *to flex the hip.*
- The practitioner resists both efforts and an isometric contraction of the psoas and associated muscles therefore takes place.
- After an approximately 7 second isometric contraction, and complete relaxation of effort, the thigh should, on an exhalation, be taken without force into slight stretch. This stretch position is held for 30 seconds.
- Repeat once.

Quadratus lumborum

A positional release procedure (PRT) is described here.

PRT for quadratus lumborum
- The client/patient is prone and the practitioner stands on the side contralateral to that being treated.
- The tender points for quadratus lie close to the transverse processes of L1–L5. Medial pressure (toward the spine) is usually required to access the tender points, which should be pressed lightly as pain in the area is often exquisite.

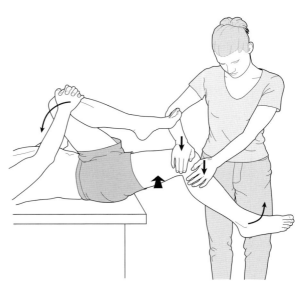

Figure 9.12 MET of psoas using Grieve's position – isometric contraction phase.

- Once the most sensitive tender point has been identified this should be lightly compressed and the client/patient asked to register the discomfort as a 10.
- While the practitioner maintains the monitoring contact on the tender point, the client/patient is asked to externally rotate, abduct, and flex the hip on the side being treated to a position that reduces the score significantly.
- The limb, flexed at hip and knee, should lie supported on the treatment table.
- The client/patient turns his/her head ipsilaterally and slides the ipsilateral hand beneath the flexed thigh, easing the hand very slowly toward the foot of the treatment table, until a further reduction in the pain score is noted.
- This combination of hip flexion/abduction/rotation and arm movement effectively laterally flexes the lumbar spine, so slackening quadratus fibers.
- If further reduction is required in the pain score (i.e. if it is not already at 3 or less), the practitioner's caudad hand should apply gentle cephalad pressure from the ipsilateral ischial tuberosity.
- This final compressive force usually reduces the score to 0. This position should be held for at least 30, and ideally up to 90, seconds before a slow return to the starting position.

Scalenes (and other upper fixators of the shoulder/accessory breathing muscles)

The scalene and other upper fixators of the shoulder/accessory breathing muscles (for example, levator

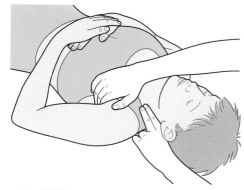

Figure 9.13 PRT for scalenes.

scapulae, upper trapezius, sternocleidomastoid) are amenable to soft tissue manipulation methods. Positional release technique methods are described here.

PRT for scalenes

- The tender points relating to the scalene muscles lie on the transverse processes (sometimes on the very tips of these) of C2–C6.
- The patient lies supine and the practitioner sits at the head of the table, palpating a tender point with sufficient pressure to allow the discomfort to be ascribed a value of no more than 7/10 (where 10 is extreme pain on a VAS).
- The patient is then told, for the purpose of the technique, to change this value to 10.
- For the anterior and medial scalene, the head and neck are flexed and sideflexed toward the affected side.
- For the posterior scalene, a neutral position may be employed.
- The head and neck may be supported on a small cushion or rolled towel.
- The nonpalpating hand engages the 2nd and 3rd ribs close to the axilla and eases them cephalad, until the reported discomfort reduces from 10 to 3 or less. (See Fig. 9.13.)
- This is held for 30–90 seconds, after which a slow release of the tissues being held is allowed.

Thoracic and costal mobilization

A wide range of mobilization and manipulation approaches exist by means of which restricted thoracic spine and rib structures can be encouraged towards more normal function. These include high velocity, low amplitude (HVLA) thrust techniques, MET, PRT, and general mobilization methods.

An effective MET procedure for mobilizing the thoracic spine is described here (Lenehan et al 2003).

MET for thoracic spine

- The patient is seated on a treatment table, with arms folded, hands on shoulders, elbows forward.
- The practitioner stands behind and to the side, one hand cupping the patient's elbows, and the other palpating or stabilizing the thoracic spine.
- The ability of the trunk to rotate left and right is assessed.
- It is then taken into rotation, to its *easy end of range*, in the direction of greatest restriction.
- In that position the patient is asked to attempt, using no more than 20% of available strength, to sideflex (either direction) for 5 seconds while the practitioner prevents any movement.
- Following this isometric contraction, the patient should be taken into a new easy end of range of rotation – commonly (Lenehan et al 2003) around 10% further than previously.
- This process is repeated once in the same direction, and is then performed with the trunk rotated in the opposite direction.

Scar tissue release

Kobesova et al (2007) suggest that scars may develop adhesive properties that compromise tissue tensioning, altering proprioceptive input, behaving in much the same way as active myofascial trigger points. It is suggested that faulty afferent input can result in disturbed efferent output leading to – for example – protective postural patterns, increased neurovascular activity, and pain syndromes. The term *active scar* is designated to describe the ongoing additional neural activity associated with adhesive scar formations.

Lewit and Olanska (2004) report a series of 51 such cases in which postsurgical scar tissue was found to be the primary pain generator for a multitude of locomotor system pain syndromes. On palpation (light stretching) of dysfunctional tissues, the patient commonly reports sensations of 'burning, prickling, or lightning-like jabs of pain.'

Valouchova and Lewit (2009) report that active scars in the abdomen and pelvis commonly restrict back flexion, which the patient feels as low back pain.

Treatment methods are simple, involving 'minimyofascial release' methods – where skin alongside scars is treated initially, with subsequent attention to deeper layers. Treatment involves 'engaging the pathologic barrier and waiting; after a short delay, a release gradually occurs until the normal barrier is restored.'

Assessment for breathing

A simple questionnaire (Nijmegen Questionnaire) is internationally accepted as being over 90% accurate in suggesting that hyperventilation exists as a contributory feature of a person's symptom picture. This noninvasive test is a simple and accurate indicator of acute and chronic hyperventilation (see Box 9.4).

Signs indicating breathing pattern disorder (BPD) (See Fig. 7.5)

- Restlessness (type A, 'neurotic'): look for rapid, fidgety behavior and movement.
- 'Air hunger' and sighing: 'air hunger' describes an attempted inhalation performed almost as a gasping effort, trying to force air into lungs that have not exhaled.
- A rapid swallowing rate (aerophagia) often resulting in bloating.
- Poor breath-holding times: shown by an inability to comfortably (i.e. without strain) hold the breath out for more than 10–15 seconds. This suggests poor carbon dioxide tolerance because 'normal' is considered to be around 30 seconds.
- A perceptible rise of the shoulders on inhalation suggests chronic overactivity and shortening of the accessory respiratory muscles and the likelihood they will contain active trigger points.
- Obvious paradoxical breathing ('hi-lo' test) with a hand on the chest and a hand on stomach (the upper hand moves first on inhalation, demonstrating an inappropriate pattern). Abdomen moves out on inhale and in during exhale.
- Visible 'cord-like' sternomastoid muscles, suggesting overuse of the accessory breathing muscles.
- A rapid breathing rate: over 18 per minute (although this may not be obvious).
- Symptoms including muscular stiffness and aching (particularly of the neck and shoulders), fatigue, brain fog, irritable bowel syndrome, chronic pain, anxiety, panic, phobias, cold extremities, paraesthesia, photophobia/hyperacusis, and comments such as, 'I can't take a deep breath.'
- A positive Nijmegen Questionnaire test.

Observe and palpate for overuse of upper chest breathing muscles during normal relaxed breathing. In addition, the following assessments are easily incorporated into the massage:

- The massage therapist stands behind the seated client and places his/her hands over the upper trapezius area so that the tips of the fingers rest on the top of the clavicles.
- As the client breathes, determine if the accessory muscles are being used for relaxed breathing. If the shoulders move up and down as the client breathes, it is likely that accessory muscles are being recruited. In normal relaxed breathing the shoulders should not move in this way. The client will be using accessory muscles to breathe if the chest movement is concentrated in the upper chest instead of the lower ribs and abdomen.

Box 9.4 Nijmegen Questionnaire

	Never	Rare	Some-times	Often	Very often
	0	1	2	3	4
Chest pain					
Feeling tense					
Blurred vision					
Dizzy spells					
Feeling confused					
Faster or deeper breathing					
Short of breath					
Tight feelings in chest					
Bloated feeling in stomach					
Tingling fingers					
Unable to breathe deeply					
Stiff fingers or arms					
Tight feelings around mouth					
Cold hands or feet					
Palpitations					
Feelings of anxiety					
			Total		*/64

*Patients mark with a tick how often they suffer from the symptoms listed. A score above 23/64 is diagnostic of hyperventilation syndrome.

- Using any of the accessory muscles for breathing results in an increase in tension and tendency toward the development of trigger points. These situations can be identified with palpation. Connective tissue changes are common since this breathing dysfunction is often chronic. The connective tissues are palpated as thick, dense, and shortened in this area.
- Have the client inhale and exhale and observe for a consistent exhale that is longer than the inhale. Normal relaxed breathing consists of a shorter inhalation phase in relationship to a longer exhalation phase. The ratio of inhalation time to exhalation is one count inhale to four counts exhale. A reverse of this pattern indicates a breathing pattern disorder. The ideal pattern would range between 2–4 counts during the inhalation and 8–10 counts for the exhalation. Targeted massage and breathing retraining methods can be used to restore normal relaxed breathing.
- Have the client hold his/her breath without strain to assess for tolerance to carbon dioxide levels. He/she should be able to comfortably hold the breath for at least 15 seconds, with 30 seconds being ideal.
- Palpate and gently mobilize the thorax to assess for rib mobility. This is done in supine, prone, sidelying, and seated position. The ribs should have a springy feel, and be a bit more mobile from the 6th rib to the 10th rib.

Suggested strategies and treatment sequence for HVS/BPD

The following sequence is based on the professional practice of Dr Chaitow and while it represents only one approach for treatment of disordered breathing, it does contain the elements necessary for a successful restoration of normal breathing. Treatment and retraining commonly involves 8–12 weekly sessions, followed by treatment every 2–3 weeks, for approximately 6 months. An educational component should be included at each session.

Massage therapists can increase the effectiveness of massage by incorporating the strategies into the general full body massage approach.

- *First two treatments (not less than weekly):* Release and/or stretch of upper fixators of the shoulders/accessory breathing muscle (upper traps, levator, scalenes/SCS, pecs, lats) as well as attention to trigger points in these; soft tissue (NMT, MET, PRT, etc.); attention to the diaphragm area (anterior intercostals, sternum, abdominal attachments costal margin, quadratus lumborum/psoas), as well as attention to trigger points in these.
  - *Retraining:* Pursed lip breathing, as well as guidance as to restricting shoulder rise during inhalation.
- *Sessions (weeks) 3 and 4:* As above, plus mobilization of thoracic spine and ribs (as well as lymphatic pump/drainage methods), plus address fascial and osseous links (cranial, pelvic, limbs).
  - *Retraining:* Antiarousal breathing, plus specific relaxation methods, stress management, autogenic training, visualization, meditation, counseling.
- *Sessions (weeks) 5–12:* As above, plus focus on other body influences (ergonomics, posture).
  - *Retraining:* Additional exercises as appropriate.
- *Sessions (weeks) 13–26:* Review and treat residual dysfunctional patterns/tissues.
- *Throughout:* As indicated, incorporate nutrition, psychotherapy, and adjunctive methods, such as hydrotherapy, tai chi, yoga, Pilates, massage, acupuncture, etc.

KEY POINTS

- The objective is to 'lighten the adaptive load' and to enhance functionality – better mobility, flexibility, stability, balance – and of course to relieve or remove unpleasant symptoms.
- The more fragile and sensitive the person, the less that should be done at any time.
- Stress management may play a part in easing the adaptation load in conditions such as recurrent or chronic head/neck pain.
- There are a variety of methods to treat pain: acupuncture, relaxation methods, manipulation, essential oils, and hydrotherapy.
- Lifestyle changes can be used to manage pain: exercise, sleep, diet.
- Breathing function relates to the pain experience.
- Breathing retraining can help manage pain.
- Methods to normalize the breathing function can be integrated into the full body massage.

References

Balaban C, Thayer J: Neurological bases for balance – anxiety links, *J Anxiety Disord* 15(1–2):53–79, 2001.

Banzett RB, Lanzing RW, Brown R, Topulos GP, Yagar D, Steel SM: 'Air hunger' from increased PCO_2 persists after complete neuromuscular block in humans, *Respir Physiol* 81:1–17, 1990.

Bernardon M, Limone A, Businelli C: Diabetic ketoacidosis in pregnancy, *Gazzetta Medica Italiana Archivio per le Scienze Mediche* 168(1):45–49, 2009.

Blake E: Constitutional hydrotherapy: a workbook of clinical lessons, Portland, 2006, Holistic Health.

Blake E: Hydrotherapy. In Chaitow L, editor: Naturopathic physical medicine, Edinburgh, 2008, Churchill Livingstone.

Bockenhauer S, Chen H, Julliard K, et al: Measuring thoracic excursion: reliability of the cloth tape measure technique, *J Am Osteopath Assoc* 107:191–196, 2007.

Bohannon RW, Larkin PA, Cook A, et al: Decrease in timed balance test scores with aging, *Phys Ther* 64(7):1067–1070, 1984.

Botella De Maglia J, Real Soriano R: Arterial oxygen saturation during ascent of a mountain higher than 8,000 meters, *Med Intensiva* 32(6):277–281, 2008.

Bradley D: Hyperventilation syndrome, Auckland, 1998, Tandem Press.

Bradley D: Self-help for hyperventilation syndrome, ed 3, Alameda, 2001, Hunter House.

Brashear R: Hyperventilation syndrome, *Lung* 161(1): 257–273, 1983.

Brotto L, Klein C, Gorzalka B: Laboratory induced hyperventilation differentiates female sexual arousal disorder subtypes, *Arch Sex Behav* 38(4):463–475, 2009.

Brügger A: Lehrbuch der Funktionellen Storungen des Bewegungssystems, Zollikon, Benglen, 2000, Brügger-Verlag.

Burkill G, Healy J: Anatomy of the retroperitoneum, *Imaging* 12(1):10–20, 2000.

Buteyko K: Buteyko method: experience of application in medical practice, Moscow, 1990, Patriot.

Cappo B, Holmes D: Utility of prolonged respiratory exhalation for reducing physiological and psychological arousal in non-threatening and threatening situations, *J Psychosomatic Res* 28(4):265–273, 1984.

Carrière B: Interdependence of posture and the pelvic floor. In Carrière B, Feldt C, editors: The pelvic floor, New York, 2006, Thieme Verlag, pp 68–80.

Carrière B: The pelvic floor, New York, 2006, Thieme, p 68.

Carroll D, Seers K: Relaxation for the relief of chronic pain: a systematic review, *J Adv Nurs* 27:476–487, 1998.

Chaitow B: My healing secrets, Bradford, 1980, Health Science Press.

Chaitow L: Integrated neuromuscular inhibition technique, *Br J Osteopath* 13:17–20, 1994.

Chaitow L: Breathing pattern disorders, motor control, and low back pain, *J Osteop Med* 7(1):34–41, 2004.

Chaitow L: Breathing patterns, connective tissue and soft-shelled eggs, *Naturopathy Digest*, January, 2006. Online at http://www.naturopathydigest.com/archives/2006/jan/chaitow.php

Chaitow L: Chronic pelvic pain: pelvic floor problems, sacroiliac dysfunction and the trigger point connections, *J Bodyw Mov Ther* 11(4):327–339, 2007.

Chaitow L: Positional release techniques, ed 3, Edinburgh, 2007, Churchill Livingstone.

Chaitow L, Bradley D, Gilbert C: Multidisciplinary approaches to breathing pattern disorders, Edinburgh, 2006, Churchill Livingstone.

Chaitow L, DeLany J: Clinical applications of neuromuscular techniques, vol 1 – the upper body, ed 2, Edinburgh, 2008, Churchill Livingstone, p 298.

Chalaye P, Goffaux P, Lafrenaye S, Marchand S: Respiratory effects on experimental heat pain and cardiac activity, *Pain Med* 10(8):1334–1340, 2009.

Chaulier K, Chalumeau S, Ber C-E: Metabolic acidosis in a context of acute severe asthma, *Annales Françaises d'Anesthésie et de Réanimation* 26(4):352–355, 2007.

Cimino R, Farella M, Michelotti A: Does the ovarian cycle influence the pressure-pain threshold of the masticatory muscles in symptom-free women? *J Orofac Pain* 14(2):105–111, 2000.

Conway AV, Freeman LJ, Nixon PGF: Hypnotic examination of trigger factors in the hyperventilation syndrome, *Am J Clin Hypn* 30:296–304, 1988.

Coulter I, Hurwitz E, Adamas A, et al: The appropriateness of manipulation and mobilization of the cervical spine, Santa Monica, 1996, Rand.

Courtney R, Cohen M, Reece J: Comparison of the Manual Assessment of Respiratory Motion (MARM) and the Hi Lo Breathing Assessment in determining a simulated breathing pattern, *Int J Ost Med* 12:86–91, 2009.

Courtney R, Greenwood KM: Preliminary investigation of a measure of dysfunctional breathing symptoms: the Self Evaluation of Breathing Questionnaire (SEBQ), *Int J Ost Med* 12:121–127, 2009.

Courtney R, van Dixhoorn J, et al: Evaluation of breathing pattern: comparison of a manual assessment of respiratory motion (MARM) and respiratory induction plethysmography, *Appl Psychophysiol Biofeedback* 33: 91–100, 2008.

Cox JM, Bakkum BW: Possible generators of retrotrochanteric gluteal and thigh pain, *J Manipulative Physiol Ther* 28(7):534–538, 2005. 537.

Cresswell A: The influence of sudden perturbations on trunk muscle activity and intra-abdominal pressure while standing, *Exp Brain Res* 98:336–344, 1994.

Damas-Mora J, Davies L, Taylor W, et al: Menstrual respiratory changes and symptoms, *Br J Psychiatr* 136:492–497, 1980.

Debreczeni R, Amrein I, Kamondi A, et al: Hypocapnia induced by involuntary hyperventilation during mental arithmetic reduces cerebral blood flow velocity, *Tohoku J Exp Med* 217(2):147–154, 2009.

Dempsey J, Sheel A, St, Croix C: Respiratory influences on sympathetic vasomotor outflow in humans, *Respir Physiol Neurobiol* 130(1):3–20, 2002.

Downey LV, Zun LS: The effects of deep breathing training on pain management in the emergency department, *South Med J* 102(7):688–692, 2009.

Evans D, Lum L, Dart A: Chest pain with normal coronary arteries, *Lancet* 315(8163):311.

Faling L: Controlled breathing techniques and chest physical therapy in chronic obstructive pulmonary disease. In Casabur R, editor: Principles and practices of pulmonary therapy, Philadelphia, 1995, WB Saunders.

Fitzgerald M, et al: Randomized feasibility trial of myofascial physical therapy for the treatment of urologic chronic pelvic pain syndromes, *J Urol* 182:570–580, 2009.

Flink IK, Nicholas MK, Boersma K, Linton SJ: Reducing the threat value of chronic pain: a preliminary replicated single-case study of interoceptive exposure versus distraction in six individuals with chronic back pain, *Behav Res Ther* 47(8):721–728, 2009.

Ford M, Camilleri M, Hanson R: Hyperventilation, central autonomic control, and colonic tone in humans, *Gut* 37:499–504, 1995.

Freeman LJ, Nixon P: Chest pain and the hyperventilation syndrome. Some aetiological considerations, *Postgrad Med J* 61(721):957–961, 1985.

Gardner W: The pathophysiology of hyperventilation disorders, *Chest* 109:516–534, 1996.

Garland W: Somatic changes in hyperventilating subject. Presentation at International Society for the Advancement of Respiratory Psychophysiology Congress, Paris, 1994.

Gibbons SGT: The model of psoas major stability function. Proceedings of 1st International Conference on Movement Dysfunction, Edinburgh, 2001, Sept 21–23.

Gilbert C: Emotional sources of dysfunctional breathing, *J Bodyw Mov Ther* 2:224–230, 1998.

Grewar H, McLean L: The integrated continence system: a manual therapy approach to the treatment of stress urinary incontinence, *Manual Therapy* 13:375–386, 2008.

Grieve G. In Boyling JD, Palastanga N, editors: The masqueraders in Grieve's modern manual therapy, ed 2, Edinburgh, 1994, Churchill Livingstone.

Grossman P, De Swart J CG, Defares PB: A controlled study of breathing therapy for treatment of hyperventilation syndrome, *J Psychosom Res* 29(1):49–58, 1985.

Haldeman S, Kohlbeck FJ, McGregor M: Stroke, cerebral artery dissection and cervical spine manipulative therapy, *J Neurol* 249:1098–1104, 2002.

Han J, Gayan-Ramirez G, Dekhuijzen R: Respiratory function of the rib cage muscles, *Europ Respir J* 6(5): 722–728, 1993.

Haugstad GK, Haugstad TS, Kirste UM, et al: Mensendieck somatocognitive therapy as treatment approach to chronic pelvic pain: results of a randomized controlled intervention study, *Am J Obstetric Gynecol* 194:1303–1310, 2006.

Hides JA, Richardson CA, Jull GA: Multifidus muscle recovery is not automatic after resolution of acute, first-episode low back pain, *Spine* 21:2763–2769, 1996.

Hill M: Cervical artery dissection, imaging, trauma and causal inference, *Can J Neurol Sci* 30(4):302–304, 2003.

Hochstetter J, et al: An investigation into the immediate impact of breathlessness management on the breathless patient: randomised controlled trial, *Physiotherapy* 91: 178–185, 2005.

Hodges PW, Heinjnen I, Gandevia SC: Postural activity of the diaphragm is reduced in humans when respiratory demand increases, *J Physiol* 537(3):999, 2001.

Hodges P, Sapsford R, Pengel L: Postural and respiratory functions of the PFMs, *Neurourol Urodyn* 26(3):362–371, 2007.

Hodges, Richardson: 1996, 1998, 1999

Hudson A, Gandevia S, Butler J: The effect of lung volume on the co-ordinated recruitment of scalene and sternomastoid muscles in humans, *J Physiol* 584(1): 261–270, 2007.

Hurwitz BE: The effect of inspiration and posture on cardiac rate and T-wave amplitude during apneic breathholding in man, *Psychophysiology* 18:179–180, 1981. (Abstract)

Janda V: Introduction to functional pathology of the motor system. Proceedings of the VII Commonwealth and International Conference on Sport, *Physiotherapy in Sport* 3:39, 1982.

Janda V, Frank C, Liebenson C: Evaluation of muscular imbalance. In Liebenson C, editor: Rehabilitation of the spine: a practitioner's manual, ed 2, Philadelphia, 2007, Lippincott Williams and Wilkins.

Jensen D, Duffin J, Lam Y-M: Physiological mechanisms of hyperventilation during human pregnancy, *Respir Physiol Neurobiol* 161(1):76–86, 2008.

Jones R: Pelvic floor muscle rehabilitation, *Urology News* 5(5):2–4, 2001.

Kapreli E, Vourazanis E, Strimpakos N: Neck pain causes respiratory dysfunction, *Med Hypotheses* 70(5):1009–1013, 2008.

Key J: The pelvic crossed syndromes: a reflection of imbalanced function in the myofascial envelope; a further exploration of Janda's work, *J Bodyw Mov Ther* 14:3, 2010.

Key J, et al: A model of movement dysfunction provides a classification system guiding diagnosis and therapeutic care in spinal pain and related musculo-skeletal syndromes: a paradigm shift, *J Bodyw Mov Ther* 12(2): 105–120, 2007.

Kitabchi AE, Umpierrez GE, Murphy M, et al: Hyperglycemic crises in adult patients with diabetes: a consensus statement from the American Diabetes Association, *Diabetes Care* 29(12):2739–2748, 2006.

Kobesova A, et al: Twenty-year-old pathogenic 'active' postsurgical scar: a case study of a patient with persistent right lower quadrant pain, *J Manipulative Physiol Ther* 30(3):234–238, 2007.

Kuligowska E, Deeds L III, Lu K III: Pelvic pain: overlooked and underdiagnosed gynecologic conditions, *RadioGraphics* 25(1):3–20, 2005.

Lansing RW: The perception of respiratory work and effort can be independent of the perception of air hunger, *Am J Respir Crit Care Med* 162:1690–1696, 2001.

Lawless J: Aromatherapy and the mind, London, 1994, Thorsons.

Lee D: An integrated approach for the management of low back and pelvic girdle pain. In Vleeming A, Mooney V, Stoekart R, editors: Movement stability & lumbopelvic pain, Edinburgh, 2007, Elsevier, pp 593–620.

Lee D, Lee L: Stress urinary incontinence – a consequence of failed load transfer through the pelvis. Presented at the

5th World Interdisciplinary Congress on Low Back and Pelvic Pain Melbourne, November, 2004.

Lee D, Lee LJ, McLaughlin L: Stability, continence and breathing: the role of fascia following pregnancy and delivery, *J Bodyw Mov Ther* 12:333–348, 2008.

Lemon K: An assessment of treating depression and anxiety with aromatherapy, *Int J Aromatherapy* 14(2):63–69, 2004.

Lenehan KL, Fryer G, McLaughlin P: The effect of muscle energy technique on gross trunk range of motion, *Int J Osteopath Med* 6(1):13–18, 2003.

Levitsky MG: Pulmonary physiology, ed 6, Toronto, 2003, McGraw-Hill.

Lewit K: Manipulative therapy in rehabilitation of the locomotor system, ed 3, London, 1999, Butterworth-Heinemann.

Lewit K: Relationship of faulty respiration to posture, with clinical implications, *J Am Osteopath Assoc* 79:525–528, 1980.

Lewit K, Olšanská Š: Clinical importance of active scars as a cause of myofascial pain, *JMPT* 27(6):399–402, 2004.

Lewthwaite R: Motivational considerations in physical therapy involvement, *Phys Ther* 70(12):808–819, 1990.

Ley R, Timmons BH: Behavioral and psychological approaches to breathing disorders, New York, 1994, Plenum Press.

Liebenson C: Active rehabilitation protocols. In Liebenson C, editor: Rehabilitation of the spine, Baltimore, 1996, Williams and Wilkins.

Liebenson C: Self-management of shoulder disorders – Part 3: Treatment, *J Bodyw Mov Ther* 10:65–70, 2006.

Lum LC: Hyperventilation: the tip and the iceberg, *J Psychosom Res* 19(5–6):375–383, 1975.

Lum L: Hyperventilation and anxiety states (Editorial), *J Roy Soc Med* January:1–4, 1984.

Lum L: Treatment difficulties and failures: causes and clinical management, *Biological Psychology* 43(3):24, 1996.

Malone D, Baldwin N, Tomecek F, et al: Complications of spinal manipulation: a comprehensive review of the literature, *J Fam Pract* 42:475–480, 2002.

Masubuchi Y, Abe T, Yokoba M: Relation between neck accessory inspiratory muscle electromyographic activity and lung volume, *J Japanese Respiratory Society* 39(4):244–249, 2001.

Mazur M, Furgała A, Jabłoński K, et al: Dysfunction of the autonomic nervous system activity is responsible for gastric myoelectric disturbances in the irritable bowel syndrome patients, *J Physiol Pharmacol* 58(Suppl 3):131–139, 2007.

McLaughlin L: Breathing evaluation and retraining in body work, *J Bodyw Mov Ther* 13(3):276–282, 2009.

Mehling WE, Hamel KA, et al: Randomized, controlled trial of breath therapy for patients with chronic low-back pain, *Altern Ther Health Med* 11(4):44–52, 2005.

Newell R: Anatomy of the post-laryngeal airways, lungs and diaphragm, *Surgery* 23(11):393–397, 2005.

Nishino T, Shimoyama N, Ide T, et al: Experimental pain augments experimental dyspnea, but not vice versa in human volunteers, *Anesthesiology* 91(6):1633–1638, 1999.

Nixon P, Andrews J: A study of anaerobic threshold in chronic fatigue syndrome (CFS), *Bio Psychol* 43(3):264, 1996.

Olsen A, Rao S: Clinical neurophysiology and electrodiagnostic testing of the pelvic floor, *Gastroenterol Clin North Am* 30(1):33–54, v–vi, 2001.

O'Sullivan P, Beales D: Changes in pelvic floor and diaphragm kinematics and respiratory patterns in subjects with sacroiliac joint pain following a motor learning intervention: A case series, *Manual Therapy* 12:209–218, 2007.

O'Sullivan P, Beales D, Beetham J, et al: Altered motor control strategies in subjects with sacroiliac joint pain during the active straight-leg-raise test, *Spine* 27(1):E1–8, 2002.

Palanjian K: *Shiatsu Seminars in Integrative Medicine* 2(3):107–115, 2004.

Perri M, Halford E: Pain and faulty breathing: a pilot study, *J Bodyw Mov Ther* 8(4):297–306, 2004.

Pleidelová J, Baláziová M, Porubská V: Frequency of scalene muscle disorders, *Rehabilitacia* 35(4):203–207, 2002.

Prather H, Dugan S, Fitzgerald C, et al: Review of anatomy, evaluation, and treatment of musculoskeletal pelvic floor pain in women, *Physical Medicine and Rehabilitation* 1(4):346–358, 2009.

Pryor JA, Prasad SA: Physiotherapy for respiratory and cardiac problems, ed 3, Edinburgh, 2002, Churchill Livingstone, p 81.

Renggli A, Verges S, Notter D: Development of respiratory muscle contractile fatigue in the course of hyperpnoea, *Respir Physiol Neurobiol* 164:366–372, 2008.

Rhudy J, Meagher M: Fear and anxiety: divergent effects on human pain thresholds, *Pain* 84:65–75, 2000.

Rucco V, Feruglio C, Genco F, et al: Autogenic training versus Erickson's analogical technique in treatment of fibromyalgia syndrome, *Rivista Europea per le Scienze Mediche e Farmacologiche* 17:41, 1995.

Ryan S, McNicholas M, Eustace S: Anatomy for diagnostic imaging, Sydney, 2004, Saunders, p 191.

Schleifer L, Ley R, Spalding T: A hyperventilation theory of job stress and musculoskeletal disorders, *Am J Ind Med* 41(5):420–432, 2002.

Scott DJ, Stohler CS, Egnatuk CM, Wang H, Koeppe RA, Zubieta JK: Individual differences in reward responding explain placebo-induced expectations and effects, *Neuro* 19 55(2):325–336, 2007.

Shekelle PG, Adamas AH, Chassin RM, et al: Spinal manipulation for low back pain, *Ann Intern Med* 117:590–598, 1992.

Simon P, Schwartzstein M, Weiss J, et al: Distinguishable sensations of breathlessness induced in normal volunteers, *Am Rev Respir Dis* 140:1021–1027, 1989.

Simons D, Travell J, Simons L: Myofascial pain and dysfunction: the trigger point manual, vol 1: upper half of body, ed 2, Baltimore, 1999, Williams and Wilkins.

Slatkovska L, Jensen D, Davies G, et al: Phasic menstrual cycle effects on the control of breathing in healthy women, *Respir Physiol Neurobiol* 154(3):379–388, 2006.

Suwa K: Ischemia may be less detrimental than anemia for O_2 transport because of CO_2 transport: A model analysis, *J Anesth* 9(1):61–64, 1995.

Tan G, Fink B, Dao TK, et al: Associations among pain, PTSD, mTBI, and heart rate variability in veterans of Operation Enduring and Iraqi Freedom: a pilot study, *Pain Med* 10(7):1237–1245, 2009.

Ternesten-Hasséus E, Johansson E-L, Bende M: Dyspnea from exercise in cold air is not always asthma, *J Asthma* 45(8):705–709, 2008.

Tiep B, Burns M, Kro D, et al: Pursed lip breathing using ear oximetry, *Chest* 90:218–221, 1986.

Travell J, Simons D: Myofascial pain and dysfunction: the trigger point manual, vol 1: upper body, Baltimore, 1983, Williams and Wilkins, p 671.

Travell J, Simons D: Myofascial pain and dysfunction: the trigger point manual, vol. 2: the lower extremities, Baltimore, 1992, Williams and Wilkins.

Troosters T, Verstraete A, Ramon K: Physical performance of patients with numerous psychosomatic complaints suggestive of hyperventilation, *Eur Respir J* 14(6): 1314–1319, 1999.

Valouchová P, Lewit K: Surface electromyography of abdominal and back muscles in patients with active scars, *J Bodyw Mov Ther* 13:262–267, 2009.

Van Dieën J, Selen L, Cholewicki J: Trunk muscle activation in low-back pain patients, an analysis of the literature, *J Electromyogr Kinesiol* 13:333–351, 2003.

Van Dixhoorn J, Duivenvoorden HJ: Efficacy of Nijmegen Questionnaire in recognition of the hyperventilation syndrome, *J Psychom Res* 29(2):199–206, 1985.

Vanhecke T, Franklin B, Ajluni S, et al: Cardiorespiratory fitness and sleep-related breathing disorders, *Expert Rev Cardiovasc Ther* 6(5):745–758, 2008.

Wager TD, Scott DJ, Zubieta JK: Placebo effects on human mu-opioid activity during pain, *Proc Natl Acad Sci USA Jun 26* 104(26):11056–11061, 2007.

Watier A: Irritable bowel syndrome and bladder-sphincter dysfunction, *Pelvi-perineologie* 4(2):136–141, 2009.

Watrous L: From nature cure to advanced naturopathic medicine, *J Naturopath Med* 7(2):72–79, 1996.

Wilke A, Noll B, Maisch B: Angina pectoris caused by extra-coronary diseases, *Herz* 24(2):132–139, 1999.

Yokoyama I, Inoue Y, Kinoshita T, et al: Heart and brain circulation and CO_2 in healthy men, *Acta Physiologica* 193(3):202–330, 2008.

Zautra AJ, Fasman R, Davis MC, Craig AD: The effects of slow breathing on affective responses to pain stimuli: An experimental study, *Pain* 149(1): 1–2, 2010.

Zubieta JK, Stohler CS: Neurobiological mechanisms of placebo responses, *Ann N Y Acad Sci* 1156:198–210, 2009.

Index

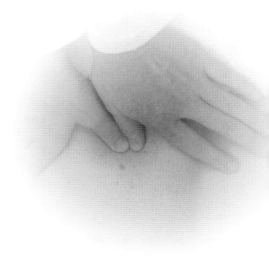

abdominal massage, for
    constipation, 29
aromatherapy, 156
heart surgery, massage therapy
    following, 32, 33
labor pain relief, 27
low back pain, 24
myalgia, 29
postoperative cancer patients, 35–36
shoulder, musculoskeletal disorders
    of, 23
Range of motion, 83, 143–144
Rapid breathing, 164, 169, 180
Rate of breathing, 164, 174
Raynaud's phenomenon, 21
Reciprocal inhibition (RI), 115, 117
Rectus femoris, 147, 149
Referred pain, 5, 98, 127
Reflex sympathetic dystrophy
    syndrome (RSDS), 56
Reflexology, 151
Regional cerebral blood flow (rCBF), 8
Rehabilitation exercise methods, 124
Rejection levels, 83
Repetitive stress injuries, 56
Research, massage, 13
    benefits and safety factors, 15–22
    cancer care, 22, 23
    chair massage for carers, 37
    culture of massage therapy, 36–37
    delayed onset muscle soreness, 37
    evaluation of, 14–15
    hospice environment, 27
    labor pain, 27, 28
    musculoskeletal pain, chronic, 23,
        24, 25, 26
    pain, 22, 28, 29, 30–31
    pain syndromes, 31
    palliative care, 35
    postoperative pain, 32–34
    preterm infants, heart rate
        responses, 36
    symptom management, 34
Respiratory alkalosis, 50, 169
Retroperitoneal space, 168
Reward or pleasure network, 46
Reye's syndrome, 64
Rheumatoid arthritis, 55
Rhomboids, 140
Rhythm, massage, 94
Ribcage, 132
Riluzole, 35
Rotation or torsion loading, 98–99

S

Sacroiliac (SI) joint, 144
Safety factors, 14–22

Salicylates, 64
Salicylism, 64
Sartorius, 147
Scalenes, 130, 132, 178–179
    dysfunction, 170
Scalp, 128
Scapula, 138–139, 139f
Scar tissue release, 179
Schleip, R., 18, 19
Sciatica, 55, 56
Seated position
    ergonomics, 158f
    shoulder massage, 139
Second somatic (SII) region, 8
Self-care, breathing pattern disorders,
    163
Self-Evaluation Breathing
    Questionnaire (SEBQ), 165
Selye, H., 105–106, 106f
Semispinalis muscle, 130
Sensation of pain, 2–4
Sensitization
    central, 43–44, 107
    defined, 43–45
    model, 107–110
Serotonin, 15, 65
Severe pain, 7
Shear loading, 97–98
Sherman, K., 110
Shiatsu, 156
Shingles, 56
Short McGill Questionnaire, 73, 76f
Shortness, 114, 116–117
Shoulder compression, 131f
Shoulder impingement syndrome
    (SIS), 22, 23
Shoulder massage, 138–141, 153
Sidelying position
    anterior torso, 133, 153
    arm massage, 141
    foot massage, 151
    head/facial massage, 128–130
    hip massage, 146–147
    neck massage, 131, 152f
    shoulder massage, 139, 139f
    thigh massage, 148f
Single leg stance balance test, 163
Sinuses, massage of, 129f
Skin assessment and palpation, 84–86,
    136f
Skin disorders, 56
Skin reddening, 137, 141–142,
    148–149
Sleep disorders, 48, 167
Slow breathing, 164
Slow-stroke massage, 16
Smiling, 128
Smooth muscle cells (SMCs), 19, 50
Social attachment system, 45–46

Soft tissue manipulations, 93
Soft tissue pain, 2, 14
Somatic pain, 2, 5, 48
Somatosensory cortex, 7, 46
Spatial summation, 8
Specific adaptation concept, 158
Speed, massage, 94
Spinal cord
    pain messages reaching, 7, 14
    spinal stenosis affecting, 56–57
Spinal cord injury (SCI), 34–35, 57
Spinal manipulation, 66
Spinal nerve blocks, 58
Spinal stenosis, 56–57
Spinalis, 130
Spindle cells, 96, 129, 130
Splenius capitis muscle, 130
Spondylolisthesis, 55
Sports injuries, 57
    see also Delayed onset muscle
        soreness (DOMS)
Spray-and-stretch methods, 122–124
STAR acronym, trigger point
    palpation, 87–88
Static touch, vs massage, 30–31
Stecco, A., 17–18
Stecco, C., 17–18
Stecco, L., 18
Sternoclavicular (SC) joints, 138–139
Sternocleidomastoid (SCM) muscles,
    130, 132, 170
Sternomastoid muscles, 180
Strain-counterstrain (SCS) approach,
    118–121
Stress
    and acute pain, 47
    and breathing, 164
    defined, 10
    response to stressors, 17
    therapeutic, 110
Stress management/relaxation
    methods, 156–158
Stretching
    local stretch, 122
    massage application with, 78, 78f
    releasing skin changes by, 85–86
    skin stretching assessment, 84–85
Stump pain, 55
Suboccipitals, 130–132
Subscapularis muscle, 140
Substance abuse see Addiction
Substance P, 2, 7, 14, 25
Suffering, 45–46
Supine position
    anterior torso, 133, 153
    arm massage, 141, 142f
    head/facial massage, 128–130
    shoulder massage, 139
Surface level, 83